Polycystic Ovary Syndrome (PCOS): State of the Art

Polycystic Ovary Syndrome (PCOS): State of the Art

Editor

Enrico Carmina

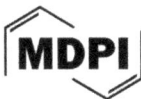

Basel • Beijing • Wuhan • Barcelona • Belgrade • Novi Sad • Cluj • Manchester

Editor
Enrico Carmina
University of Palermo
Palermo
Italy

Editorial Office
MDPI
St. Alban-Anlage 66
4052 Basel, Switzerland

This is a reprint of articles from the Special Issue published online in the open access journal *Journal of Clinical Medicine* (ISSN 2077-0383) (available at: https://www.mdpi.com/journal/jcm/special_issues/80X5Y60K25).

For citation purposes, cite each article independently as indicated on the article page online and as indicated below:

Lastname, A.A.; Lastname, B.B. Article Title. *Journal Name* **Year**, *Volume Number*, Page Range.

ISBN 978-3-7258-1133-5 (Hbk)
ISBN 978-3-7258-1134-2 (PDF)
doi.org/10.3390/books978-3-7258-1134-2

© 2024 by the authors. Articles in this book are Open Access and distributed under the Creative Commons Attribution (CC BY) license. The book as a whole is distributed by MDPI under the terms and conditions of the Creative Commons Attribution-NonCommercial-NoDerivs (CC BY-NC-ND) license.

Contents

About the Editor vii

Preface ix

Daniel A. Dumesic, David H. Abbott and Gregorio D. Chazenbalk
An Evolutionary Model for the Ancient Origins of Polycystic Ovary Syndrome
Reprinted from: *J. Clin. Med.* 2023, 12, 6120, doi:10.3390/jcm12196120 1

Magdalena Boegl, Didier Dewailly, Rodrig Marculescu, Johanna Steininger, Johannes Ott
and Marlene Hager
The LH:FSH Ratio in Functional Hypothalamic Amenorrhea: An Observational Study
Reprinted from: *J. Clin. Med.* 2024, 13, 1201, doi:10.3390/jcm13051201 17

María Elena Espinosa, Angélica Melo, Marion Leon, Estefanía Bautista-Valarezo,
Fabiola Zambrano, Pamela Uribe, et al.
Vaginal Microbiota and Proinflammatory Status in Patients with Polycystic Ovary Syndrome:
An Exploratory Study
Reprinted from: *J. Clin. Med.* 2024, 13, 2278, doi:10.3390/jcm13082278 28

Anna Warchala, Paweł Madej, Marta Kochanowicz and Marek Krzystanek
Sexual Function in Women with Polycystic Ovary Syndrome Living in Stable Heterosexual
Relationships: A Cross-Sectional Study
Reprinted from: *J. Clin. Med.* 2024, 13, 2227, doi:10.3390/jcm13082227 41

Geranne Jiskoot, Sara Somers, Chloë De Roo, Dominic Stoop and Joop Laven
Translation of the Modified Polycystic Ovary Syndrome Questionnaire (mPCOSQ) and the
Polycystic Ovary Syndrome Quality of Life Tool (PCOSQOL) in Dutch and Flemish Women
with PCOS
Reprinted from: *J. Clin. Med.* 2023, 12, 3927, doi:10.3390/jcm12123927 56

Alexandra Dietz de Loos, Geranne Jiskoot, Rita van den Berg-Emons, Yvonne Louwers,
Annemerle Beerthuizen, Jan van Busschbach and Joop Laven
The Effect of Tailored Short Message Service (SMS) on Physical Activity: Results from a
Three-Component Randomized Controlled Lifestyle Intervention in Women with PCOS
Reprinted from: *J. Clin. Med.* 2023, 12, 2466, doi:10.3390/jcm12072466 65

Lucie Huyghe, Camille Robin, Agathe Dumont, Christine Decanter, Maeva Kyheng,
Didier Dewailly, et al.
How to Choose the Optimal Starting Dose of Clomiphene Citrate (50 or 100 mg per Day) for a
First Cycle of Ovulation Induction in Anovulatory PCOS Women?
Reprinted from: *J. Clin. Med.* 2023, 12, 4943, doi:10.3390/jcm12154943 80

Alexandra Dietz de Loos, Geranne Jiskoot, Yvonne Louwers, Annemerle Beerthuizen,
Jan Busschbach and Joop Laven
Pregnancy Outcomes in Women with PCOS: Follow-Up Study of a Randomized Controlled
Three-Component Lifestyle Intervention
Reprinted from: *J. Clin. Med.* 2023, 12, 426, doi:10.3390/jcm12020426 94

Maria-Elina Mosorin, Terhi Piltonen, Anni S. Rantala, Marika Kangasniemi, Elisa Korhonen,
Risto Bloigu, et al.
Oral and Vaginal Hormonal Contraceptives Induce Similar Unfavorable Metabolic Effects in
Women with PCOS: A Randomized Controlled Trial
Reprinted from: *J. Clin. Med.* 2023, 12, 2827, doi:10.3390/jcm12082827 109

Sidika E. Karakas
Reactive Hypoglycemia: A Trigger for Nutrient-Induced Endocrine and Metabolic Responses in Polycystic Ovary Syndrome
Reprinted from: *J. Clin. Med.* **2023**, *12*, 7252, doi:10.3390/jcm12237252 . . . . **122**

Rachel Porth, Karina Oelerich and Mala S. Sivanandy
The Role of Sodium-Glucose Cotransporter-2 Inhibitors in the Treatment of Polycystic Ovary Syndrome: A Review
Reprinted from: *J. Clin. Med.* **2024**, *13*, 1056, doi:10.3390/jcm13041056 . . . . **135**

Enrico Carmina and Rosa Alba Longo
Semaglutide Treatment of Excessive Body Weight in Obese PCOS Patients Unresponsive to Lifestyle Programs
Reprinted from: *J. Clin. Med.* **2023**, *12*, 5921, doi:10.3390/jcm12185921 . . . . **147**

About the Editor

Enrico Carmina

Enrico Carmina is a clinical scientist with extensive experience in diagnosing and treating endocrine patients and a special interest in female endocrinology. He is well-recognized as one of the world's leading clinical scientists in the field of androgen and PCOS research with an extensive publication record that includes 435 publications, 28,211 citations (Google scholar), and a citation h-index of 72 (Google Scholar). He has been a Full Professor of Endocrinology at the University of Palermo and Chairman of Systematic Medicine IV at the same University. Previously, he was a Professor of Clinical Research in the USA, initially in Los Angeles at USC and later in New York at Columbia University. He served as President in 2004–2005 and then Executive Director of the Androgen Excess and PCOS Society, Inc. for 13 years from 2007 to November 2020. During this time, the Society grew significantly, becoming one the main international societies in the field of endocrinology and reproductive endocrinology.

Preface

This Special Issue of the *Journal of Clinical Medicine* is dedicated to polycystic ovary syndrome (PCOS), a very common disorder that affects about 10% of all women during their adult life.

The aim of this Special Issue was to present new information about the different aspects of the syndrome that may improve our understanding of the pathogenesis, diagnosis, and treatment of PCOS. Experts from all around the world have contributed to this Special Issue.

The first paper presents an evolutionary model of PCOS that has profound consequences on our methods of preventing and treating this syndrome. The second paper describes the importance of a normal LH/FSH ratio in the differential diagnosis of PCOS versus hypothalamic amenorrhea. Other papers analyze the validity of questionnaires for detecting alterations in quality of life in these women and analyze vaginal microbiota and the sexual function of women with PCOS.

Many papers analyze the treatment of PCOS. The first of these papers describes promotion of physical activity in women with PCOS. Another paper analyzes possible differences in the metabolic effects of oral versus intravaginal contraceptives. Two studies are dedicated to infertility in PCOS, with the first trying to solve a common clinical problem related to the initial dose of clomiphene for induction of ovulation and the second evaluating the effects of lifestyle programs on pregnancy outcomes.

One interesting paper analyzes the importance of hypoglycemia induction in reducing the long-term effects of a simple carbohydrate diet and suggests the benefits of protein supplements. Finally, two important papers report the results of new treatments for high body weight in women with PCOS. The first of these papers is dedicated to the use of sodium-glucose cotransporter-2 (SGLT-2) inhibitors in patients with the syndrome. In fact, SGLT-2 inhibitors appear to be effective in improving menstrual frequency, reducing body weight, lowering total testosterone, and improving some glycemic indices in women with PCOS. The final paper reports a very promising initial experience with the use of low doses of semaglutide, a GLP-1 analog, on body weight and diabetic risk in obese PCOS patients who were not responsive to a lifestyle program.

We believe that this reprint of important papers dedicated to PCOS will be very useful to both researchers and clinicians interested in finding new ways to improve the life of women with PCOS.

Enrico Carmina
Editor

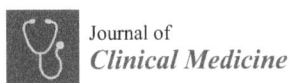

Article

An Evolutionary Model for the Ancient Origins of Polycystic Ovary Syndrome

Daniel A. Dumesic [1,*], David H. Abbott [2] and Gregorio D. Chazenbalk [1]

1. Department of Obstetrics and Gynecology, David Geffen School of Medicine at UCLA, 10833 Le Conte Ave, Los Angeles, CA 90095, USA; gchazenbalk@gmail.com
2. Department of Obstetrics and Gynecology, Wisconsin National Primate Research Center, University of Wisconsin, 1223 Capitol Court, Madison, WI 53715, USA; abbott@primate.wisc.edu
* Correspondence: ddumesic@mednet.ucla.edu; Tel.: +1-310-794-5542; Fax: +1-310-206-2057

Abstract: Polycystic ovary syndrome (PCOS) is a common endocrinopathy of reproductive-aged women, characterized by hyperandrogenism, oligo-anovulation and insulin resistance and closely linked with preferential abdominal fat accumulation. As an ancestral primate trait, PCOS was likely further selected in humans when scarcity of food in hunter–gatherers of the late Pleistocene additionally programmed for enhanced fat storage to meet the metabolic demands of reproduction in later life. As an evolutionary model for PCOS, healthy normal-weight women with hyperandrogenic PCOS have subcutaneous (SC) abdominal adipose stem cells that favor fat storage through exaggerated lipid accumulation during development to adipocytes in vitro. In turn, fat storage is counterbalanced by reduced insulin sensitivity and preferential accumulation of highly lipolytic intra-abdominal fat in vivo. This metabolic adaptation in PCOS balances energy storage with glucose availability and fatty acid oxidation for optimal energy use during reproduction; its accompanying oligo-anovulation allowed PCOS women from antiquity sufficient time and strength for childrearing of fewer offspring with a greater likelihood of childhood survival. Heritable PCOS characteristics are affected by today's contemporary environment through epigenetic events that predispose women to lipotoxicity, with excess weight gain and pregnancy complications, calling for an emphasis on preventive healthcare to optimize the long-term, endocrine-metabolic health of PCOS women in today's obesogenic environment.

Keywords: polycystic ovary syndrome; hyperandrogenism; insulin resistance; adipocyte; adipose stem cells; evolution; body fat distribution; metabolic adaptation

1. Introduction

As the most common endocrinopathy of reproductive-aged women, polycystic ovary syndrome (PCOS) is characterized by hyperandrogenism, oligo-anovulation and insulin resistance and closely linked with preferential abdominal fat accumulation [1]. Its clinical manifestations of hirsutism, menstrual irregularity, glucose intolerance and dyslipidemia worsen with obesity to increase the risks of developing subfertility, diabetes, metabolic syndrome and/or cardiovascular disease [2]. Almost one half of women with PCOS in the United States have metabolic syndrome (i.e., increased abdominal (android) obesity, hyperglycemia, dyslipidemia and/or hypertension), with a prevalence higher than that of age-matched women without PCOS in this country [1,3] and of PCOS women in other countries where obesity is less common [4,5].

Through an evolutionary perspective, the high worldwide prevalence of PCOS in today's environment should have disappeared over millennia, unless a beneficial effect favored both survival and reproduction [6]. Perhaps not surprisingly, therefore, ancestral traits resembling PCOS have been reported throughout antiquity [7] and in a non-human primate (i.e., the female rhesus macaque) [8–10] that shares a common ancestor with humans [11]. One explanation is that an ancient female primate trait resembling PCOS may have been favored originally in the cooling, increasingly arid and less forested African environments of the Oligocene before ancestors of humans diverged from those of macaques [12,13], as the isolated continent of Africa contacted Euroasia [14], enabling intercontinental migration [15] (Figure 1).

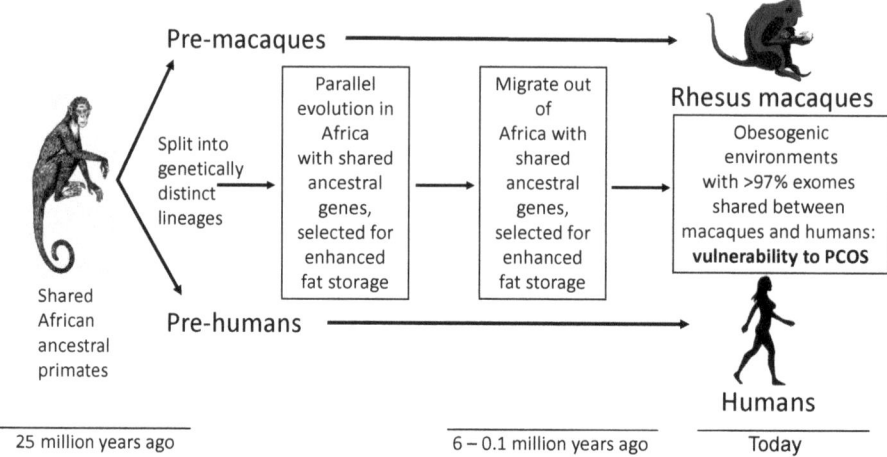

Figure 1. Polycystic ovary syndrome as an ancient metabolic-reproductive adaptation that originally enhanced fat storage for survival of humans during ancient times of food deprivation and also favored fewer offspring with a greater likelihood of childhood survival, but now predisposes women to endocrine-reproductive dysfunction in today's obesogenic environment (16). Ancestral traits resembling PCOS also exist in female rhesus macaques [8–10], which share a common ancestor with humans through parallel evolution.

Such an ancestral trait may have been additionally favored in human hunter–gatherers of the late Pleistocene, or in more ancient human populations, when scarcity of food further selected for programming of enhanced fat storage to meet the metabolic demands of reproduction in later life (i.e., metabolic thrift) [7,16–18]. Parallel evolution in macaques, particularly rhesus macaques living in semi-desert and high-altitude environments [13], may have emulated selection in humans for programming of enhanced fat storage (Figure 1). Such evolutionary metabolic adaptations in female primates, including women, would complement the ancient sympathoadrenal response to stress, whereby altered glucocorticoid and catecholamine activities mobilize hepatic glucose and FFAs from visceral fat to act in concert with insulin resistance and ensure sufficient energy during a "fight or flight" response for survival [19–21].

Through this evolutionary perspective, the present review examines PCOS as an ancient metabolic adaptation that underwent additional selection pressure for survival of humans during ancient times of food deprivation, but now predisposes to metabolic-endocrine-reproductive dysfunction in today's obesogenic environment [17,18,22]. A parallel obesogenic environmental change experienced by female rhesus macaques in their natural habitat [13], as well as by macaques removed from their natural habitat decades ago and housed in United States National Primate Research Centers (NPRCs) [23,24], may emulate the current obesogenic environmental challenge confronting humans (Figure 1). Consistent with this notion, approximately 15% of adult female rhesus macaques at the Wisconsin NPRC are naturally hyperandrogenic and exhibit PCOS-like traits [9,10]. Polycystic ovarian syndrome and PCOS-like phenotypes may thus form a continuum of ancient primate traits. Understanding trait-related molecular mechanisms, including genetic, epigenetic, protein and lipid interactions leading to optimal energy utilization, along with the perspective of providing benefits for survival and reproduction in both humans and rhesus macaques, offers novel insight into more effective clinical management for women with PCOS.

2. Genetics and Epigenetics of PCOS

The heritability of PCOS has been established by family and twin studies [25–28]; the prevalence of PCOS in female first-degree relatives of affected women is 20–40% [25,27,29], with monozygotic versus dizygotic twin studies showing the heritability of PCOS as high as 70% [26]. Large genome-wide association studies (GWAS) in cohorts of PCOS women and controls have identified several PCOS-susceptible loci in candidate genes involving gonadotropin secretion/action, androgen biosynthesis/gonadal function, insulin action/metabolism and follicle development [1,30–38]. Several PCOS candidate genes are shared among women with differing PCOS phenotypes (i.e., Rotterdam, National Institutes of Health (NIH) criteria, or self-reported) [36]. Some, such as thyroid adenoma associated (*THADA*) and insulin receptor (*INSR*), are associated with metabolic disorders in PCOS and type 2 diabetes mellitus (T2DM) [39], and others with high bioavailable (unbound) circulating T levels [40]. Genetic correlations between PCOS status and components of metabolic syndrome, including childhood obesity, T2DM, and fasting insulin, high-density lipoprotein-cholesterol (HDL-C) as well as triglyceride (TG) levels, further suggest shared genetic and biological origins between these parameters and PCOS [36,38]. That similar PCOS risk genes are expressed in women with PCOS from Chinese and European populations points to the ancient human origins of PCOS [37,38], potentially dating back before the migration of humans out of sub-Saharan Africa 300,000–50,000 years ago or earlier [41,42].

Importantly, women with NIH-defined PCOS have two distinct PCOS subtypes with different genetic heterogeneity: one defined as a "reproductive" group (23% of cases), characterized by higher luteinizing hormone (LH) and sex hormone binding globulin (SHBG) levels with relatively low body mass index (BMI) and insulin levels; the other defined as a "metabolic" group (37% of cases), characterized by higher BMI, glucose and insulin levels, with lower SHBG and LH levels [38,43]. These PCOS subtypes may differ in their developmental origins [43], with their heritability variably interacting with risk-increasing environmental factors to fully explain its prevalence.

Alternatively, rare variants in *DENND1A*, a gene encoding a 1009 amino acid protein with a clathrin-binding domain regulating endosome-mediated endocytosis, receptor cycling and calcium-dependent signaling cascades [44,45], also have been associated with endocrine-metabolic traits in families of daughters with PCOS [46]. A post-transcription form of *DENND1A*, namely DENND1A.v2, is over-expressed in some PCOS women [47,48], with DENND1A.v2 over-expression in human theca cells increasing androgen biosynthesis/release, potentially through PCOS-candidate gene *ZNF217* diminishing the theca cell expression of microRNA mIR-130b-3p, a noncoding microRNA transcriptional repressor [49].

Genetic variants of anti-mullerian hormone (AMH) and its type 2 receptor (AMHR2) also have been identified in about 7% of women with PCOS by NIH criteria, with 37 such variants having reduced in vitro bioactivity and diminished AMH inhibition of CYP17A1 as a risk factor for PCOS [50,51]. Both AMH and AMHR2 gene variants regulate intraovarian follicle development and hypothalamic GnRH function, and possibly ovarian androgen production [52], and may underlie elevated circulating AMH levels and ovarian hyperandrogenism in PCOS women [51].

Considered together, the current understanding of the genetics of PCOS suggests multiple contributing risk genes within which different variants can contribute to a PCOS phenotype. Given the heterogeneity of PCOS phenotypic expression, the high prevalence of PCOS, and its complex gene associations that account for some PCOS cases, PCOS may have multiple molecular underpinnings that arise from common or varied developmental origins.

Epigenetic changes coexist with many of these PCOS candidate genes [53,54]. In SC abdominal adipose, over-expression of the LHCG receptor and under-expression of the insulin receptor in non-obese and obese PCOS women, respectively, accompany reciprocal DNA methylation patterns [55], while reciprocal changes of gene expression and DNA methylation also coexist in adipogenic pathways of overweight PCOS women [56]. In PCOS theca cells, moreover, decreased expression of miR-130b-3b (i.e., a noncoding microRNA transcriptional repressor) correlates with increased DENND1A.V2 and CYP17A1 expression as well as with androgen synthesis [49,57], while three PCOS-specific gene variants of AMHR2 occur in regions of higher methylation and acetylation activity [51]. PCOS-susceptible loci alone, however, do not fully explain the majority of PCOS phenotypic expression [58], so that heritability of PCOS likely involves one or more PCOS candidate genes that have interacted with environmental factors throughout antiquity to modify the target tissue phenotype through epigenetic events [5].

3. PCOS Phenotypic Expression

Most women with PCOS have systemic insulin resistance from perturbed insulin receptor/post-receptor signaling, altered adipokine secretion and/or abnormal steroid metabolism [2], in combination with preferential abdominal fat accumulation worsened by obesity [1,59–61]. Most women with PCOS also have increased adiposity [62–64], which interacts with hyperandrogenism to worsen PCOS phenotypic expression [1–3,65–67] and insulin resistance [2,68,69]. Different PCOS phenotypes according to the Rotterdam criteria also vary in endocrine-metabolic dysfunction [70], with NIH-defined PCOS women (i.e., hyperandrogenism with oligo-anovulation) having the greatest risk of developing menstrual irregularity, anovulatory infertility, T2DM and metabolic syndrome [1]. Furthermore, women with PCOS from a referral population have a more severe phenotype than those from the general population [71,72].

To understand the origins of PCOS, the above variables underlying endocrine-metabolic dysfunction in PCOS need to be eliminated when comparing the clinical characteristics of healthy, normal-weight PCOS women according to the NIH criteria with age/BMI-balanced controls [68,69,71,73,74]. In doing so, healthy normal-weight PCOS women as defined by the NIH criteria show low-normal insulin sensitivity (Si) in frequently sampled intravenous glucose tolerance testing (FSIVGTT) in combination with preferential abdominal fat accumulation (i.e., android fat) as determined by total body dual-energy x-ray absorptiometry (DXA) [59,75,76]. Compared to age- and BMI-matched controls, normal-weight PCOS women as determined by the NIH criteria also exhibit adipose insulin resistance (adipose-IR; defined by the product of fasting circulating free fatty acid (FFA) and insulin levels) [73,76,77].

4. Total Abdominal (Android) Fat Mass

Abdominal fat mass comprises two major adipose depots: subcutaneous (SC) and intra-abdominal adipose. In humans, SC abdominal adipose normally stores lipid as protection against insulin resistance, while intra-abdominal adipose has the opposite effect [78]. Total body dual-energy x-ray absorptiometry studies confirm that android fat mass and the percent android fat relative to total body fat are greater in normal-weight PCOS women than age- and BMI-matched controls [59,75]. In all women combined, android fat mass positively correlates with circulating levels of total testosterone (T), free T, androstenedione (A4) and fasting insulin, as does the percent android fat mass relative to total body fat with circulating levels of total T, free T, A4 and fasting insulin [59,76]. Android fat mass in these individuals also negatively correlates with circulating cortisol levels, demonstrating an opposing system interplay of testosterone with cortisol in the control of android fat mass in women with PCOS [76].

Adjusting for fasting insulin levels, android fat mass remains positively correlated with circulating total T levels, as does the percent android fat mass relative to total body fat with circulating levels of total T, free T and A4 [59]. In these normal-weight PCOS women, moreover, androgen receptor blockade by low-dose flutamide simultaneously decreases percent android fat and increases fasting glucose levels, supporting the role of androgen excess in the metabolic adaptation of PCOS through body fat distribution [16,79].

4.1. Intra-Abdominal Adipose

Intra-abdominal (visceral) adipose in humans is normally highly lipolytic and resists androgen inhibition of catecholamine-induced lipolysis (lipid breakdown) despite expressing androgen receptors [80]. Intra-abdominal fat mass in normal-weight NIH-defined PCOS women is increased in proportion to circulating androgen concentrations and fasting levels of insulin, TG and non-high-density lipoprotein (non-HDL) cholesterol [59]; it also exhibits exaggerated catecholamine-induced lipolysis in non-obese PCOS women [81,82]. These intra-abdominal fat characteristics favor enhanced FFA availability for hepatic lipid storage and utilization [83]. However, they also promote insulin resistance with obesity when increased FFA availability exceeds the capacity of target tissues to oxidize fat or convert diacylglycerols to triacylglycerols [81,82,84].

4.2. Subcutaneous Abdominal Adipose

Subcutaneous abdominal adipose normally protects against insulin resistance by balancing lipogenesis (lipid formation) with lipolysis (lipid breakdown) in mature adipocytes in combination with adipogenesis (whereby adipose stem cells [ASCs] initially commit to preadipocytes and then differentiate into newly formed adipocytes) (Figure 2) [85–89].

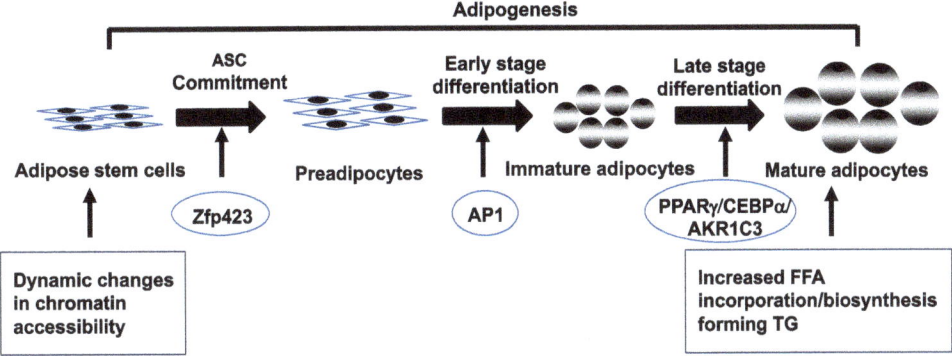

Figure 2. Schematic representation of adipogenesis in subcutaneous abdominal adipose stem cells (ASCs) from normal-weight women with polycystic ovary syndrome. Adipogenesis involves ASC commitment to preadipocytes, followed by an early/late stage preadipocyte differentiation to immature/mature adipocytes [85–87]. Dynamic changes in chromatin accessibility of SC abdominal ASCs during adipogenesis activate different transcriptional factors/genes (zinc-finger protein 423 (Zfp423), activator protein-1 (AP-1), peroxisome proliferator-activated receptor γ (PPARγ), CCAAT enhancer binding protein a (CEBPα) and aldo-ketoreductase type 1C3 (AKR1C3), leading to increased free fatty acid (FFA) incorporation/biosynthesis, thus forming triglycerides (TGs) in newly-formed mature adipocytes. In this manner, SC adipose can increase its fat storage through enlargement of mature adipocytes (i.e., hypertrophy) and development of new adipocytes (i.e., hyperplasia) to buffer fatty acid influx as energy intake exceeds its expenditure [88,89].

Within SC adipose, androgen normally diminishes insulin-stimulated glucose uptake and impairs catecholamine-stimulated lipolysis through reduced β2-adrenergic receptor and hormone-sensitive lipase (HSL) protein expression [80,81,90]. Women with PCOS have similar SC abdominal adipose characteristics of diminished insulin-mediated glucose uptake, reduced glucose transporter type 4 (GLUT-4) expression [91] and catecholamine lipolytic resistance [92,93]. Importantly, catecholamine lipolytic resistance in normal-weight

PCOS women [92,93] can be counterbalanced by impaired insulin suppression of lipolysis in overweight PCOS women [94].

Within SC adipose, an aldo-ketoreductase enzyme, namely aldo-ketoreductase type 1C3 (AKR1C3), generates local T from A4 [95,96]. AKR1C3 gene expression and activity are greater in SC gluteal than omental fat, with SC gluteal fat favoring androgen activation (i.e., AKR1C3), and omental cells favoring androgen inactivation (i.e., aldo-ketoreductase type 1C2 (AKR1C2)) [96]. In PCOS women, increased AKR1C3-mediated androgen activation enhances lipid storage through increased lipogenesis and decreased lipolysis [97,98], promoting fat accretion [75,98,99] despite diminished insulin-stimulated glucose uptake [90].

4.3. Subcutaneous Abdominal Stem Cells and Cellular Reprogramming

Subcutaneous abdominal ASCs from normal-weight PCOS women exhibit altered dynamic chromatin accessibility during adipogenesis compared to control ASCs and are characterized by limited chromatin accessibility in undifferentiated ASCs (quiescent stage) followed by exaggerated availability (active stage) in newly-formed adipocytes [100]. These chromatin remodeling patterns of PCOS stem cells accompany enrichment of binding motifs for transcription factors (TFs) of the activator protein-1 (AP-1) subfamily during early cell differentiation, with altered gene expression of adipogenic/angiogenic functions involving androgen–insulin interactions through transforming growth factor (TGF)-ß1 signaling [77].

In these SC abdominal ASCs of normal-weight PCOS women, an exaggerated commitment to preadipocytes via zinc-finger protein 423 (*ZFP423*) overexpression negatively correlates with fasting circulating glucose levels [99] and accompanies a greater proportion of small SC abdominal adipocytes [59,77], presumably to buffer against fatty acid influx [89,101]. Similar small SC abdominal adipocytes occur in other individuals [101–103], in whom they protect against insulin resistance through stem cell *ZFP423* upregulation from epigenetic modifications [104].

Following exaggerated commitment to preadipocytes, these same abdominal ASCs from normal-weight PCOS exhibit accelerated lipid accumulation in newly-formed adipocytes in vitro that predicts reduced serum FFA levels and improved systemic insulin sensitivity in vivo [75,99]. These differentiating PCOS stem cells can overexpress the genes, peroxisome proliferator-activated receptor γ (*PPARγ*) and CCAAT enhancer binding protein *a* (*CEBPa*), in combination with increased *AKR1C3* gene expression during adipocyte maturation in vitro (Figure 2) [79,98,100].

From a causal perspective, administration of flutamide (an androgen receptor blocker) to healthy normal-weight PCOS women attenuates accelerated lipid accumulation within these newly-formed adipocytes in vitro and increases fasting circulating glucose levels (but within the normal range) [79]. In addition to intrinsic changes in PCOS stem cell characteristics, therefore, local androgen excess in PCOS appears to enhance lipid storage in SC abdominal adipocytes [79,98,99] and favor insulin sensitivity [75,105,106].

5. Lipotoxicity

Lipotoxicity refers to the ectopic lipid accumulation in non-adipose tissue, where it induces oxidative/endoplasmic reticulum stress linked with insulin resistance and inflammation [107]. Overweight/obese PCOS women, with greater preferential abdominal fat accumulation, hyperandrogenism and insulin resistance [2], are at particular risk of developing lipotoxicity due to excess FFA uptake into non-adipose cells, in part from increased highly lipolytic intra-abdominal fat with impaired insulin suppression of lipolysis [81,82,94,108–110]. In these individuals, excess fatty acid influx in the skeletal muscle and liver promotes diacylglycerol-induced insulin resistance, impairs insulin signaling via increased insulin receptor serine phosphorylation, and disrupts mitochondrial oxidative phosphorylation [84,111]. Enlarged SC abdominal mature adipocytes in overweight compared to normal-weight PCOS women also fosters a pro-inflammatory lipid depot environment [59,94].

Within today's contemporary lifestyle, NIH-defined PCOS women have a two- to threefold higher prevalence of metabolic syndrome (33–47%) than age-matched women without PCOS [3,112–114], which is reduced by diminished abdominal fat accumulation [114]. Beginning in adolescence, an increased risk for developing metabolic syndrome [115] is evident in hyperandrogenic women [116], who preferentially increase abdominal adiposity with weight gain [61].

Increased abdominal fat in PCOS women also increases the risk of developing nonalcoholic fatty liver disease (NAFLD) [117–119], with non-alcoholic hepatic steatosis varying in inflammation and fibrosis [120]. Obesity in PCOS women is an important risk factor for hepatic steatosis [117], as is androgen excess per se, since the probability of hepatic steatosis (37%) and elevated serum aminotransferase levels is greater in hyperandrogenic women with PCOS than age- and weight-matched controls [121,122]. Magnetic resonance spectroscopy further confirms greater liver fat content in women with hyperandrogenic PCOS than non-hyperandrogenic PCOS [123].

6. Parallel Evolution of PCOS-like Traits in Naturally Hyperandrogenic Female Rhesus Macaques

Ancestors of macaques migrated out of Africa before humans (Figure 1), about 5–6 million years ago [12,15]. Second only to humans, contemporary rhesus macaques occupy the largest habitat range of any primate, somewhat emulating humans in their diversity of habitats, including obesogenic urban environments [13]. Such close evolutionary history to humans bestows considerable similarities in genomic, developmental, physiological, anatomical, neurological, behavioral and aging characteristics, as well as comparable breadth of natural disease susceptibility [10], including female hyperandrogenism, PCOS [8,9] and obesity [124]. Obesity in rhesus macaques is heritable [125], emulates that in humans [126–128] and may associate with human obesity risk genes [125], increased risk of T2DM [127,129], dyslipidemia [12,126,128,130] and cardiometabolic disease [131,132]. In female rhesus macaques, as in women, hyperandrogenism enhances obesity outcomes [128,130,133]. Examining the etiology for female rhesus macaque hyperandrogenism and accompanying PCOS-like traits, including metabolic dysfunction, may thus provide supportive evidence for parallel evolution of these traits to humans and for a shared vulnerability to PCOS (Figure 1). In addition, female rhesus macaques and humans share menstrual cycle traits, including a relatively lengthy follicular or preovulatory phase, exposing selection of a single preovulatory follicle to hyperandrogenic anovulatory consequences of prolonged LH hypersecretion, FSH hyposecretion [134] and hyperinsulinemia [10].

Hyperandrogenic female rhesus monkeys with increased adiposity also emulate the metabolic dysfunction seen in women with PCOS. They exhibit increased abdominal subcutaneous and visceral adiposity [128,133,135], adipose insulin resistance and impaired insulin secretion [136], and an increased incidence of T2DM [137]. Their SC abdominal adipocytes demonstrate an altered ability to store fat relative to BMI [128,130,135,138], with impaired preadipocyte differentiation into adipocytes accompanying a decrease in C/EBPα mRNA. An associated enhancement of SC abdominal ASC commitment to preadipocytes through increased ZFP423 mRNA expression may indicate a compensatory mechanism for impaired preadipocyte differentiation [138]. Those with the highest testosterone values demonstrate increased BMI, central adiposity and insulin resistance [8,128].

Hyperandrogenism in female rhesus monkeys may have developmental origins, emulating PCOS in women. A positive correlation of adult anogenital distance with circulating testosterone levels in naturally hyperandrogenic adult female rhesus monkeys suggests mid-gestational hyperandrogenic origins [9]. Increased anogenital distance has also been reported for girls born to women with PCOS [139], in women with PCOS [140] and in adult female PCOS-like rhesus monkeys previously exposed to early-to-mid, but not late, gestational testosterone excess [141]. Elevated maternal circulating levels of AMH from polycystic ovaries may enhance maternal hyperandrogenism and amplify epigenetic transgenerational transmission of hyperandrogenic and metabolic phenotypes in female offspring through altered placental function [142,143]. Consistent with these findings, gestational hyperandrogenism in rhesus monkeys induces maternal hyperinsulinemia and hyperglycemia and reliably generates 75% of female offspring with heterogenous PCOS-like reproductive and metabolic phenotypes [144], along with gestational hyperinsulinemia inducing ectopic pericardial and perirenal fetal lipid accumulation [145]. Commonly occurring placental structure and function alterations found in women with PCOS [146–149] and in hyperandrogenic adult female rhesus monkeys [150] can alter nutrient delivery to the fetus [146,151], with subsequent hyperandrogenism, insulin resistance and pancreatic beta cell dysfunction in prepubertal daughters [152–155], predisposing them to preferential fat storage [138,153]. Given these findings implicating hyperandrogenic developmental origins in the etiology of preferential fat storage, female rhesus monkeys may provide unique insight into the proximate mechanisms amplifying outcomes from the inheritance of PCOS risk genes, calling for gene editing studies of monkey embryos/cells to express female phenotypes generated by specific PCOS risk genes in individuals of known genetic backgrounds [10,156].

7. Conclusions

Polycystic ovary syndrome has persisted from antiquity to become the most common endocrine-metabolic disorder of reproductive-aged women. While its ancestral traits once favored abdominal fat deposition and increased energy availability through hyperandrogenism and insulin resistance for reproduction within hostile environments of food deprivation, these same traits now underlie different PCOS phenotypes, with various risks for endocrine-metabolic dysfunction, which are worsened by obesity. Normal-weight women with NIH-defined PCOS who are otherwise healthy have SC abdominal adipose characteristics that favor lipid storage in combination with low-normal insulin sensitivity accompanied by increased highly lipolytic intra-abdominal fat deposition. As an ancestral trait programmed by genetic inheritance and epigenetic amplification during gestation, such an evolutionary metabolic adaptation in normal-weight PCOS women balances enhanced SC adipose storage with increased circulating glucose availability and free fatty acid oxidation as energy substrate for the brain, muscle and other crucial target tissues. This metabolic adaptation in hyperandrogenic PCOS women also favors oligo-ovulation, which allowed women from antiquity sufficient time for childrearing of fewer offspring, who in turn had a greater likelihood of childhood survival [6].

Important strengths of this review paper are the inclusion of normal-weight PCOS women as defined by the NIH criteria, who were otherwise healthy and who were also age- and BMI-matched to controls whenever possible to eliminate the confounding effects of age and obesity on outcomes of interest. It is important to recognize, however, that this review is not intended to be a comprehensive review of the field of PCOS. Rather, it explores the hypothesis, based on the available (epi)genetic and physiological data, that the phenotypic expression of PCOS represents an evolutionary metabolic adaptation that balances preferential abdominal fat accumulation with increased energy availability through hyperandrogenism and insulin resistance to optimize energy use for reproduction during ancient times of food deprivation.

8. Future Directions

These heritable PCOS characteristics are now adversely affected by today's contemporary environment through epigenetic events that predispose women to lipotoxicity, with excess weight gain and pregnancy complications. Understanding the evolutionary origins of PCOS emphasizes the need for a greater focus on preventive healthcare, with early and appropriate lifestyle as well as therapeutic choices to optimize the long-term, endocrine-metabolic health of PCOS women in today's obesogenic environment.

Author Contributions: Conceptualization, D.A.D., G.D.C. and D.H.A.; methodology, D.A.D., G.D.C. and D.H.A.; formal analysis, D.A.D., G.D.C. and D.H.A.; writing—original draft preparation, D.A.D., G.D.C. and D.H.A.; writing—review and editing, D.A.D., G.D.C. and D.H.A.; funding acquisition, D.A.D., G.D.C. and D.H.A. All authors have read and agreed to the published version of the manuscript.

Funding: This work was supported by a grant from the Eunice Kennedy Shriver National Institute of Child Health & Human Development (NICHD), National Institutes of Health (NIH), under awards P50 HD071836 and P51 ODO11092 for the Endocrine Technologies Support Core (ETSC) through the Oregon National Primate Research Center; statistical analyses by the NIH National Center for Advancing Translational Science (NCATS) UCLA CTSI, Grant Number UL1TR001881; and the Santa Monica Bay Woman's Club. Nonhuman primate research was supported by awards R01 DK121559 (National Institute of Diabetes and Digestive and Kidney Diseases), R21 HD102172 (NICHD) and P51 OD011106 for the Office of Research Infrastructure Programs (ORIP) through the Wisconsin National Primate Research Center. The content is solely the responsibility of the authors and does not necessarily represent the official views of the NIH.

Institutional Review Board Statement: All studies were performed according to the Declaration of Helsinki after approval by the UCLA Institutional Review Board and signed informed consent by each subject (IRB number 12-001780; approval date 18 January 2013).

Informed Consent Statement: Informed consent was obtained from all subjects involved in the study. Written informed consent was obtained from the patient(s) to publish this paper.

Data Availability Statement: Not applicable.

Acknowledgments: We thank Karla Largaespada at UCLA for subject recruitment strategies and administrative responsibilities, which were crucial for the successful study of the PCOS and control subjects; the veterinary, pathology, animal care and assays staff at the Wisconsin National Primate Research Center (WNPRC); and Jon Levine (WNPRC) for his highly valued contributions to refining and enabling our research into the developmental origins of PCOS.

Conflicts of Interest: D.A.D. has consulted for Spruce Biosciences, Inc.; Precede Biosciences, Inc.; Ferring Research Institute; and Organon LLC. The funders had no role in the design of the study; in the collection, analysis or interpretation of data; in the writing of the manuscript; or in the decision to publish the results. G.D.C. and D.H.A. have nothing to disclose.

References

1. Chang, R.J.; Dumesic, D.A. Polycystic Ovary Syndrome and Hyperandrogenic States. In *Yen and Jaffe's Reproductive Endocrinology: Physiology, Pathophysiology and Clinical Management*, 9th ed.; Strauss, J.F., III, Barbieri, R.L., Dokras, A., Williams, C.J., Williams, S.Z., Eds.; Elsevier Saunders: Philadelphia, PA, USA, 2024; pp. 517–547.
2. Dumesic, D.A.; Oberfield, S.E.; Stener-Victorin, E.; Marshall, J.C.; Laven, J.S.; Legro, R.S. Scientific Statement on the Diagnostic Criteria, Epidemiology, Pathophysiology, and Molecular Genetics of Polycystic Ovary Syndrome. *Endocr. Rev.* **2015**, *36*, 487–525. [CrossRef]
3. Moran, L.J.; Misso, M.L.; Wild, R.A.; Norman, R.J. Impaired glucose tolerance, type 2 diabetes and metabolic syndrome in polycystic ovary syndrome: A systematic review and meta-analysis. *Hum. Repro. Update* **2010**, *16*, 347–363. [CrossRef]
4. Carmina, E.; Napoli, N.; Longo, R.A.; Rini, G.B.; Lobo, R.A. Metabolic syndrome in polycystic ovary syndrome (PCOS): Lower prevalence in southern Italy than in the USA and the influence of criteria for the diagnosis of PCOS. *Eur. J. Endocrinol.* **2006**, *154*, 141–145. [CrossRef] [PubMed]
5. Dumesic, D.A.; Hoyos, L.R.; Chazenbalk, G.D.; Naik, R.; Padmanabhan, V.; Abbott, D.H. Mechanisms of Intergenerational Transmission of Polycystic Ovary Syndrome. *Reproduction* **2020**, *159*, R1–R13. [CrossRef]
6. Corbett, S.; Morin-Papunen, L. Polycystic ovary syndrome and recent human evolution. *Mol. Cell. Endocrinol.* **2013**, *373*, 39–50. [CrossRef]
7. Azziz, R.; Dumesic, D.A.; Goodarzi, M. Polycystic Ovary Syndrome: An ancient disorder? *Fertil. Steril.* **2011**, *95*, 1544–1548. [CrossRef]
8. Arifin, E.; Shively, C.A.; Register, T.C.; Cline, J.M. Polycystic ovary syndrome with endometrial hyperplasia in a cynomolgus monkey (*Macaca fascicularis*). *Vet. Pathol.* **2008**, *45*, 512–515. [CrossRef] [PubMed]
9. Abbott, D.H.; Rayome, B.H.; Dumesic, D.A.; Lewis, K.C.; Edwards, A.K.; Wallen, K.; Wilson, M.E.; Appt, S.E.; Levine, J.E. Clustering of PCOS-like traits in naturally hyperandrogenic female rhesus monkeys. *Hum. Reprod.* **2017**, *32*, 923–936. [CrossRef] [PubMed]

10. Abbott, D.H.; Rogers, J.; Dumesic, D.A.; Levine, J.E. Naturally Occurring and Experimentally Induced Rhesus Macaque Models for Polycystic Ovary Syndrome: Translational Gateways to Clinical Application. *Med. Sci.* **2019**, *7*, 107. [CrossRef]
11. Perelman, P.; Johnson, W.E.; Roos, C.; Seuánez, H.N.; Horvath, J.E.; Moreira, M.A.; Kessing, B.; Pontius, J.; Roelke, M.; Rumpler, Y.; et al. A molecular phylogeny of living primates. *PLoS Genet.* **2011**, *7*, e1001342. [CrossRef]
12. Raaum, R.L.; Sterner, K.N.; Noviello, C.M.; Stewart, C.B.; Disotell, T.R. Catarrhine primate divergence dates estimated from complete mitochondrial genomes: Concordance with fossil and nuclear DNA evidence. *J. Hum. Evol.* **2005**, *48*, 237–257. [CrossRef]
13. Cooper, E.B.; Brent, L.J.N.; Snyder-Mackler, N.; Singh, M.; Sengupta, A.; Khatiwada, S.; Malaivijitnond, S.; Qi Hai, Z.; Higham, J.P. The rhesus macaque as a success story of the Anthropocene. *Elife* **2022**, *11*, e78169. [CrossRef] [PubMed]
14. Leakey, M.; Grossman, A.; Gutiérrez, M.; Fleagle, J.G. Faunal change in the Turkana Basin during the late Oligocene and Miocene. *Evol. Anthropol.* **2011**, *20*, 238–253. [CrossRef] [PubMed]
15. Stewart, C.B.; Disotell, T.R. Primate evolution—In and out of Africa. *Curr. Biol.* **1998**, *8*, R582–R588. [CrossRef] [PubMed]
16. Dumesic, D.A.; Padmanabhan, V.; Levine, J.; Chazenbalk, G.D.; Abbott, D.H. Polycystic Ovary Syndrome as a Plausible Evolutionary Metabolic Adaptation. *Repro. Biol. Endocrinol.* **2022**, *20*, 12. [CrossRef]
17. Parker, J.; O'Brien, C.; Hawrelak, J.; Gersh, F.L. Polycystic Ovary Syndrome: An Evolutionary Adaptation to Lifestyle and the Environment. *Int. J. Environ. Res. Public Health* **2022**, *19*, 1336. [CrossRef]
18. Parker, J. Pathophysiological Effects of Contemporary Lifestyle on Evolutionary-Conserved Survival Mechanisms in Polycystic Ovary Syndrome. *Life* **2023**, *13*, 1056. [CrossRef] [PubMed]
19. Tsatsoulis, A.; Mantzaris, M.D.; Bellou, S.; Andrikoula, M. Insulin resistance: An adaptive mechanism becomes maladaptive in the current environment—An evolutionary perspective. *Metabolism* **2013**, *62*, 622–633. [CrossRef] [PubMed]
20. Björntorp, P. Metabolic implications of body fat distribution. *Diabetes Care* **1991**, *14*, 1132–1143. [CrossRef]
21. Björntorp, P. Visceral obesity: A "civilization syndrome". *Obes. Res.* **1993**, *1*, 206–222. [CrossRef]
22. López-Otín, C.; Kroemer, G. Hallmarks of Health. *Cell* **2021**, *184*, 33–63. [CrossRef]
23. Klimentidis, Y.C.; Beasley, T.M.; Lin, H.Y.; Murati, G.; Glass, G.E.; Guyton, M.; Newton, W.; Jorgensen, M.; Heymsfield, S.B.; Kemnitz, J.; et al. Canaries in the coal mine: A cross-species analysis of the plurality of obesity epidemics. *Proc. Biol. Sci.* **2011**, *278*, 1626–1632. [CrossRef]
24. Terasawa, E.; Kurian, J.R.; Keen, K.L.; Shiel, N.A.; Colman, R.J.; Capuano, S.V. Body weight impact on puberty: Effects of high-calorie diet on puberty onset in female rhesus monkeys. *Endocrinology* **2012**, *153*, 1696–1705. [CrossRef] [PubMed]
25. Legro, R.S.; Driscoll, D.; Strauss, J.F., 3rd; Fox, J.; Dunaif, A. Evidence for a genetic basis for hyperandrogenemia in polycystic ovary syndrome. *Proc. Natl. Acad. Sci. USA* **1998**, *95*, 14956–14960. [CrossRef]
26. Vink, J.M.; Sadrzadeh, S.; Lambalk, C.B.; Boomsma, D.I. Heritability of polycystic ovary syndrome in a Dutch twin-family study. *J. Clin. Endocrinol. Metab.* **2006**, *91*, 2100–2104. [CrossRef]
27. Risal, S.; Pei, Y.; Lu, H.; Manti, M.; Fornes, R.; Pui, H.P.; Zhao, Z.; Massart, J.; Ohlsson, C.; Lindgren, E.; et al. Prenatal androgen exposure and transgenerational susceptibility to polycystic ovary syndrome. *Nat. Med.* **2019**, *25*, 1894–1904. [CrossRef]
28. Shan, D.; Han, J.; Cai, Y.; Zou, L.; Xu, L.; Shen, Y. Reproductive Health in First-degree Relatives of Patients with Polycystic Ovary Syndrome: A Review and Meta-analysis. *J. Clin. Endocrinol. Metab.* **2022**, *107*, 273–295. [CrossRef]
29. Kahsar-Miller, M.D.; Nixon, C.; Boots, L.R.; Go, R.C.; Azziz, R. Prevalence of polycystic ovary syndrome (PCOS) in first-degree relatives of patients with PCOS. *Fertil. Steril.* **2001**, *75*, 53–58. [CrossRef] [PubMed]
30. Chen, Z.J.; Zhao, H.; He, L.; Shi, Y.; Qin, Y.; Shi, Y.; Li, Z.; You, L.; Zhao, J.; Liu, J.; et al. Genome-wide association study identifies susceptibility loci for polycystic ovary syndrome on chromosome 2p16.3, 2p21 and 9q33.3. *Nat. Genet.* **2011**, *43*, 55–59. [CrossRef] [PubMed]
31. Shi, Y.; Zhao, H.; Shi, Y.; Cao, Y.; Yang, D.; Li, Z.; Zhang, B.; Liang, X.; Li, T.; Chen, J.; et al. Genome-wide association study identifies eight new risk loci for polycystic ovary syndrome. *Nat. Genet.* **2012**, *44*, 1020–1025. [CrossRef]
32. Goodarzi, M.O.; Jones, M.R.; Li, X.; Chua, A.K.; Garcia, O.A.; Chen, Y.D.; Krauss, R.M.; Rotter, J.I.; Ankener, W.; Legro, R.S.; et al. Replication of association of DENND1A and THADA variants with polycystic ovary syndrome in European cohorts. *J. Med. Genet.* **2012**, *49*, 90–95. [CrossRef] [PubMed]
33. Mutharasan, P.; Galdones, E.; Penalver Bernabe, B.; Garcia, O.A.; Jafari, N.; Shea, L.D.; Woodruff, T.K.; Legro, R.S.; Dunaif, A.; Urbanek, M. Evidence for chromosome 2p16.3 polycystic ovary syndrome susceptibility locus in affected women of European ancestry. *J. Clin. Endocrinol. Metab.* **2013**, *98*, E185–E190. [CrossRef]
34. Hayes, M.G.; Urbanek, M.; Ehrmann, D.A.; Armstrong, L.L.; Lee, J.Y.; Sisk, R.; Karaderi, T.; Barber, T.M.; McCarthy, M.I.; Franks, S.; et al. Genome-wide association of polycystic ovary syndrome implicates alterations in gonadotropin secretion in European ancestry populations. *Nat. Commun.* **2015**, *6*, 7502. [CrossRef]
35. Day, F.R.; Hinds, D.A.; Tung, J.Y.; Stolk, L.; Styrkarsdottir, U.; Saxena, R.; Bjonnes, A.; Broer, L.; Dunger, D.B.; Halldorsson, B.V.; et al. Causal mechanisms and balancing selection inferred from genetic associations with polycystic ovary syndrome. *Nat. Commun.* **2015**, *6*, 8464. [CrossRef]
36. Day, F.; Karaderi, T.; Jones, M.R.; Meun, C.; He, C.; Drong, A.; Kraft, P.; Lin, N.; Huang, H.; Broer, L.; et al. Large-scale genome-wide meta-analysis of polycystic ovary syndrome suggests shared genetic architecture for different diagnosis criteria. *PLoS Genet.* **2018**, *14*, e1007813. [CrossRef]

37. Dapas, M.; Dunaif, A. The contribution of rare genetic variants to the pathogenesis of polycystic ovary syndrome. *Curr. Opin. Endocr. Metab. Res.* **2020**, *12*, 26–32. [CrossRef] [PubMed]
38. Dapas, M.; Dunaif, A. Deconstructing a Syndrome: Genomic Insights into PCOS Causal Mechanisms and Classification. *Endocr. Rev.* **2022**, *43*, 927–965. [CrossRef] [PubMed]
39. Tian, Y.; Li, J.; Su, S.; Cao, Y.; Wang, Z.; Zhao, S.; Zhao, H. PCOS-GWAS Susceptibility Variants in *THADA*, *INSR*, *TOX3*, and *DENND1A* Are Associated with Metabolic Syndrome or Insulin Resistance in Women with PCOS. *Front. Endocrinol.* **2020**, *11*, 274. [CrossRef] [PubMed]
40. Ruth, K.S.; Day, F.R.; Tyrrell, J.; Thompson, D.J.; Wood, A.R.; Mahajan, A.; Beaumont, R.N.; Wittemans, L.; Martin, S.; Busch, A.S.; et al. Using human genetics to understand the disease impacts of testosterone in men and women. *Nat. Med.* **2020**, *26*, 252–258. [CrossRef] [PubMed]
41. Shriner, D.; Tekola-Ayele, F.; Adeyemo, A.; Rotimi, C.N. Ancient Human Migration after Out-of-Africa. *Sci. Rep.* **2016**, *6*, 26565. [CrossRef] [PubMed]
42. Nielsen, R.; Akey, J.M.; Jakobsson, M.; Pritchard, J.K.; Tishkoff, S.; Willerslev, E. Tracing the peopling of the world through genomics. *Nature* **2017**, *541*, 302–310. [CrossRef]
43. Dapas, M.; Lin, F.T.J.; Nadkarni, G.N.; Sisk, R.; Legro, R.S.; Urbanek, M.; Hayes, M.G.; Dunaif, A. Distinct subtypes of polycystic ovary syndrome with novel genetic associations: An unsupervised, phenotypic clustering analysis. *PLoS Med.* **2020**, *17*, e1003132. [CrossRef] [PubMed]
44. Strauss, J.F., 3rd; McAllister, J.M.; Urbanek, M. Persistence pays off for PCOS gene prospectors. *J. Clin. Endocrinol. Metab.* **2012**, *97*, 2286–2288. [CrossRef]
45. Tee, M.K.; Speek, M.; Legeza, B.; Modi, B.; Teves, M.E.; McAllister, J.M.; Strauss, J.F., 3rd; Miller, W.L. Alternative splicing of DENND1A, a PCOS candidate gene, generates variant 2. *Mol. Cell. Endocrinol.* **2016**, *434*, 25–35. [CrossRef] [PubMed]
46. Dapas, M.; Sisk, R.; Legro, R.S.; Urbanek, M.; Dunaif, A.; Hayes, M.G. Family-based quantitative trait meta-analysis implicates rare noncoding variants in DENND1A in polycystic ovary syndrome. *J. Clin. Endocrinol. Metab.* **2019**, *104*, 3835–3850. [CrossRef] [PubMed]
47. McAllister, J.M.; Modi, B.; Miller, B.A.; Biegler, J.; Bruggeman, R.; Legro, R.S.; Strauss, J.F., 3rd. Overexpression of a DENND1A isoform produces a polycystic ovary syndrome theca phenotype. *Proc. Natl. Acad. Sci. USA* **2014**, *111*, E1519–E1527. [CrossRef]
48. McAllister, J.M.; Legro, R.S.; Modi, B.P.; Strauss, J.F., 3rd. Functional genomics of PCOS: From GWAS to molecular mechanisms. *Trends Endocrinol. Metab.* **2015**, *26*, 118–124. [CrossRef]
49. Waterbury, J.S.; Teves, M.E.; Gaynor, A.; Han, A.X.; Mavodza, G.; Newell, J.; Strauss, J.F., 3rd; McAllister, J.M. The PCOS GWAS Candidate Gene *ZNF217* Influences Theca Cell Expression of *DENND1A.V2*, *CYP17A1*, and Androgen Production. *J. Endocr. Soc.* **2022**, *6*, bvac078. [CrossRef]
50. Gorsic, L.K.; Kosova, G.; Werstein, B.; Sisk, R.; Legro, R.S.; Hayes, M.G.; Teixeira, J.M.; Dunaif, A.; Urbanek, M. Pathogenic Anti-Mullerian Hormone Variants in Polycystic Ovary Syndrome. *J. Clin. Endocrinol. Metab.* **2017**, *102*, 2862–2872. [CrossRef]
51. Gorsic, L.K.; Dapas, M.; Legro, R.S.; Hayes, M.G.; Urbanek, M. Functional Genetic Variation in the Anti-Mullerian Hormone Pathway in Women with Polycystic Ovary Syndrome. *J. Clin. Endocrinol. Metab.* **2019**, *104*, 2855–2874. [CrossRef]
52. Barbotin, A.L.; Peigné, M.; Malone, S.A.; Giacobini, P. Emerging Roles of Anti-Müllerian Hormone in Hypothalamic-Pituitary Function. *Neuroendocrinology* **2019**, *109*, 218–229. [CrossRef]
53. Nilsson, E.; Benrick, A.; Kokosar, M.; Krook, A.; Lindgren, E.; Källman, T.; Martis, M.M.; Højlund, K.; Ling, C.; Stener-Victorin, E. Transcriptional and epigenetic changes influencing skeletal muscle metabolism in women with polycystic ovary syndrome. *J. Clin. Endocrinol. Metab.* **2018**, *103*, 4465–4477. [CrossRef] [PubMed]
54. Vázquez-Martínez, E.R.; Gómez-Viais, Y.I.; García-Gómez, E.; Reyes-Mayoral, C.; Reyes-Muñoz, E.; Camacho-Arroyo, I.; Cerbón, M. DNA methylation in the pathogenesis of polycystic ovary syndrome. *Reproduction* **2019**, *158*, R27–R40. [CrossRef] [PubMed]
55. Jones, M.R.; Brower, M.A.; Xu, N.; Cui, J.; Mengesha, E.; Chen, Y.D.; Taylor, K.D.; Azziz, R.; Goodarzi, M.O. Systems Genetics Reveals the Functional Context of PCOS Loci and Identifies Genetic and Molecular Mechanisms of Disease Heterogeneity. *PLoS Genet.* **2015**, *11*, e1005455. [CrossRef]
56. Kokosar, M.; Benrick, A.; Perfilyev, A.; Fornes, R.; Nilsson, E.; Maliqueo, M.; Behre, C.J.; Sazonova, A.; Ohlsson, C.; Ling, C.; et al. Epigenetic and Transcriptional Alterations in Human Adipose Tissue of Polycystic Ovary Syndrome. *Sci. Rep.* **2016**, *6*, 22883. [CrossRef] [PubMed]
57. McAllister, J.M.; Han, A.X.; Modi, B.P.; Teves, M.E.; Mavodza, G.R.; Anderson, Z.L.; Shen, T.; Christenson, L.K.; Archer, K.J.; Strauss, J.F. miRNA Profiling Reveals miRNA-130b-3p Mediates DENND1A Variant 2 Expression and Androgen Biosynthesis. *Endocrinology* **2019**, *160*, 1964–1981. [CrossRef] [PubMed]
58. Abbott, D.H.; Dumesic, D.A.; Levine, J.E. Hyperandrogenic Origins of Polycystic Ovary Syndrome—Implications for Pathophysiology and Therapy. *Expert Rev. Endocrinol. Metab.* **2019**, *14*, 131–143. [CrossRef]
59. Dumesic, D.A.; Akopians, A.L.; Madrigal, V.K.; Ramirez, E.; Margolis, D.J.; Sarma, M.K.; Thomas, A.M.; Grogan, T.R.; Haykal, R.; Schooler, T.A.; et al. Hyperandrogenism Accompanies Increased Intra-Abdominal Fat Storage in Normal Weight Polycystic Ovary Syndrome Women. *J. Clin. Endocrinol. Metab.* **2016**, *101*, 4178–4188. [CrossRef]

60. Tosi, F.; Di Sarra, D.; Kaufman, J.M.; Bonin, C.; Moretta, R.; Bonoro, E.; Zanolin, E.; Mogetti, P. Total body fat and central fat mass independently predict insulin resistance but not hyperandrogenemia in women with polycystic ovary syndrome. *J. Clin. Endocrinol. Metab.* **2015**, *100*, 661–669. [CrossRef]
61. Holte, J.; Bergh, T.; Berne, C.; Berglund, L.; Lithell, H. Enhanced early insulin response to glucose in relation to insulin resistance in women with polycystic ovary syndrome and normal glucose tolerance. *J. Clin. Endocrinol. Metab.* **1994**, *78*, 1052–1058. [CrossRef]
62. Rosenzweig, J.L.; Ferrannini, E.; Grundy, S.M.; Haffner, S.M.; Heine, R.J.; Horton, E.S.; Kawamori, R. Primary prevention of cardiovascular disease and type 2 diabetes in patients at metabolic risk: An endocrine society clinical practice guideline. *J. Clin. Endocrinol. Metab.* **2008**, *93*, 3671–3689. [CrossRef] [PubMed]
63. Wyatt, H.R. Update on treatment strategies for obesity. *J. Clin. Endocrinol. Metab.* **2013**, *98*, 1299–1306. [CrossRef]
64. Pasquali, R.; Pelusi, C.; Genghini, S.; Cacciari, M.; Gambineri, A. Obesity and reproductive disorders in women. *Hum. Reprod. Update* **2003**, *9*, 359–372. [CrossRef]
65. Diamanti-Kandarakis, E.; Dunaif, A. Insulin resistance and the polycystic ovary syndrome revisited: An update on mechanisms and implications. *Endocr. Rev.* **2012**, *33*, 981–1030. [CrossRef] [PubMed]
66. Lim, S.S.; Norman, R.J.; Davies, M.J.; Moran, L.J. The effect of obesity on polycystic ovary syndrome: A systematic review and meta-analysis. *Obes. Rev.* **2013**, *14*, 95–109. [CrossRef] [PubMed]
67. Yildiz, B.O.; Knochenhauer, E.S.; Azziz, R. Impact of obesity on the risk for polycystic ovary syndrome. *J. Clin. Endocrinol. Metab.* **2008**, *93*, 162–168. [CrossRef]
68. Kakoly, N.S.; Khomami, M.B.; Joham, A.E.; Corray, S.D.; Misso, M.L.; Norman, R.J.; Harrison, C.L.; Ranasinha, S.; Teede, H.J.; Moran, L.J. Ethnicity, obesity and the prevalence of impaired glucose tolerance and type 2 diabetes in PCOS: A systematic review and meta-regression. *Hum. Reprod. Update* **2018**, *24*, 455–467. [CrossRef]
69. Palaniappan, L.P.; Carnethon, M.R.; Fortmann, S.P. Heterogeneity in the relationship between ethnicity, BMI, and fasting insulin. *Diabetes Care* **2002**, *25*, 1351–1357. [CrossRef]
70. Teede, H.J.; Tay, C.T.; Laven, J.; Dokras, A.; Moran, L.J.; Piltonen, T.T.; Costello, M.F.; Boivin, J.; Redman, L.M.; Boyle, J.A.; et al. Recommendations from the 2023 International Evidence-based Guideline for the Assessment and Management of Polycystic Ovary Syndrome. *Fertil. Steril.* **2023**. Epub ahead of print. [CrossRef]
71. Ezeh, U.; Yildiz, B.O.; Azziz, R. Referral bias in defining the phenotype and prevalence of obesity in polycystic ovary syndrome. *J. Clin. Endocrinol. Metab.* **2013**, *98*, E1088–E1096. [CrossRef]
72. Lizneva, D.; Kirubakaran, R.; Mykhalchenko, K.; Suturina, L.; Chernukha, G.; Diamond, M.P.; Azziz, R. Phenotypes and body mass in women with polycystic ovary syndrome identified in referral versus unselected populations: Systematic review and meta-analysis. *Fertil. Steril.* **2016**, *106*, 1510–1520.e2. [CrossRef]
73. Søndergaard, E.; Espinosa De Ycaza, A.E.; Morgan-Bathke, M.; Jensen, M.D. How to measure adipose tissue insulin sensitivity. *J. Clin. Endocrinol. Metab.* **2017**, *102*, 1193–1199. [CrossRef] [PubMed]
74. Hershkop, K.; Besor, O.; Santoro, N.; Pierpont, B.; Caprio, S.; Weiss, R. Adipose insulin resistance in obese adolescents across the spectrum of glucose tolerance. *J. Clin. Endocrinol. Metab.* **2016**, *101*, 2423–2431. [CrossRef] [PubMed]
75. Dumesic, D.A.; Tulberg, A.; Leung, K.L.; Fisch, S.C.; Grogan, T.R.; Abbott, D.H.; Naik, R.; Chazenbalk, G.D. Accelerated subcutaneous abdominal stem cell adipogenesis predicts insulin sensitivity in normal-weight women with polycystic ovary syndrome. *Fertil. Steril.* **2021**, *116*, 232–242. [CrossRef] [PubMed]
76. Dumesic, D.A.; Turcu, A.F.; Liu, H.; Grogan, T.R.; Abbott, D.H.; Lu, G.; Dharanipragada, D.; Chazenbalk, G.D. Interplay of Cortisol, Testosterone, and Abdominal Fat Mass in Normal-weight Women with Polycystic Ovary Syndrome. *J. Endocr. Soc.* **2023**, *7*, bvad079. [CrossRef]
77. Dumesic, D.A.; Phan, J.D.; Leung, K.L.; Grogan, T.R.; Ding, X.; Li, X.; Hoyos, L.R.; Abbott, D.H.; Chazenbalk, G.D. Adipose Insulin Resistance in Normal-Weight Polycystic Ovary Syndrome Women. *J. Clin. Endocrinol. Metab.* **2019**, *104*, 2171–2183. [CrossRef]
78. McLaughlin, T.; Lamendola, C.; Liu, A.; Abbasi, F. Preferential fat deposition in subcutaneous versus visceral depots is associated with insulin sensitivity. *J. Clin. Endocrinol. Metab.* **2011**, *969*, E1756–E1760. [CrossRef]
79. Dumesic, D.A.; Winnett, C.; Lu, G.; Grogan, T.R.; Abbott, D.H.; Naik, R.; Chazenbalk, G.D. Randomized Clinical Trial: Effect of Low-Dose Flutamide on Abdominal Adipogenic Function in Normal-Weight Polycystic Ovary Syndrome Women. *Fertil. Steril.* **2023**, *119*, 116–126. [CrossRef]
80. Dicker, A.; Ryden, M.; Naslund, E.; Muehlen, I.E.; Wiren, M.; Lafontan, M.; Arner, P. Effect of testosterone on lipolysis in human pre-adipocytes from different fat depots. *Diabetologia* **2004**, *47*, 420–428. [CrossRef]
81. Arner, P. Effects of testosterone on fat cell lipolysis. Species differences and possible role in polycystic ovarian syndrome. *Biochimie* **2005**, *87*, 39–43. [CrossRef]
82. Ek, I.; Arner, P.; Rydén, M.; Holm, C.; Thörne, A.; Hoffstedt, J.; Wahrenberg, H. A unique defect in the regulation of visceral fat cell lipolysis in the polycystic ovary syndrome as an early link to insulin resistance. *Diabetes* **2002**, *51*, 484–492. [CrossRef]
83. Zhou, M.S.; Wang, A.; Yu, H. Link between insulin resistance and hypertension: What is the evidence from evolutionary biology? *Diabetol. Metab. Syndr.* **2014**, *6*, 12. [CrossRef]
84. Samuel, V.T.; Petersen, K.F.; Shulman, G.I. Lipid-induced insulin resistance: Unraveling the mechanism. *Lancet* **2010**, *375*, 2267–2277. [CrossRef] [PubMed]

85. Chazenbalk, G.D.; Singh, P.; Irge, D.; Shah, A.; Abbott, D.H.; Dumesic, D.A. Androgens inhibit adipogenesis during human adipose stem cell commitment to predipocyte formation. *Steroids* **2013**, *78*, 920–926. [CrossRef]
86. Cristancho, A.G.; Lazar, M.A. Forming functional fat: A growing understanding of adipocyte differentiation. *Nat. Rev. Mol. Cell Biol.* **2011**, *12*, 722–734. [CrossRef] [PubMed]
87. Tang, Q.Q.; Lane, M.D. Adipogenesis: From stem cell to adipocyte. *Annu. Rev. Biochem.* **2012**, *81*, 715–736. [CrossRef] [PubMed]
88. Saponaro, C.; Gaggini, M.; Carli, F.; Gastaldelli, A. The subtle balance between lipolysis and lipogenesis: A critical point in metabolic homeostasis. *Nutrients* **2015**, *7*, 9453–9474. [CrossRef] [PubMed]
89. Romacho, T.; Elsen, M.; Rohrborn, D.; Eckel, J. Adipose tissue and its role in organ crosstalk. *Acta Physiol.* **2014**, *210*, 733–753. [CrossRef] [PubMed]
90. Corbould, A. Chronic testosterone treatment induces selective insulin resistance in subcutaneous adipocytes of women. *J. Endocrinol.* **2007**, *192*, 585–594. [CrossRef]
91. Rosenbaum, D.; Harber, R.S.; Dunaif, A. Insulin resistance in polycystic ovary syndrome: Decreased expression of GLUT-4 glucose transporters in adipocytes. *Am. J. Physiol.* **1993**, *264 Pt 1*, E197–E202. [CrossRef]
92. Faulds, G.; Rydén, M.; Ek, I.; Wahrenberg, H.; Arner, P. Mechanisms behind lipolytic catecholamine resistance of subcutaneous fat cells in the polycystic ovarian syndrome. *J. Clin. Endocrinol. Metab.* **2003**, *88*, 2269–2273. [CrossRef] [PubMed]
93. Ek, I.; Arner, P.; Bergqvist, A.; Carlstrom K Wahrenberg, H. Impaired adipocyte lipolysis in nonobese women with the polycystic ovary syndrome: A possible link to insulin resistance? *J. Clin. Endocrinol. Metab.* **1997**, *82*, 1147–1153. [CrossRef]
94. Manneråas-Holm, L.; Leonhardt, H.; Kullberg, J.; Jennische, E.; Odén, A.; Holm, G.; Hellström, M.; Lönn, L.; Olivecrona, G.; Stener-Victorin, E.; et al. Adipose tissue has aberrant morphology and function in PCOS: Enlarged adipocytes and low serum adiponectin, but not circulating sex steroids, are strongly associated with insulin resistance. *J. Clin. Endocrinol. Metab.* **2011**, *96*, E304–E311. [CrossRef] [PubMed]
95. Blouin, K.; Veilleux, A.; Luu-The, V.; Tchernof, A. Androgen metabolism in adipose tissue: Recent advances. *Mol. Cell. Endocrinol.* **2009**, *301*, 97–103. [CrossRef]
96. Quinkler, M.; Sinha, B.; Tomlinson, J.W.; Bujalska, I.J.; Stewart, P.M.; Arlt, W. Androgen generation in adipose tissue in women with simple obesity—A site-specific role for 17beta-hydroxysteroid dehydrogenase type 5. *J. Endocrinol.* **2004**, *183*, 331–342. [CrossRef] [PubMed]
97. O'Reilly, M.W.; Kempegowda, P.; Walsh, M.; Taylor, A.E.; Manolopoulos, K.N.; Allwood, J.W.; Semple, R.K.; Hebenstreit, D.; Dunn, W.B.; Tomlinson, J.W.; et al. AKR1C3-Mediated Adipose Androgen Generation Drives Lipotoxicity in Women with Polycystic Ovary Syndrome. *J. Clin. Endocrinol. Metab.* **2017**, *102*, 3327–3339. [CrossRef]
98. Dumesic, D.A.; Tulberg, A.; McNamara, M.; Grogan, T.R.; Abbott, D.H.; Naik, R.; Lu, G.; Chazenbalk, G.D. Serum Testosterone to Androstenedione Ratio Predicts Metabolic Health in Normal-Weight Polycystic Ovary Syndrome Women. *J. Endocr. Soc.* **2021**, *5*, bvab158. [CrossRef] [PubMed]
99. Fisch, S.C.; Nikou, A.F.; Wright, E.A.; Phan, J.D.; Leung, K.L.; Grogan, T.R.; Abbott, D.H.; Chazenbalk, G.D.; Dumesic, D.A. Precocious Subcutaneous Abdominal Stem Cell Development to Adipocytes in Normal-Weight Polycystic Ovary Syndrome Women. *Fertil. Steril.* **2018**, *110*, 1367–1376. [CrossRef] [PubMed]
100. Leung, K.L.; Sanchita, S.; Pham, C.T.; Davis, B.A.; Okhovat, M.; Ding, X.; Dumesic, P.; Grogan, T.R.; Williams, K.J.; Morselli, M.; et al. Dynamic changes in chromatin accessibility, altered adipogenic gene expression, and total versus de novo fatty acid synthesis in subcutaneous adipose stem cells of normal-weight polycystic ovary syndrome (PCOS) women during adipogenesis: Evidence of cellular programming. *Clin. Epigenetics* **2020**, *12*, 181. [CrossRef]
101. Spalding, K.L.; Arner, E.; Westermark, P.O.; Bernard, S.; Buchholz, B.A.; Bergmann, O.; Blomqvist, L.; Hoffsted, J.; Naslund, E.; Britton, T.; et al. Dynamics of fat cell turnover in humans. *Nature* **2008**, *453*, 783–787. [CrossRef]
102. Tandon, P.; Wafer, R.; Minchin, J.E. Adipose morphology and metabolic disease. *J. Exp. Biol.* **2018**, *221* (Suppl. S1), jeb164970. [CrossRef]
103. Arner, E.; Westermark, P.O.; Spalding, K.L.; Britton, T.; Ryden, M.; Frisen, J.; Bernard, S.; Arner, P. Adipocyte turnover: Relevance to human adipose tissue morphology. *Diabetes* **2010**, *59*, 105–109. [CrossRef] [PubMed]
104. Longo, M.; Raciti, G.A.; Zatterale, F.; Parrillo, L.; Desiderio, A.; Spinelli, R.; Hammarstedt, A.; Hedjazifar, S.; Hoffmann, J.M.; Nigro, C.; et al. Epigenetic modifications of the Zfp/ZNF423 gene control murine adipogenic commitment and are dysregulated in human hypertrophic obesity. *Diabetologia* **2018**, *61*, 369–380. [CrossRef]
105. Nouws, J.; Fitch, M.; Mata, M.; Santoro, N.; Galuppo, B.; Kursawe, R.; Narayan, D.; Vash-Margita, A.; Pierpont, B.; Shulman, G.I.; et al. Altered In Vivo Lipid Fluxes and Cell Dynamics in Subcutaneous Adipose Tissues Are Associated with the Unfavorable Pattern of Fat Distribution in Obese Adolescent Girls. *Diabetes* **2019**, *68*, 1168–1177. [CrossRef]
106. Umano, G.R.; Shabanova, V.; Pierpont, B.; Mata, M.; Nouws, J.; Tricò, D.; Galderisi, A.; Santoro, N.; Caprio, S. A low visceral fat proportion, independent of total body fat mass, protects obese adolescent girls against fatty liver and glucose dysregulation: A longitudinal study. *Int. J. Obes.* **2019**, *43*, 673–682. [CrossRef]
107. Brennan, K.M.; Kroener, L.L.; Chazenbalk, G.D.; Dumesic, D.A. Polycystic Ovary Syndrome: Impact of Lipotoxicity on Metabolic and Reproductive Health. *Obstet. Gynecol. Surv.* **2019**, *74*, 223–231. [CrossRef] [PubMed]
108. Virtue, S.; Vidal-Puig, A. It's not how fat you are, it's what you do with it that counts. *PLoS Biol.* **2008**, *6*, e237. [CrossRef]

109. Unger, R.H.; Clark, G.O.; Scherer, P.E.; Orci, L. Lipid homeostasis, lipotoxicity and the metabolic syndrome. *Biochim. Biophys. Acta* **2010**, *1801*, 209–214. [CrossRef] [PubMed]
110. de Zegher, F.; Lopez-Bermejo, A.; Ibáñez, L. Adipose tissue expandability and the early origins of PCOS. *Trends Endocrinol. Metab.* **2009**, *20*, 418–423. [CrossRef]
111. Shulman, G.I. Ectopic fat in insulin resistance, dyslipidemia, and cardiometabolic disease. *N. Eng. J. Med.* **2014**, *371*, 1131–1141. [CrossRef]
112. Apridonidze, T.; Essah, P.A.; Iuorno, M.J.; Nestler, J.E. Prevalence and characteristics of the metabolic syndrome in women with polycystic ovary syndrome. *J. Clin. Endocrinol. Metab.* **2005**, *90*, 1929–1935. [CrossRef] [PubMed]
113. Dokras, A.; Bochner, M.; Hollinrake, E.; Markham, S.; Vanvoorhis, B.; Jagasia, D.H. Screening women with polycystic ovary syndrome for metabolic syndrome. *Obstet. Gynecol.* **2005**, *106*, 131–137. [CrossRef] [PubMed]
114. Ehrmann, D.A.; Liljenquist, D.R.; Kasza, K.; Azziz, R.; Legro, R.S.; Ghazzi, M.N.; PCOS/Troglitazone Study Group. Prevalence and predictors of the metabolic syndrome in women with polycystic ovary syndrome. *J. Clin. Endocrinol. Metab.* **2006**, *91*, 48–53. [CrossRef] [PubMed]
115. Fazleen, N.E.; Whittaker, M.; Mamun, A. Risk of metabolic syndrome in adolescents with polycystic ovarian syndrome: A systematic review and meta-analysis. *Diabetes Metab. Syndr.* **2018**, *12*, 1083–1090. [CrossRef] [PubMed]
116. Yang, R.; Yang, S.; Li, R.; Liu, P.; Qiao, J.; Zhang, Y. Effects of hyperandrogenism on metabolic abnormalities in patients with polycystic ovary syndrome: A meta-analysis. *Reprod. Biol. Endocrinol.* **2016**, *14*, 67. [CrossRef]
117. Gambarin-Gelwan, M.; Kinkhabwala, S.V.; Schiano, T.D.; Bodian, C.; Yeh, H.C.; Futterweit, W. Prevalence of nonalcoholic fatty liver disease in women with polycystic ovary syndrome. *Clin. Gastroenterol. Hepatol.* **2007**, *5*, 496–501. [CrossRef] [PubMed]
118. Macut, D.; Tziomalos, K.; Božić-Antić, I.; Bjekić-Macut, J.; Katsikis, I.; Papadakis, E.; Andrić, Z.; Panidis, D. Non-alcoholic fatty liver disease is associated with insulin resistance and lipid accumulation product in women with polycystic ovary syndrome. *Hum. Reprod.* **2016**, *31*, 1347–1353. [CrossRef]
119. Vassilatou, E.; Vassiliadi, D.A.; Salambasis, K.; Lazaridou, H.; Koutsomitopoulos, N.; Kelekis, N.; Kassanos, D.; Hadjidakis, D.; Dimitriadis, G. Increased prevalence of polycystic ovary syndrome in premenopausal women with nonalcoholic fatty liver disease. *Eur. J. Endocrinol.* **2015**, *173*, 739–747. [CrossRef] [PubMed]
120. Browning, J.D.; Horton, J.D. Molecular mediators of hepatic steatosis and liver injury. *J. Clin. Investig.* **2004**, *114*, 147–152. [CrossRef]
121. Vassilatou, E.; Lafoyianni, S.; Vryonidou, A.; Ioannidis, D.; Kosma, L.; Katsoulis, K.; Papavassiliou, E.; Tzavara, I. Increased androgen bioavailability is associated with non-alcoholic fatty liver disease in women with polycystic ovary syndrome. *Hum. Reprod.* **2010**, *25*, 212–220. [CrossRef]
122. Petta, S.; Ciresi, A.; Bianco, J.; Geraci, V.; Boemi, R.; Galvano, L.; Magliozzo, F.; Merlino, G.; Craxì, A.; Giordano, C. Insulin resistance and hyperandrogenism drive steatosis and fibrosis risk in young females with PCOS. *PLoS ONE* **2017**, *12*, e0186136. [CrossRef]
123. Jones, H.; Sprung, V.S.; Pugh, C.J.; Daousi, C.; Irwin, A.; Aziz, N.; Adams, V.L.; Thomas, E.L.; Bell, J.D.; Kemp, G.J.; et al. Polycystic ovary syndrome with hyperandrogenism is characterized by an increased risk of hepatic steatosis compared to nonhyperandrogenic PCOS phenotypes and healthy controls, independent of obesity and insulin resistance. *J. Clin. Endocrinol. Metab.* **2012**, *97*, 3709–3716. [CrossRef]
124. Schwartz, S.M.; Kemnitz, J.W.; Howard, C.F., Jr. Obesity in free-ranging rhesus macaques. *Int. J. Obes. Relat. Metab. Disord.* **1993**, *17*, 1–9. [PubMed]
125. Raboin, M.J.; Letaw, J.; Mitchell, A.D.; Toffey, D.; McKelvey, J.; Roberts, C.T., Jr.; Curran, J.E.; Vinson, A. Genetic Architecture of Human Obesity Traits in the Rhesus Macaque. *Obesity* **2019**, *27*, 479–488. [CrossRef] [PubMed]
126. Kemnitz, J.W.; Goy, R.W.; Flitsch, T.J.; Lohmiller, J.J.; Robinson, J.A. Obesity in male and female rhesus monkeys: Fat distribution, glucoregulation, and serum androgen levels. *J. Clin. Endocrinol. Metab.* **1989**, *69*, 287–293. [CrossRef]
127. Pound, L.D.; Kievit, P.; Grove, K.L. The nonhuman primate as a model for type 2 diabetes. *Curr. Opin. Endocrinol. Diabetes Obes.* **2014**, *21*, 89–94. [CrossRef]
128. True, C.; Abbott, D.H.; Roberts, C.T., Jr.; Varlamov, O. Sex Differences in Androgen Regulation of Metabolism in Nonhuman Primates. *Adv. Exp. Med. Biol.* **2017**, *1043*, 559–574. [CrossRef]
129. Bodkin, N.L.; Alexander, T.M.; Ortmeyer, H.K.; Johnson, E.; Hansen, B.C. Mortality and morbidity in laboratory-maintained Rhesus monkeys and effects of long-term dietary restriction. *J. Gerontol. A Biol. Sci. Med. Sci.* **2003**, *58*, 212–219. [CrossRef]
130. Bishop, C.V.; Takahashi, D.; Mishler, E.; Slayden, O.D.; Roberts, C.T.; Hennebold, J.; True, C. Individual and combined effects of 5-year exposure to hyperandrogenemia and Western-style diet on metabolism and reproduction in female rhesus macaques. *Hum. Reprod.* **2021**, *36*, 444–454. [CrossRef]
131. Brown, E.; Ozawa, K.; Moccetti, F.; Vinson, A.; Hodovan, J.; Nguyen, T.A.; Bader, L.; López, J.A.; Kievit, P.; Shaw, G.D.; et al. Arterial Platelet Adhesion in Atherosclerosis-Prone Arteries of Obese, Insulin-Resistant Nonhuman Primates. *J. Am. Heart Assoc.* **2021**, *10*, e019413. [CrossRef]
132. Newman, L.E.; Testard, C.; DeCasien, A.R.; Chiou, K.L.; Watowich, M.M.; Janiak, M.C.; Pavez-Fox, M.A.; Sanchez Rosado, M.R.; Cooper, E.B.; Costa, C.E.; et al. The biology of aging in a social world: Insights from free-ranging rhesus macaques. *bioRxiv* **2023**, preprint. [CrossRef]

133. Eisner, J.R.; Dumesic, D.A.; Kemnitz, J.W.; Colman, R.J.; Abbott, D.H. Increased adiposity in female rhesus monkeys exposed to androgen excess during early gestation. *Obes. Res.* **2003**, *11*, 279–286. [CrossRef]
134. Barnett, D.K.; Abbott, D.H. Reproductive adaptations to a large-brained fetus open a vulnerability to anovulation similar to polycystic ovary syndrome. *Am. J. Hum. Biol.* **2003**, *15*, 296–319. [CrossRef] [PubMed]
135. Bruns, C.M.; Baum, S.T.; Colman, R.J.; Dumesic, D.A.; Eisner, J.R.; Jensen, M.D.; Whigham, L.D.; Abbott, D.H. Prenatal androgen excess negatively impacts body fat distribution in a nonhuman primate model of polycystic ovary syndrome. *Int. J. Obes.* **2007**, *31*, 1579–1585. [CrossRef] [PubMed]
136. Zhou, R.; Bruns, C.M.; Bird, I.M.; Kemnitz, J.W.; Goodfriend, T.L.; Dumesic, D.A.; Abbott, D.H. Pioglitazone improves insulin action and normalizes menstrual cycles in a majority of prenatally androgenized female rhesus monkeys. *Reprod. Toxicol.* **2007**, *23*, 438–448. [CrossRef] [PubMed]
137. Abbott, D.H.; Barnett, D.K.; Bruns, C.M.; Dumesic, D.A. Androgen excess fetal programming of female reproduction: A developmental aetiology for polycystic ovary syndrome? *Hum. Reprod. Update* **2005**, *11*, 357–374. [CrossRef] [PubMed]
138. Keller, E.; Chazenbalk, G.D.; Aguilera, P.; Madrigal, V.; Grogan, T.; Elashoff, D.; Dumesic, D.A.; Abbott, D.H. Impaired preadipocyte differentiation into adipocytes in subcutaneous abdominal adipose of PCOS-like female rhesus monkeys. *Endocrinology* **2014**, *155*, 2696–2703. [CrossRef] [PubMed]
139. Barrett, E.S.; Hoeger, K.M.; Sathyanarayana, S.; Abbott, D.H.; Redmon, J.B.; Nguyen, R.H.N.; Swan, S.H. Anogenital distance in newborn daughters of women with polycystic ovary syndrome indicates fetal testosterone exposure. *J. Dev. Orig. Health Dis.* **2018**, *9*, 307–314. [CrossRef]
140. Sánchez-Ferrer, M.L.; Mendiola, J.; Hernández-Peñalver, A.I.; Corbalán-Biyang, S.; Carmona-Barnosi, A.; Prieto-Sánchez, M.T.; Nieto, A.; Torres-Cantero, A.M. Presence of polycystic ovary syndrome is associated with longer anogenital distance in adult Mediterranean women. *Hum. Reprod.* **2017**, *32*, 2315–2323. [CrossRef]
141. Abbott, A.D.; Colman, R.J.; Tiefenthaler, R.; Dumesic, D.A.; Abbott, D.H. Early-to-mid gestation fetal testosterone increases right hand 2D:4D finger length ratio in polycystic ovary syndrome-like monkeys. *PLoS ONE* **2012**, *7*, e42372. [CrossRef]
142. Tata, B.; Mimouni, N.E.H.; Barbotin, A.L.; Malone, S.A.; Loyens, A.; Pigny, P.; Dewailly, D.; Catteau-Jonard, S.; Sundström-Poromaa, I.; Piltonen, T.T.; et al. Elevated prenatal anti-Müllerian hormone reprograms the fetus and induces polycystic ovary syndrome in adulthood. *Nat. Med.* **2018**, *24*, 834–846. [CrossRef] [PubMed]
143. Mimouni, N.E.H.; Paiva, I.; Barbotin, A.L.; Timzoura, F.E.; Plassard, D.; Le Gras, S.; Ternier, G.; Pigny, P.; Catteau-Jonard, S.; Simon, V.; et al. Polycystic ovary syndrome is transmitted via a transgenerational epigenetic process. *Cell Metab.* **2021**, *33*, 513–530.e8. [CrossRef] [PubMed]
144. Abbott, D.H.; Tarantal, A.F.; Dumesic, D.A. Fetal, infant, adolescent and adult phenotypes of polycystic ovary syndrome in prenatally androgenized female rhesus monkeys. *Am. J. Primatol.* **2009**, *71*, 776–784. [CrossRef]
145. Susa, J.B.; Neave, C.; Sehgal, P.; Singer, D.B.; Zeller, W.P.; Schwartz, R. Chronic hyperinsulinemia in the fetal rhesus monkey. Effects of physiologic hyperinsulinemia on fetal growth and composition. *Diabetes* **1984**, *33*, 656–660. [CrossRef] [PubMed]
146. Filippou, P.; Homburg, R. Is foetal hyperexposure to androgens a cause of PCOS? *Hum. Reprod. Update* **2017**, *23*, 421–432. [CrossRef]
147. Palomba, S.; Russo, T.; Falbo, A.; Di Cello, A.; Tolino, A.; Tucci, L.; La Sala, G.B.; Zullo, F. Macroscopic and microscopic findings of the placenta in women with polycystic ovary syndrome. *Hum. Reprod.* **2013**, *28*, 2838–2847. [CrossRef]
148. Zhang, Q.; Bao, Z.K.; Deng, M.X.; Xu, Q.; Ding, D.D.; Pan, M.M.; Xi, X.; Wang, F.F.; Zou, Y.; Qu, F. Fetal growth, fetal development, and placental features in women with polycystic ovary syndrome: Analysis based on fetal and placental magnetic resonance imaging. *J. Zhejiang Univ. Sci. B* **2020**, *21*, 977–989. [CrossRef]
149. Hochberg, A.; Mills, G.; Volodarsky-Perel, A.; Nu, T.N.T.; Machado-Gedeon, A.; Cui, Y.; Shaul, J.; Dahan, M.H. The impact of polycystic ovary syndrome on placental histopathology patterns in in-vitro fertilization singleton live births. *Placenta* **2023**, *139*, 12–18. [CrossRef] [PubMed]
150. Kuo, K.; Roberts, V.H.J.; Gaffney, J.; Takahashi, D.L.; Morgan, T.; Lo, J.O.; Stouffer, R.L.; Frias, A.E. Maternal High-Fat Diet Consumption and Chronic Hyperandrogenemia Are Associated with Placental Dysfunction in Female Rhesus Macaques. *Endocrinology* **2019**, *160*, 1937–1949. [CrossRef] [PubMed]
151. Abbott, D.H.; Bruns, C.R.; Barnett, D.K.; Dunaif, A.; Goodfriend, T.L.; Dumesic, D.A.; Tarantal, A.F. Experimentally induced gestational androgen excess disrupts glucoregulation in rhesus monkey dams and their female offspring. *Am. J. Physiol. Endocrinol. Metab.* **2010**, *299*, E741–E751. [CrossRef]
152. Harnois-Leblanc, S.; Hernandez, M.I.; Codner, E.; Cassorla, F.; Oberfield, S.E.; Leibel, N.I.; Mathew, R.P.; Ten, S.; Magoffin, D.A.; Lane, C.J.; et al. Profile of Daughters and Sisters of Women with Polycystic Ovary Syndrome: The Role of Proband's Glucose Tolerance. *J. Clin. Endocrinol. Metab.* **2022**, *107*, e912–e923. [CrossRef] [PubMed]
153. Hanem, L.G.E.; Salvesen, Ø.; Madsen, A.; Sagen, J.V.; Mellgren, G.; Juliusson, P.B.; Carlsen, S.M.; Vanky, E.; Ødegård, R. Maternal PCOS status and metformin in pregnancy: Steroid hormones in 5–10 years old children from the PregMet randomized controlled study. *PLoS ONE* **2021**, *16*, e0257186. [CrossRef] [PubMed]
154. Maliqueo, M.; Galgani, J.E.; Pérez-Bravo, F.; Echiburú, B.; de Guevara, A.L.; Crisosto, N.; Sir-Petermann, T. Relationship of serum adipocyte-derived proteins with insulin sensitivity and reproductive features in pre-pubertal and pubertal daughters of polycystic ovary syndrome women. *Eur. J. Obstet. Gynecol. Reprod. Biol.* **2012**, *161*, 56–61. [CrossRef]

155. Sir-Petermann, T.; Maliqueo, M.; Codner, E.; Echiburú, B.; Crisosto, N.; Pérez, V.; Pérez-Bravo, F.; Cassorla, F. Early metabolic derangements in daughters of women with polycystic ovary syndrome. *J. Clin. Endocrinol. Metab.* **2007**, *92*, 4637–4642. [CrossRef] [PubMed]
156. Warren, W.C.; Harris, R.A.; Haukness, M.; Fiddes, I.T.; Murali, S.C.; Fernandes, J.; Dishuck, P.C.; Storer, J.M.; Raveendran, M.; Hillier, L.W.; et al. Sequence diversity analyses of an improved rhesus macaque genome enhance its biomedical utility. *Science* **2020**, *370*, eabc6617. [CrossRef]

Disclaimer/Publisher's Note: The statements, opinions and data contained in all publications are solely those of the individual author(s) and contributor(s) and not of MDPI and/or the editor(s). MDPI and/or the editor(s) disclaim responsibility for any injury to people or property resulting from any ideas, methods, instructions or products referred to in the content.

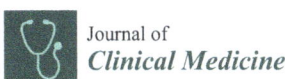 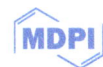

Article

The LH:FSH Ratio in Functional Hypothalamic Amenorrhea: An Observational Study

Magdalena Boegl [1], Didier Dewailly [2], Rodrig Marculescu [3], Johanna Steininger [1], Johannes Ott [1],*
and Marlene Hager [1]

[1] Clinical Division of Gynecological Endocrinology and Reproductive Medicine, Department of Obstetrics and Gynecology, Medical University of Vienna, 1090 Vienna, Austria; magdalena.boegl@meduniwien.ac.at (M.B.); johanna.steininger@meduniwien.ac.at (J.S.); marlene.hager@meduniwien.ac.at (M.H.)
[2] Faculty of Medicine Henri Warembourg, University of Lille, CEDEX, 59045 Lille, France; didier.dewailly@orange.fr
[3] Department of Laboratory Medicine, Medical University of Vienna, 1090 Vienna, Austria; rodrig.marculescu@meduniwien.ac.at
* Correspondence: johannes.ott@meduniwien.ac.at; Tel.: +43-1-40-400-28130

Citation: Boegl, M.; Dewailly, D.; Marculescu, R.; Steininger, J.; Ott, J.; Hager, M. The LH:FSH Ratio in Functional Hypothalamic Amenorrhea: An Observational Study. *J. Clin. Med.* **2024**, *13*, 1201. https://doi.org/10.3390/jcm13051201

Academic Editor: Błażej Męczekalski

Received: 29 January 2024
Revised: 12 February 2024
Accepted: 16 February 2024
Published: 20 February 2024

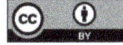

Copyright: © 2024 by the authors. Licensee MDPI, Basel, Switzerland. This article is an open access article distributed under the terms and conditions of the Creative Commons Attribution (CC BY) license (https://creativecommons.org/licenses/by/4.0/).

Abstract: Background: In functional hypothalamic amenorrhea (FHA), luteinizing hormone and follicle-stimulating hormone levels show high interindividual variability, which significantly limits their diagnostic value in differentiating FHA from polycystic ovary syndrome (PCOS). Our aim was to profile the LH:FSH ratio in a large sample of patients with well-defined FHA. Methods: This observational study included all consecutive patients with FHA presenting to the Department of Gynecologic Endocrinology and Reproductive Medicine, Medical University of Vienna, between January 2017 and August 2023. The main parameters of interest were the LH level, the FSH level, and the LH:FSH ratio. In a subgroup analysis, we compared the LH:FSH ratio of patients with PCO morphology (PCOM) on ultrasound with that of patients without PCOM. Results: A total of 135 patients were included. Only a minority of patients revealed FSH and LH levels ≤ 2.0 mIU/mL (13% and 39%, respectively). Most patients (81.5%) had an LH:FSH ratio ≤ 1.0, while a minority (2.2%) had a ratio ≥ 2.1. The LH:FSH ratio was similar in patients with and without PCOM. Conclusion: In a well-defined FHA sample, the LH:FSH ratio was ≤ 1 in most patients. The LH:FSH ratio may prove useful in distinguishing FHA from PCOS but needs further investigation.

Keywords: hypogonadotropic hypogonadism; functional hypothalamic amenorrhea; gonadotropin-releasing hormone; polycystic ovary syndrome; LH:FSH ratio

1. Introduction

Secondary amenorrhea is defined as the cessation of previously regular menstruation for a period of more than three months or previously irregular menstruation longer than six months [1] and affects about 4% of women in the general population [2]. Functional hypothalamic amenorrhea (FHA) and polycystic ovary syndrome (PCOS) are two of the most common underlying conditions [3]. FHA is commonly associated with stress [4], vigorous exercise, weight loss, and psychological disorders [5], leading to suppression of the hypothalamic–pituitary–ovarian (HPO) axis [6], which in turn disrupts follicular growth and ovulation. The resulting hypoestrogenism has profound effects on cardiovascular health [7], bone density, and fatigue and decreases libido [8]. In many cases, the onset is attributed to the interplay of various etiologies, which are potentially influenced by genetic or epigenetic predispositions [9]. However, correcting or ameliorating the stressors can fully restore ovulatory ovarian function [10].

PCOS is an important and sometimes difficult differential diagnosis [11]. PCOS is diagnosed using the Rotterdam criteria as recommended in the "International evidence-based guideline for the assessment and management of polycystic ovary syndrome 2018" [12]. The Rotterdam criteria require the presence of two of the following features: oligo-anovulation, signs of hyperandrogenism, and polycystic ovaries (≥12 follicles measuring 2–9 mm in diameter and/or an ovarian volume >10 mL in at least one ovary) visible on ultrasound [12,13]. However, according to the recently published "International Evidence-based Guideline for the assessment and management of Polycsytic Ovary Syndrome (PCOS) 2023", anti-Muellerian hormone (AMH) levels in plasma can be determined instead of sonographic measurement of the follicular cysts [14]. Anti-Muellerian hormone is commonly used to assess the ovarian follicular reserve and to identify PCOM in adults.

Since up to 50% of women with FHA reveal polycystic ovarian morphology on ultrasound [4,15], which is also accompanied by increased AMH levels, these patients can easily be misdiagnosed as PCOS [16]. To date, four different PCOS phenotypes have been identified: Phenotypes A, B, C, and D. Non-hyperandrogenic phenotype D (PCOS-D) requires only anovulation and PCO morphology and remains the most difficult to distinguish from FHA with PCOM [15]. Recent data show that with an AMH threshold of 3.2 ng/mL, 34.8% are classified as phenotype D [17]. The similarities such as secondary amenorrhea, PCO morphology on ultrasound/increased AMH levels, and infertility make it very difficult to differentiate between the two conditions. The fact that there are no highly reliable parameters for the differential diagnosis between FHA and PCOS has been underlined by a recent review [11].

In FHA, the imminent cause of amenorrhea is a disrupted frequency pattern of gonadotropin-releasing hormone (GnRH) secretion [18]. Exposure to stress activates the hypothalamic–pituitary–adrenal axis, leading to an elevated secretion of corticotropin-releasing hormone (CRH) and glucocorticoids such as cortisol [19], which inhibit GnRH secretion and release. As a result, LH (luteinizing hormone) and FSH (follicle-stimulating hormone) levels decrease and then are no longer sufficient to maintain folliculogenesis and ovulatory ovarian function [10]. Thus, it seems reasonable to use LH and FSH as parameters to diagnose FHA and differentiate between FHA and PCOS. According to several studies, this seems feasible for LH [11,16] but controversies exist for the use of FSH [11,16]. Generally, while the LH profile has been extensively studied in FHA women, less is known about the role of FSH in women with FHA [20,21]. The pattern of GnRH secretion appears to be an important factor in regulating gonadotropin subunit gene expression, gonadotropin synthesis, and hormone secretion [22]. It is thought that in hypothalamic–pituitary–ovarian axis dysfunction, an inadequate production of GnRH by the hypothalamus (i.e., slow frequency of GnRH pulses) leads to a decreased secretion of LH and, to a lesser extent, of FSH, since reduced GnRH pulsatility favors FSH secretion [23]. Consequently, the LH:FSH ratio would theoretically be lower in FHA than in other situations and could be used as a diagnostic criterion. We have indeed previously reported that a threshold of 0.96 has a very high specificity to discriminate between women with FHA and PCOM and women with phenotype D of PCOS [16].

However, since FSH levels in FHA patients vary from one study to the other and since no one has previously primarily focused on the LH:FSH ratio, we aimed to investigate this parameter in our large patient population with well-defined FHA. Our goal was to define its distribution and to search for relationships with various hormones in women with FHA to shed some new light on the pathophysiologic aspects of FHA.

2. Materials and Methods

Study design: we conducted a single-center, retrospective observational study to investigate the LH:FSH ratio in patients with well-defined FHA.

Study population: This observational study included 135 consecutive patients with FHA presenting to the Clinical Department of Gynecological Endocrinology and Reproductive Medicine, Medical University of Vienna, Austria, from January 2017 to August 2023. The FHA definition includes the presence of secondary amenorrhea for at least six consecutive months and a negative progestogen challenge test. Women with pregnancy, hypothyroidism, acne and hirsutism, hyperprolactinemia, and other organ-related pituitary dysfunctions (by MRI) were excluded from study participation.

Reasons causing amenorrhea were extensively described in previous studies [4,21,24–26]. In detail, all women presenting with FHA had experienced reasonably regular menstrual cycles prior to the manifestation of amenorrhea. A weight loss exceeding 10 kg prior to the onset of amenorrhea was considered significant. Furthermore, a body mass index (BMI) below 18.5 kg per square meter, as per the established criteria for classifying underweight individuals, indicated a likelihood of FHA due to underweight status. Diagnoses of eating disorders were made in accordance with the ICD-10 criteria. Each participant classified as an "exerciser" when engaged in physical activity for a minimum of 10 h per week, which encompassed various forms of exercise including dancing, aerobics, biking, and more, or running at least 30 miles per week. It is imperative to acknowledge the presence of emotionally distressing events leading to the onset of amenorrhea, including familial, scholastic, occupational, or psychosocial stressors (psychiatric disorders were ruled out using DSM IV criteria). None of the women displayed clinical manifestations of hirsutism or acne.

Parameters analyzed: The AKIM software (SAP-based patient management system at the Medical University of Vienna) was used for data acquisition. In addition, the following serum parameters were analyzed: anti-Müllerian hormone (AMH), total testosterone, sex hormone-binding globulin (SHBG), prolactin, estradiol, and thyroid-stimulating hormone. The data was retrieved from the electronical medical database AKIM (based on SAP ERP Release 2005, V33 (01/2021), Walldorf, Baden Würtenberg, Germany).

Blood samples were collected from a peripheral vein during the early follicular phase (cycle days 2–5) after bleeding induction with oral estradiol (2 mg per day) and dydrogesterone (20 mg/day) for 10 days. Laboratory analyses were performed at the Department of Laboratory Medicine, Medical University of Vienna, in compliance with ISO 15189 quality standards acc (International ISO standard, number 15189, Akkreditierung Austria, Stubenring 1, 1010 Vienna, Austria, 2012) ording to previous publications [4,16,27,28]: estradiol, follicle-stimulating hormone (FSH), luteinizing hormone (LH), anti-Mullerian hormone (AMH) and sex hormone-binding globulin (SHBG) were measured by the corresponding Cobas electrochemiluminescence immunoassays (ECLIAs) on Cobas e 602 analyzers (Roche, Mannheim, Germany). All specific tests used were described previously by Beitl et al. [16].

The baseline patient characteristics collected included age at admission, body mass index (BMI), gravidity, parity, and follicle number per ovary (FNPO), which was determined by ultrasound using an "Aloka Prosound 6" ultrasound machine and an "UST-9124 Intra Cavity transducer" (frequency range 2.0–7.5 MHz; Hitachi, Wiener Neudorf, Austria). The threshold for defining follicular excess was set at 12 follicles per ovary, as recommended for an ultrasound machine with probe frequency range < 8 MHz [29].

Statistical Analysis: We present categorical data as numbers and frequencies, and continuous data as median and interquartile range (IQR). We used the analysis of variance (ANOVA) for between-group comparisons. Univariate correlations between some variables were sought using Spearman's non-parametric test. To evaluate possibly associated factors with categorical data, univariable binary regression models were used. All significant parameters were then entered into a multivariable binary regression model. For these models, odds ratios (ORs), their 95% confidence intervals (95% CI), and p-values are provided. The IBM Statistical Package for Social Science software (SPSS 28.0) was used for all statistical tests. p-values < 0.05 were considered significant.

3. Results

A total of 135 consecutive patients with FHA were included in this study. Table 1 shows the baseline characteristics of the study patients.

Table 1. Basic patient characteristics.

Age (years), median (IQR) [1]	26 (22;29)
BMI (kg/m^2), median (IQR) [1]	20.3 (18.6;22.0)
Gravidity: n (%) [2]	
0	134 (99.3)
1	1 (0.7)
Parity: n (%) [2]	
0	134 (99.3)
1	1 (0.7)
Causes for FHA: n (%) [2,3]	
Stress	44 (32.6)
Excessive exercise	55 (40.7)
Anorexia nervosa	30 (22.2)
Acute weight loss	33 (24.4)
Underweight	24 (17.8)
Duration since last menstrual bleeding (months), median (IQR) [1]	14 (10;24)
Hormones, median (IQR) [1]	
TSH (IU/mL)	1.57 (1.12;2.03)
Prolactin (ng/mL)	8.9 (6.6;12.9)
FSH (mIU/mL)	4.7 (3.3;6.5)
LH (mIU/mL)	2.6 (1.3;4.7)
Estradiol (pg/mL)	23 (12;31)
Testosterone (ng/mL)	0.20 (0.13;0.29)
DHEAS (µg/mL)	2.03 (1.40;2.73)
SHBG (nmol/L)	73.0 (55.1;101.8)
AMH (ng/mL)	3.1 (1.6;6.2)
Polycystic ovarian morphology on ultrasound, n (%) [2]	58 (43.0)

Note: [1] Continuous data are provided as median and interquartile range; [2] categorical data are presented as absolute numbers (n) and relative frequencies (percent); [3] since more than one cause of FHA (e.g., excessive exercise + stress) was identified in some patients, the sum of the cause distribution exceeds the total number of study patients. BMI = body mass index, TSH = thyroid-stimulating hormone, FSH = follicle-stimulating hormone, LH = luteinizing hormone, DHEAS = dehydroepiandrosterone-sulfate, SHBG = sex hormone-binding globulin, AMH = anti-Mullerian hormone.

The distribution of FSH and LH values is shown in Figure 1. FSH was ≤ 4.0 mIU/mL and ≤ 2.0 mIU/mL in 38.5% and 12.6%, respectively, whereas this was the case for 68.9% and 38.5% of LH levels, respectively. The LH:FSH ratio was ≤ 1.0 in most patients (81.5%), whereas a value ≥ 2.1 was found in only 2.2% (Figure 2).

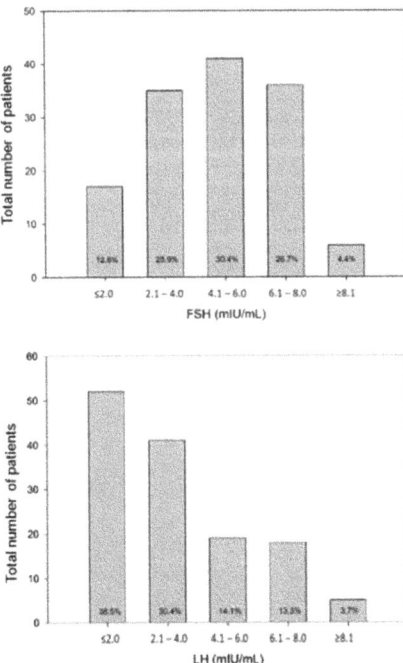

Figure 1. Distribution of FSH and LH levels (mIU/mL) at initial diagnosis of FHA.

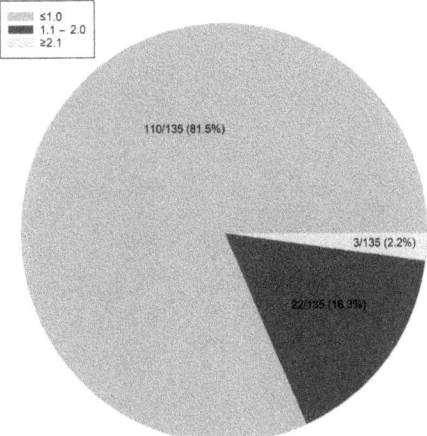

Figure 2. Distribution of the LH:FSH ratio at the initial diagnosis of FHA.

The following significant positive correlations ($p < 0.05$) between serum parameters were found (Table 2): FSH and LH; FSH and estradiol; FSH and AMH; LH and the LH:FSH ratio; LH and estradiol; LH and testosterone; LH and prolactin; the LH:FSH ratio and prolactin; the LH:FSH ratio and estradiol; the LH:FSH ratio and prolactin; estradiol and testosterone; estradiol and prolactin; as well as testosterone and prolactin.

Table 2. Correlation analyses.

		FSH	LH	LH:FSH Ratio	Estradiol	Testosterone	AMH	Prolactin
FSH	r2	-	0.556	−0.141	0.291	0.045	0.221	0.323
	p		<0.001	0.103	<0.001	0.604	*0.010*	0.134
LH	r2	0.556	-	0.633	0.387	0.218	0.060	0.315
	p	<0.001		<0.001	<0.001	*0.011*	0.134	<0.001
LH:FSH ratio	r2	−0.141	0.633	-	0.271	0.159	−0.076	0.261
	p	0.103	<0.001		*0.002*	0.066	0.385	*0.002*
Estradiol	r2	0.291	0.387	0.271	-	0.243	0.076	0.182
	p	<0.001	<0.001	*0.002*		*0.005*	0.386	*0.037*
Testosterone	r2	0.045	0.218	0.159	0.243	-	0.126	0.268
	p	0.604	*0.011*	0.066	*0.005*		0.134	*0.002*
AMH	r2	0.221	0.060	−0.076	0.076	0.126	-	−0.051
	p	*0.010*	0.134	0.385	0.386	0.134		0.555
Prolactin	r2	0.323	0.315	0.261	0.182	0.268	−0.051	-
	p	0.134	<0.001	*0.002*	*0.037*	*0.002*	0.555	

Correlation coefficients and *p*-values for Spearman correlations are provided; italic numbers indicate statistical significance.

In order to detect possible confounders, we then conducted a univariable followed using a multivariable binary regression model using the LH:FSH ratio as the dependent variable (≤ 1 versus >1; Table 3). In the univariable models, higher estradiol and higher LH were associated with an LH:FSH ratio >1, whereas this was only the case for LH in the multivariable analysis (OR 0.520, 95%CI: 0.400–0.675; $p < 0.001$).

Table 3. Parameters associated with an LH:FSH ratio ≤ 1 in women with FHA. Univariable followed by a multivariable binary regression model.

	LH:FSH Ratio ≤ 1 (n = 110)	LH:FSH Ratio > 1 (n = 25)	OR (95%CI)	p	OR (95%CI)	p
Age (years) [1]	26 (22;29)	24 (22;28)	1.047 (0.956;1.147)	0.321	-	-
BMI (kg/m^2) [1]	19.9 (18.6;21.7)	21.2 (18.6;22.3)	0.880 (0.740;1.047)	0.149	-	-
Causes for FHA:						
Stress [2,3]	33 (30.0)	11 (44.0)	0.545 (0.224;1.327)	0.181	-	-
Excessive exercise [2,3]	45 (40.9)	10 (40.0)	1.038 (0.428;2.518)	0.933	-	-
Anorexia nervosa [2,3]	22 (20.0)	8 (32.0)	0.531 (0.203;1.389)	0.197	-	-
Acute weight loss [2,3]	27 (24.5)	6 (24.0)	1.030 (0.373;2.844)	0.954	-	-
Underweight [2,3]	19 (17.3)	5 (20.0)	0.835 (0.279;2.503)	0.748	-	-
Duration since last bleeding (months) [1]	14 (12;24)	12 (8;16)	1.039 (0.998;1.082)	0.065	-	-
FSH (mIU/mL) [1]	4.7 (3.4;6.3)	4.7 (2.6;6.5)	1.056 (0.868;1.284)	0.588	-	-
LH (mIU/mL) [1]	2.2 (1.2;3.5)	6.3 (4.0;7.7)	0.499 (0.385;0.647)	<0.001	0.520 (0.400;0.675)	<0.001
Prolactin (ng/mL) [1]	8.1 (6.4;12.4)	12.0 (8.8;14.2)	0.960 (0.894;1.031)	0.260	-	-
Estradiol (pg/mL) [1]	21 (11;28)	25 (22;39)	0.956 (0.928;0.986)	0.004	0.975 (0.939;1.013)	0.196
Testosterone (ng/mL) [1]	0.19 (0.13;0.29)	0.25 (0.14;0.33)	0.015 (0.000;1.030)	0.052	-	-
SHBG (nmol/L) [1]	74.0 (57.4;99.1)	70.0 (48.6;113.0)	0.998 (0.986;1.010)	0.720	-	-
AMH (ng/mL) [1]	2.8 (1.6;6.1)	4.5 (2.2;6.2)	0.955 (0.863;1.087)	0.486	-	-
PCOM [2]	42 (38.2)	13 (52.0)	0.570 (0.238;1.366)	0.208	-	-

[1] Numerical data are provided as median (interquartile range) and [2] categorical data as number (frequency); [3] multiple mentions possible.

the quality of orgasm they experienced (r = 0.21; p = 0.041). The correlation coefficient suggested a small effect.

Table 5. Demographic and physical correlates of sexual functioning of women with PCOS—U Mann–Whitney test results (grouping variables: residence, acne presence, and hirsutism).

		W	p	r_{bs}
Grouping variable: Residence (alone vs. with family)	Pleasure	64.50	0.429	0.12
	Desire—frequency	72.50	0.099	0.26
	Desire—interest	77.50	0.030	0.35
	Arousal	675.50	0.255	0.19
	Orgasm	507.00	0.500	−0.11
	Total CSFQ	668.00	0.296	0.17
Grouping variable: Acne presence (yes vs. no)	Pleasure	921.50	0.560	−0.07
	Desire—frequency	866.00	0.303	−0.13
	Desire—interest	892.50	0.426	−0.10
	Arousal	926.50	0.604	−0.06
	Orgasm	947.50	0.731	−0.04
	Total CSFQ	921.00	0.578	−0.07
Grouping variable: Hirsutism (yes vs. no)	Pleasure	918.00	0.823	−0.03
	Desire—frequency	858.00	0.466	−0.09
	Desire—interest	958.50	0.906	0.02
	Arousal	853.00	0.446	−0.10
	Orgasm	92.50	0.847	−0.03
	Total CSFQ	928.50	0.901	−0.02

For effect size, rank-biserial (r_{bs}) correlation was reported.

The results of the U Mann–Whitney test did not reveal statistically significant differences between women diagnosed with PCOS: (1) with present and absent acne, (2) with and without hirsutism. The only difference was reported with respect to residence. In this case, women with PCOS who lived alone reported a higher level of desire (interest; p = 0.030) compared to those who lived with their families (for women who lived alone: median = 10.0, IQR = 3,50; for women who lived with their families: median = 8.50, IQR = 3.00).

3.6. Associations between VAS Scores and Physical Features (WHR, Acne, and Hirsutism)

To analyze the associations between VAS scores and some physical features (i.e., WHR and Ferriman–Gallwey score), we perform Pearson's r correlation (Table 6).

Table 6. Associations between VAS scores and physical features (WHR and Ferriman–Gallwey score)—Pearson's r correlation coefficients.

	1	2	3	4	5	6	7	8
1. WHR ratio	—							
2. Ferriman–Gallwey score	0.19	—						
3. Sexual satisfaction importance (VAS1)	−0.02	0.12	—					
4. Sexual thoughts and fantasies—last month (VAS2)	−0.09	−0.03	0.55 ***	—				
5. Personal sexual attractiveness (VAS3)	−0.18	0.03	0.26 *	0.27 *	—			
6. Impact of excessive hair on personal sexuality (VAS4)	0.07	0.41 ***	0.01	0.06	−0.16	—		
7. Social struggles due to appearance (VAS5)	0.23 *	0.15	0.07	0.22 *	−0.18	0.49 ***	—	
8. Painful sexual encounters (VAS6)	−0.03	−0.07	−0.02	0.03	−0.06	0.10	0.21 *	—
9. Level of sexual satisfaction—last month (VAS7)	0.30 **	0.05	0.30 **	0.27 **	0.18	−0.18	−0.04	−0.14

* $p < 0.05$; ** $p < 0.01$; *** $p < 0.001$.

$p < 0.001$) and more satisfying overall sexual functioning (r = 0.53, $p < 0.001$). All correlation coefficients suggested medium to large effects. Therefore, Hypothesis 1 was confirmed.

Moreover, as expected in Hypothesis 2, the perceived level of personal attractiveness (VAS3) experienced by women diagnosed with PCOS was positively correlated with almost all dimensions of the CSFQ. In contrast, the perceived impact of excess hair on personal sexuality (VAS4) and appearance-related social struggles (VAS5) was negatively associated with only a few CSFQ dimensions. Therefore, a higher level of subjective personal attractiveness was associated with a higher level of pleasure (r = 0.24, $p = 0.025$), desire—interest (r = 0.25, $p = 0.016$), arousal (r = 0.30, $p = 0.005$), and orgasm (r = 0.28, $p = 0.008$), and more satisfying overall sexual functioning (r = 0.34, $p < 0.001$). All correlation coefficients suggested small effects. Also, a perceived greater impact of excess hair on personal sexuality (r = −0.26, $p = 0.013$) and greater social struggles due to appearance (r = −0.27, $p = 0.009$) corresponded to lower levels of pleasure. All correlation coefficients suggested small effects. Therefore, Hypothesis 2 was partially confirmed.

As assumed in Hypothesis 3, the intensity of sexual thoughts and fantasies in the last month (VAS2) correlated positively with the dimensions of desire (for frequency: r = 0.46, $p < 0.001$; for interest: r = 0.73, $p < 0.001$). All correlation coefficients suggested medium (for frequency) or large (for percentages) effects. Therefore, Hypothesis 3 was confirmed. Interestingly, sexual fantasies were also positively associated with some other dimensions of the CSFQ, i.e., arousal (r = 0.38, $p < 0.001$) and orgasm (r = 0.25, $p = 0.016$), and with overall sexual functioning (r = 0.52, $p < 0.001$). In all cases, a higher intensity of sexual thoughts and fantasies corresponded to higher levels of desire (frequency and interest), arousal and orgasm, and more satisfying overall sexual functioning.

We also confirmed Hypothesis 4, as the analysis showed a negative correlation between the occurrence of painful sexual intercourse (VAS6) and the orgasm domain (r = −0.27, $p = 0.011$), which suggests that the frequent occurrence of painful sexual intercourse is equally significant—associated with a lower quality of orgasm. Correlation coefficients suggested a small effect. Therefore, Hypothesis 4 was confirmed. Accordingly, higher frequency of painful sexual intercourse was associated with lower levels of several other CSFQ dimensions, i.e., pleasure (r = −0.39, $p < 0.001$) and arousal (r = −0.34, $p < 0.001$), and with lower overall functioning sexual (r = −0.35, $p < 0.001$).

3.5. Demographic and Physical Correlates of Sexual Functioning of Women with PCOS

Correlations between age, WHR, Ferriman–Gallwey score, and dimensions of CSFQ were presented in Table 4. As other demographic variables were either ordinal (i.e., education) or nominal (i.e., residence, acne presence, and hirsutism), we completed the analyses with Spearman's correlation (for education—also presented in Table 4) and the U Mann–Whitney test (Table 5).

Table 4. Demographic and physical correlates of sexual functioning of women with PCOS—Pearson's correlations between age, WHR, Ferriman–Gallwey score, and dimensions of the CSFQ.

	Pleasure	Desire—Frequency	Desire—Interest	Arousal	Orgasm	Total
Age	0.01	−0.06	−0.07	0.08	0.21 *	0.09
WHR	0.07	0.02	−0.17	−0.05	0.05	−0.03
Ferriman–Gallwey score	0.03	0.07	−0.09	−0.03	−0.16	−0.07
Education	−0.03	0.02	0.13	0.02	−0.05	0.05

As the correlation matrix for CSRQ dimensions for PCOS women was presented in Table 3, we omitted this part of the current table. For education, Spearman's correlation coefficient was calculated. * $p < 0.05$.

Correlation analyses showed that neither the WHR score nor the Ferriman–Gallwey score were associated with CSFQ dimensions and overall sexual functioning in women with PCOS. Also, the level of education was not statistically significant in relation to sexual functioning. However, the analyses showed that the older the women were, the higher medium to large effects. However, the difference between PCOS participants and the control group was not statistically significant (desire—frequency: $p = 0.102$; arousal: $p = 0.938$). However, the pattern of discrepancies between women and men differed between the PCOS group and the control group (desire—frequency: $p = 0.004$; arousal: $p < 0.001$), with small effects for all variables. The results suggest that although men generally experienced higher levels of desire (frequency) compared to women (regardless of the presence or absence of a PCOS diagnosis), men in the control group reported higher levels of desire (frequency) compared to women and men who were partners of PCOS participants (mean difference was 0.61; $t = 2.81$, $p = 0.016$, Cohen's $d = 0.45$). In the case of arousal, while women from the control group declared a slightly higher level of arousal compared to women from the PCOS group (the average difference was 0.60; $t = 2.04$, $p = 0.085$, Cohen's $d = 0.33$), men from the control group declared slightly lower arousal compared to men in the PCOS group (mean difference was -0.56; $t = -1.91$, $p = 0.085$, Cohen's $d = -0.30$). Also, the discrepancy in arousal between women and men in the control group was average (the average difference was -1.16; $t = -4.91$, $p < 0.001$, Cohen's $d = -0.63$), while in the PCOS group it was very large (mean difference was -2.32, $t = -11.29$, $p < 0.001$, Cohen's $d = -1.26$).

3.4. Sexual Functioning of Women with PCOS—Correlation between CSFQ and VAS

Table 3 presents Pearson's correlation coefficients between CSFQ and VAS scores.

Table 3. Sexual functioning of woman with PCOS—Pearson's correlation coefficients between CSFQ and VAS scores.

	1	2	3	4	5	6	7	8	9	10	11	12
1. Pleasure	—											
2. Desire—frequency	0.44 ***	—										
3. Desire—interest	0.16	0.55 ***	—									
4. Arousal	0.64 ***	0.55 ***	0.49 ***	—								
5. Orgasm	0.58 ***	0.37 ***	0.35 ***	0.63 ***	—							
6. Total CSFQ	0.69 ***	0.70 ***	0.66 ***	0.89 ***	0.80 ***	—						
7. Sexual satisfaction importance (VAS1)	0.32 **	0.24 *	0.37 ***	0.30 **	0.22 *	0.35 ***	—					
8. Sexual thoughts and fantasies—last month (VAS2)	0.20	0.46 ***	0.73 ***	0.38 ***	0.25 *	0.52 ***	0.55 ***	—				
9. Personal sexual attractiveness (VAS3)	0.24 *	0.20	0.25 *	0.30 **	0.28 **	0.34 ***	0.26 *	0.27 *	—			
10. Impact of excessive hair on personal sexuality (VAS4)	−0.26 *	−0.18	−0.06	−0.11	−0.19	−0.19	0.01	0.06	−0.16	—		
11. Social struggles due to appearance (VAS5)	−0.27 **	−0.11	0.08	−0.11	−0.19	−0.17	0.07	0.22 *	−0.18	0.49 ***	—	
12. Painful sexual encounters (VAS6)	−0.39 ***	−0.13	0.05	−0.34 ***	−0.27 *	−0.35 ***	−0.02	0.03	−0.06	0.10	0.21 *	—
13. Level of sexual satisfaction—last month (VAS7)	0.67 ***	0.48 ***	0.14	0.39 ***	0.53 ***	0.53 ***	0.30 **	0.27 **	0.18	−0.18	−0.04	−0.14

* $p < 0.05$; ** $p < 0.01$; *** $p < 0.001$.

As expected in Hypothesis 1, the importance (VAS1) and level (VAS7) of sexual satisfaction felt by women diagnosed with PCOS were positively correlated with almost all dimensions of the CSFQ. Therefore, a greater importance of sexual satisfaction was associated with a higher level of pleasure ($r = 0.32$, $p = 0.002$), frequency of desire ($r = 0.24$, $p = 0.025$) and interest ($r = 0.37$, $p < 0.001$), arousal ($r = 0.30$, $p = 0.004$), and orgasm ($r = 0.22$, $p = 0.039$), and more satisfying overall sexual functioning ($r = 0.35$, $p < 0.001$). All correlation coefficients suggested small to medium effects. Accordingly, higher levels of sexual satisfaction were associated with higher levels of pleasure ($r = 0.67$, $p < 0.001$), frequency of desire ($r = 0.48$, $p < 0.001$), arousal ($r = 0.39$, $p < 0.001$), and orgasm ($r = 0.53$,

Table 1. *Cont.*

	M	SD	Min	Max	Skewness
Control group—men					
Pleasure	4.26	0.82	1.00	5.00	−1.36
Desire—frequency	8.03	1.28	4.00	10.00	−0.31
Desire—interest	10.19	1.84	6.00	15.00	0.02
Arousal	12.32	1.72	8.00	15.00	−0.44
Orgasm	12.10	1.87	7.00	15.00	−0.68
Total CSFQ	56.33	6.37	37.00	70.00	−0.74

Scoring for CSFQ-F-C (a score at or below the cut-off points indicative for sexual dysfunction) Total CSFQ: 41.0, Pleasure: 4.0, Desire/frequency: 6.0, Desire/interest: 9.0, Arousal: 12.0, Orgasm: 11.0. Scoring for CSFQ-M-C (a score at or below the cut-off points indicative for sexual dysfunction) Total CSFQ: 47.0, Pleasure: 4.0, Desire/frequency: 8.0, Desire/interest: 11.0, Arousal: 13.0, Orgasm: 13.0.

3.3. Sexual Functioning—Differences between Women with PCOS, Their Partners, and Women without PCOS

Table 2 presents the differences between women and their partners, PCOS and control groups, and the interaction between both effects.

Table 2. Differences between women with PCOS, their partners, and women without PCOS—results of mixed ANOVA.

	Effect	F	df	p	ω^2
Pleasure	Within subject	33.80	1, 158	<0.001	0.03
	Between subject	0.00	1, 158	0.971	0.00
	Within × between subject	0.02	1, 158	0.877	0.00
Desire—frequency	Within subject	59.42	1, 158	<0.001	0.07
	Between subject	2.70	1, 158	0.102	0.01
	Within × between subject	8.69	1, 158	0.004	0.01
Desire—interest	Within subject	54.71	1, 158	<0.001	0.08
	Between subject	0.19	1, 158	0.668	0.00
	Within × between subject	2.72	1, 158	0.101	0.00
Arousal	Within subject	123.57	1, 158	<0.001	0.18
	Between subject	0.01	1, 158	0.938	0.00
	Within × between subject	13.73	1, 158	<0.001	0.02
Orgasm	Within subject	42.25	1, 158	<0.001	0.07
	Between subject	0.00	1, 158	0.963	0.00
	Within × between subject	2.17	1, 158	0.143	0.00
Total CSFQ	Within subject	130.35	1, 158	<0.001	0.16
	Between subject	0.43	1, 158	0.511	0.00
	Within × between subject	0.67	1, 158	0.413	0.00

In terms of pleasure, desire (interest), orgasm, and total score, the analysis showed a statistically significant difference between women and their partners (in all cases: $p < 0.001$), which suggests small (for pleasure) to medium effects (for other variables). However, the difference between PCOS participants and the control group was not statistically significant (pleasure: $p = 0.971$, desire—interest: $p = 0.668$; orgasm: $p = 0.963$; total score: $p = 0.511$). Also, the pattern of differences between women and men was similar in both the PCOS and control groups (pleasure: $p = 0.877$; desire—interest: $p = 0.101$; orgasm: $p = 0.143$; total score: $p = 0.413$), suggesting higher levels pleasure, desire (interest), orgasm and overall sexual functioning reported by men regardless of the presence or absence of a PCOS diagnosis in their partners.

In terms of desire (frequency) and arousal, the analysis showed a statistically significant difference between women and their partners (in all cases: $p < 0.001$), suggesting

The PCR results for each of the samples analyzed are shown in Table 7. In Gram staining, yeast (blastospores) were observed in 6/33 cases; four were positive for *Candida albicans* by PCR, and two were positive for non- *C. albicans*. No positive cases were detected for *Trichomonas vaginalis*.

Table 7. Micro-organisms detected by PCR in vaginal discharge samples (n = 33).

Micro-Organisms	PCR Results	
	Positive	Negative
Gardnerella vaginalis	22(66.7)	11(33.3)
Atopobium vaginae	10(30.3)	23(69.7)
Megasphaera type 1	4(12.1)	29(87.9)
Trichomonas vaginalis	0	0
Chlamydia trachomatis	2(6.1)	31(93.9)
Candida albicans	4(12.1)	29(87.9)

4. Discussion

The presence of an altered microbiota was a frequent condition in the studied PCOS patients (69.7%), with a high prevalence of non-specific microbial vaginitis (21.2%). A significant statistical association (p-value = 0.023) was observed between the variable active STI and VM (Table 3). On the other hand, the proinflammatory state, defined as evidence of cell destruction and loose nuclei, had a high frequency (72.7%). Additionally, the VIR was present in 8/33 of PCOS patients with PMN counts greater than five per field, with the presence of NETs observed in all cases.

In this scenario of altered vaginal microbiota, it could be a particular and frequent event in women diagnosed with PCOS, where hormonal and metabolic disorders they present could play a role in NETs release [26]. Changes in the composition of the vaginal microbiota could be associated with metabolic alterations, including insulin resistance, suggesting a link between metabolic health and the vaginal microbiota. However, in this study, altered blood insulin levels were not found, and 86.7% of the patients presented normal insulin values.

Estrogens are related to the production of glycogen, which is the substrate necessary for *Lactobacilli* to grow, produce lactic acid, and maintain a low pH, which contributes to a pathogen-free vaginal environment. Elevated estrogen states, as seen during puberty and pregnancy, promote the preservation of a homeostatic (eubiotic) vaginal microenvironment by stimulating the maturation and proliferation of vaginal epithelial cells and the accumulation of glycogen [7]. However, the relationship between 17-B estradiol and Lactobacilli is not entirely understood within the context of the pathophysiology of PCOS [27,28]. In our study, the intermediate microbiota condition was the most frequent, at 33.3% in patients with PCOS. It is precisely in this condition where we begin to observe a VM with some degrees of alteration: lower presence of *Lactobacillus* and a higher presence of bacterial morphotypes of *Gardnerella vaginalis*, *Atopobium vaginae* type, and some others that usually do not cohabit in the vaginal tract. The patients in the present study presented a high frequency of *Gardnerella vaginalis* (66.7%), observed by PCR.

Regarding the epithelial damage (defined as proinflammatory state) associated with PCOS patients in the Gram reading, in over 70% of the smears, destroyed cells and naked nuclei were visualized. In cases with normal microbiota and nonspecific microbial vaginitis, 100% exhibited these characteristics with varying degrees of intensity. A similar condition is found in cytolytic vaginosis (CV), characterized by fragmented epithelial cells and abundant Lactobacilli, which causes an increase in vaginal acidity and epithelial damage [29]. These laboratory findings could help distinguish between CV and candidiasis, as these pathologies do not differ in clinical features [16]. Despite this, there is still a lack of knowledge about CV and its scope [29]. These processes associated with the pathophysiology of inflammation increase the presence of PMN-generated NETs in the vaginal discharge of women with fungal, bacterial, and parasitic infections, indicating the development of infectious foci at the vaginal level [30]. This study used identifying NETs as an indicator of activated PMNs [30,31]. Our observations showed the presence of NETs in all studied cases presenting with a VIR, which had normal microbiota (one-eighth) and non-specific microbial vaginitis (seven-eighth), as shown in Table 6. By these results, we could speculate a scenario that this syndrome by itself could trigger a proinflammatory state at the level of the vaginal epithelium, independent of the state of the vaginal microbiota.

These observations are consistent with those reported by Jin C et al. (2023) in their case-control study, where they found a higher degree of heterogeneity in the vaginal microbiome. As well as the association with other vaginal infections, *Gardnerella vaginalis* was observed more frequently (66.7%) in all stages of VM, whether accompanied by *Atopobium vaginae*, *Megasphaera phylotype* 1, or yeasts such as *Candida albicans* and a higher frequency of bacteria such as *Gardnerella vaginalis* compared to the control group [5]. Another study demonstrated a higher incidence of vaginitis in women with PCOS compared to the control group [32].

Additionally, this is the first study that shows evidence of NETotic activity at the level of the vaginal epithelium in women with PCOS. This condition, associated with amenorrhea or oligomenorrhea states, could contribute to sperm entrapment by NETs generated by activated PMNs, which could increase the risk of infertility in these patients.

5. Conclusions

In the studied series, more women with altered microbiota were noted in clinical variables, phenotypes A and B, sexual partners (>2), and oligomenorrhea. However, only the active STI and insulin variables showed a significant p-value. This is the first study to demonstrate the presence of NETs in eight cases, showing NETotic activity in women with PCOS. We also highlight the high frequency of a proinflammatory state observed across all vaginal microbiota states. These findings suggest that the syndrome itself could trigger a proinflammatory state in the vaginal epithelium, independent of the vaginal microbiota's state. Additionally, these conditions, associated with amenorrhea or oligomenorrhea, could lead to decreased fertility in these PCOS patients.

Limitations of the study. The limitations include the lack of an average population (control group) for comparisons between VM, VIR, proinflammatory status, and other variables. However, despite a small n, trends were observed when calculating the p-value. We hope that this study will serve as a basis for future studies in women with PCOS, including a more significant number of participants both with PCOS and a control group (without PCOS) in order to generate additional data to contribute to a better understanding of this pathology.

Author Contributions: M.E.E.: contributed to the conception, design, data acquisition, processing of laboratory samples, and writing of the article. R.S. and F.Z., contributed to the conception, design of the study, critical analysis of the data and writing of the article. A.M.: contributed to study conception, sample processing, Gram, Giemsa and DNA extraction and PCR readings, critical analysis of data and writing of the article. M.L.: contributed to the immunofluorescence protocol, sample preparation and scanning on the TissueFAXs microscope. E.B.-V.: contributed to study design, critical analysis of data, results and statistical analysis. P.U. and A.B.: contributed to critical analysis of data and results V.I.: contributed to review and critical analysis of data. C.H. and A.T. advised on NETS techniques and reviewed the manuscript. All authors have read and agreed to the published version of the manuscript.

Funding: This research was partially funded by the Universidad Técnica Particular de Loja PROY_INV_CS_2022_3597, and projects DI021-053 and DI19-0113 of the Universidad de La Frontera (V. Iturrieta). Support to groups to strengthen productivity in WoS journals grant DI23-3007.

Institutional Review Board Statement: The study was conducted following the Declaration of Helsinki and approved by the Human Research Ethics Committee (CEISH) 2023-006O-IE of the University of Cuenca, date of approval: 24 May 2023.

Informed Consent Statement: Informed consent was obtained from all subjects involved in the study.

Data Availability Statement: The data supporting the findings of this study are available from the corresponding author upon reasonable request.

Acknowledgments: The authors thank the women with PCOS for participating in this study. In addition, we would like to express our gratitude to ANID FONDEQUIP EQM200228 for allowing us to use the TissueFAXS i Plus Cytometer microscopy facilities to acquire of microscopy images.

Conflicts of Interest: The authors declare no conflicts of interest.

References

1. Louwers, Y.V.; Laven, J.S.E. Characteristics of Polycystic Ovary Syndrome throughout Life. *Ther. Adv. Reprod. Health* **2020**, *14*, 263349412091103. [CrossRef] [PubMed]
2. Teede, H.J.; Misso, M.L.; Costello, M.F.; Dokras, A.; Laven, J.; Moran, L.; Piltonen, T.; Health, N.; Public, M.; Health, M.; et al. Recomendaciones de La Guía Internacional Basada En La Evidencia Para La Evaluación y El Tratamiento Del Síndrome de Ovario Poliquístico. *Health Hum. Serv.* **2018**, *110*, 364–379. [CrossRef]
3. Righi, G.M.; Ferreira De Oliveira, T.; Cândida, M.; Baracat, P.; Mayumi, G.; Rua, R.; Schmidt, I.; Amaro, S.; Paulo, S. Síndrome Dos Ovários Policísticos e Sua Relação Com a Microbiota Intestinal Polycystic Ovary Syndrome and Its Relationship with the Intestinal Microbiota. *Femina* **2021**, *49*, 631–635.
4. Mora Agüero, S.d.l.Á. Microbiota y Disbiosis Vaginal. *Rev. Medica Sinerg.* **2019**, *4*, 3–13. [CrossRef]
5. Jin, C.; Qin, L.; Liu, Z.; Li, X.; Gao, X.; Cao, Y.; Zhao, S.; Wang, J.; Han, T.; Yan, L.; et al. Comparative Analysis of the Vaginal Microbiome of Healthy and Polycystic Ovary Syndrome Women: A Large Cross-Sectional Study. *Reprod. Biomed. Online* **2023**, *46*, 1005–1016. [CrossRef] [PubMed]
6. Nowak, A.; Wojtowicz, M.; Baranski, K.; Galczynska, D.; Daniluk, J.; Pluta, D. The Correlation of Vitamin D Level with Body Mass Index in Women with Polycystic Ovary Syndrome. *Ginekol. Pol.* **2023**, *94*, 883–888. [CrossRef]
7. Amabebe, E.; Anumba, D.O.C. Female Gut and Genital Tract Microbiota-Induced Crosstalk and Differential Effects of Short-Chain Fatty Acids on Immune Sequelae. *Front. Immunol.* **2020**, *11*, 553047. [CrossRef]
8. Tu, Y.; Zheng, G.; Ding, G.; Wu, Y.; Xi, J.; Ge, Y.; Gu, H.; Wang, Y.; Sheng, J.; Liu, X.; et al. Comparative Analysis of Lower Genital Tract Microbiome Between PCOS and Healthy Women. *Front. Physiol.* **2020**, *11*, 563753. [CrossRef]
9. Leliefeld, P.H.C.; Koenderman, L.; Pillay, J. How Neutrophils Shape Adaptive Immune Responses. *Front. Immunol.* **2015**, *6*, 160811. [CrossRef]
10. Zawrotniak, M.; Rapala-Kozik, M. Neutrophil Extracellular Traps (NETs)-Formation and Implications. *Acta Biochim. Pol.* **2013**, *60*, 277–284. [CrossRef]
11. Mortaz, E.; Alipoor, S.D.; Adcock, I.M.; Mumby, S.; Koenderman, L. Update on Neutrophil Function in Severe Inflammation. *Front. Immunol.* **2018**, *9*, 411381. [CrossRef]
12. Papayannopoulos, V. Neutrophil Extracellular Traps in Immunity and Disease. *Nat. Rev. Immunol.* **2018**, *18*, 134–147. [CrossRef] [PubMed]
13. Torres, P.J.; Siakowska, M.; Banaszewska, B.; Pawelczyk, L.; Duleba, A.J.; Kelley, S.T.; Thackray, V.G. Gut Microbial Diversity in Women with Polycystic Ovary Syndrome Correlates with Hyperandrogenism. *J. Clin. Endocrinol. Metab.* **2018**, *103*, 1502–1511. [CrossRef] [PubMed]
14. Guo, J.; Shao, J.; Yang, Y.; Niu, X.; Liao, J.; Zhao, Q.; Wang, D.; Li, S.; Hu, J. Gut Microbiota in Patients with Polycystic Ovary Syndrome: A Systematic Review. *Reprod. Sci.* **2022**, *29*, 69–83. [CrossRef] [PubMed]
15. Liang, Z.; Di, N.; Li, L.; Yang, D. Gut Microbiota Alterations Reveal Potential Gut–Brain Axis Changes in Polycystic Ovary Syndrome. *J. Endocrinol. Investig.* **2021**, *44*, 1727–1737. [CrossRef] [PubMed]
16. Saucedo de la Llata, E.; Moraga Sánchez, M.R.; Menchón López, M.; Obed Carmona Ruiz, I. Vaginosis Bacteriana y Candidiasis Vaginal: Análisis de Una Nueva Alternativa Terapéutica. *Rev. Iberoam. Fertil. Reprod. Hum.* **2020**, *37*, 1–7.
17. Hong, X.; Qin, P.; Yin, J.; Shi, Y.; Xuan, Y.; Chen, Z.; Zhou, X.; Yu, H.; Peng, D.; Wang, B. Clinical Manifestations of Polycystic Ovary Syndrome and Associations with the Vaginal Microbiome: A Cross-Sectional Based Exploratory Study. *Front. Endocrinol.* **2021**, *12*, 662725. [CrossRef] [PubMed]
18. Ortiz-Flores, A.E.; Luque-Ramírez, M.; Escobar-Morreale, H.F. Polycystic Ovary Syndrome in Adult Women. *Med. Clin.* **2019**, *152*, 450–457. [CrossRef] [PubMed]
19. Burgener-Kairuz, P.; Zuber, J.P.; Jaunin, P.; Buchman, T.G.; Bille, J.; Rossier, M. Rapid Detection and Identification of Candida Albicans and Torulopsis (Candida) Glabrata in Clinical Specimens by Species-Specific Nested PCR Amplification of a Cytochrome P-450 Lanosterol-α-Demethylase (L1A1) Gene Fragment. *J. Clin. Microbiol.* **1994**, *32*, 1902–1907. [CrossRef]
20. Pačes, J.; Urbánková, V.; Urbánek, P. Cloning and Characterization of a Repetitive DNA Sequence Specific for Trichomonas Vaginalis. *Mol. Biochem. Parasitol.* **1992**, *54*, 247–255. [CrossRef]
21. Zariffard, M.R.; Saifuddin, M.; Sha, B.E.; Spear, G.T. Detection of Bacterial Vaginosis-Related Organisms by Real-Time PCR for Lactobacilli, Gardnerella Vaginalis and Mycoplasma Hominis. *FEMS Immunol. Med. Microbiol.* **2002**, *34*, 277–281. [CrossRef] [PubMed]
22. Fredricks, D.N.; Fiedler, T.L.; Thomas, K.K.; Oakley, B.B.; Marrazzo, J.M. Targeted PCR for Detection of Vaginal Bacteria Associated with Bacterial Vaginosis. *J. Clin. Microbiol.* **2007**, *45*, 3270–3276. [CrossRef] [PubMed]

23. Monroy, V.S.; Mata, A.E.T.; Magdaleno, J.D.A.V. Diagnóstico de Infección Por Chlamydia Trachomatis Mediante PCR En Pacientes Que Acuden a La Clínica de Especialidades de La Mujer de La Secretaría de La Defensa Nacional. *Ginecol. Obstet. Mex.* **2009**, *77*, 13–18.
24. Palaoro, L.B. *Manual de Procedimiento Bacova Erige*; Prosar: Segunda, Argentina, 2018.
25. Nugent, R.P.; Krohn, M.A.; Hillier, S.L. Reliability of Diagnosing Bacterial Vaginosis Is Improved by a Standardized Method of Gram Stain Interpretation. *J. Clin. Microbiol.* **1991**, *29*, 297–301. [CrossRef]
26. Gu, Y.; Zhou, G.; Zhou, F.; Li, Y.; Wu, Q.; He, H.; Zhang, Y.; Ma, C.; Ding, J.; Hua, K. Gut and Vaginal Microbiomes in PCOS: Implications for Women's Health. *Front. Endocrinol.* **2022**, *13*, 808508. [CrossRef] [PubMed]
27. Clabaut, M.; Suet, A.; Racine, P.J.; Tahrioui, A.; Verdon, J.; Barreau, M.; Maillot, O.; Le Tirant, A.; Karsybayeva, M.; Kremser, C.; et al. Effect of 17β-Estradiol on a Human Vaginal *Lactobacillus Crispatus* Strain. *Sci. Rep.* **2021**, *11*, 7133. [CrossRef] [PubMed]
28. Hong, X.; Qin, P.; Huang, K.; Ding, X.; Ma, J.; Xuan, Y.; Zhu, X.; Peng, D.; Wang, B. Association between Polycystic Ovary Syndrome and the Vaginal Microbiome: A Case-Control Study. *Clin. Endocrinol.* **2020**, *93*, 52–60. [CrossRef] [PubMed]
29. Kraut, R.; Carvallo, F.D.; Golonka, R.; Campbell, S.M.; Rehmani, A.; Babenko, O.; Lee, M.C.; Vieira-Baptista, P. Scoping Review of Cytolytic Vaginosis Literature. *PLoS ONE* **2023**, *18*, e0280954. [CrossRef] [PubMed]
30. Zambrano, F.; Melo, A.; Rivera-Concha, R.; Schulz, M.; Uribe, P.; Fonseca-Salamanca, F.; Ossa, X.; Taubert, A.; Hermosilla, C.; Sánchez, R. High Presence of NETotic Cells and Neutrophil Extracellular Traps in Vaginal Discharges of Women with Vaginitis: An Exploratory Study. *Cells* **2022**, *11*, 3185. [CrossRef]
31. Papayannopoulos, V.; Metzler, K.D.; Hakkim, A.; Zychlinsky, A. Neutrophil Elastase and Myeloperoxidase Regulate the Formation of Neutrophil Extracellular Traps. *J. Cell Biol.* **2010**, *191*, 677–691. [CrossRef]
32. Lu, C.; Wang, H.; Yang, J.; Zhang, X.; Chen, Y.; Feng, R.; Qian, Y. Changes in Vaginal Microbiome Diversity in Women with Polycystic Ovary Syndrome. *Front. Cell. Infect. Microbiol.* **2021**, *11*, 1–12. [CrossRef]

Disclaimer/Publisher's Note: The statements, opinions and data contained in all publications are solely those of the individual author(s) and contributor(s) and not of MDPI and/or the editor(s). MDPI and/or the editor(s) disclaim responsibility for any injury to people or property resulting from any ideas, methods, instructions or products referred to in the content.

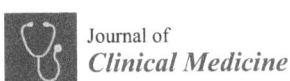
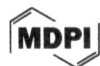

Article

Sexual Function in Women with Polycystic Ovary Syndrome Living in Stable Heterosexual Relationships: A Cross-Sectional Study

Anna Warchala [1], Paweł Madej [2], Marta Kochanowicz [3] and Marek Krzystanek [1,*]

[1] Department and Clinic of Psychiatric Rehabilitation, Faculty of Medical Sciences, Medical University of Silesia in Katowice, Ziołowa 45/47, 40-635 Katowice, Poland; awarchala@sum.edu.pl
[2] Department of Gynecological Endocrinology, Faculty of Health Science in Katowice, Medyków 14, Medical University of Silesia, 40-752 Katowice, Poland
[3] Clinical Department of Obstetrics, Gynecology and Gynecological Oncology in Kędzierzyn-Koźle, Roosvelta Str. 2, 47-200 Kędzierzyn-Koźle, Poland; marthakoch@interia.pl
* Correspondence: m.krzystanek@sum.edu.pl; Tel.: +0048-359-8020

Abstract: **Background/Objective:** The prevalence and character of female sexual dysfunction (FSD) in polycystic ovary syndrome (PCOS) have not been precisely determined. The aim of this study was to assess FSD using the Changes in Sexual Functioning Questionnaire (CSFQ-14) in women with PCOS and their partners compared to a control group, as well as correlations between five subscales, the total score of the CSFQ, and seven questions of the Visual Analogue Scale (VAS). **Methods:** The study sample ($N = 160$) comprised two groups: (1) women with PCOS and their partners ($n = 91$) and (2) women without PCOS and their partners (control group; $n = 69$). **Results:** The total scores of the CSFQ did not reveal FSD in either group of women. Regarding all subscales and the total score, the analysis showed a statistically significant difference between women and their partners (in all cases; $p < 0.001$). The discrepancy in arousal between women and men in the PCOS group was large (the mean difference was -2.32; $t = -11.29$, $p < 0.001$, Cohen's d $= -1.26$). The importance (VAS1), the level (VAS7) of sexual satisfaction, and the intensity of sexual thoughts (VAS2) correlated with almost all domains of the CSFQ. **Conclusions:** In conclusion, normal sexual function in PCOS does not mean proper sexual functioning in a sexual relationship.

Keywords: polycystic ovary syndrome; female sexual function; arousal; desire; sexual functioning of the couple

1. Introduction

Polycystic ovary syndrome (PCOS) affects 5–18% of women and is a complex condition with impacts across the lifespan [1]. It is recommended to base its diagnosis on the 2003 Rotterdam criteria and confirm with two of the three criteria: hyperandrogenism, irregular cycles, and polycystic ovary morphology [2]. The diagnostic criteria generate four phenotypes, and the clinical features are heterogeneous. This is reflected in the fact that PCOS remains the most common endocrine disease of women of reproductive age [3], the most common cause of anovulatory infertility [4], and a substantial contributor to an early onset of type 2 diabetes [5], as well as psychological disorders [6].

Numerous clinical studies have provided a greater understanding of the substantial psychological features associated with PCOS. It is reported that increased prevalences of depression, anxiety, negative body image, low self-esteem, and psychosexual dysfunction are associated with high levels of distress and adverse effects on the quality of life in women with PCOS [7,8]. Quality of life scores are often reduced in women with PCOS, with concerns around weight and infertility having the most detrimental impact [6]. However, obesity, hyperandrogenism, and infertility are weakly associated with symptoms of

depression and anxiety scores [6]. As it was shown in a 2019 community-based study, women with PCOS also have an increased prevalence of disordered eating, such as binge eating disorder, compared to controls [9].

Female sexual dysfunction (FSD) is defined in the fifth edition of the Diagnostic and Statistical Manual of Mental Disorders (DSM-5) as a frequent, long-lasting, and distressing problem concerning desire, arousal, orgasm, or pain and is associated with various conditions characterized by negative mental and physical outcomes [10]. Despite specific studies, the prevalence and character of FSD in PCOS have not been precisely determined, and the conclusions from these studies are inconsistent [11–13]. The gaps in knowledge make the condition interesting for further study. Establishing a diagnosis for sexual problems in patients with PCOS might give rise to clinical trials aimed at improving sexual disturbances in this group of patients.

2. Materials and Methods

The aim of our study was to assess sexual function in women with PCOS and their partners compared to a similar control group. We decided to use the Changes in Sexual Functioning Questionnaire (CSFQ) because it allowed us to assess sexual functions within the same domains in women and men. We wanted to examine sexual function in women with PCOS in the context of their partners. We also tried to explore the impact of self-perception in the areas of sexual satisfaction, personal attractiveness, excessive hair, social struggles, intensity of sexual thoughts and fantasies, and painful sexual encounters on specific domains in CSFQ. We decided to put forward four hypotheses. (1) The importance and level of sexual satisfaction correlates positively with specific dimensions of the CSFQ. (2) The perceived level of personal attractiveness correlates positively with specific dimensions of the CSFQ and the perceived impact of excessive hair on personal sexuality and social struggles due to appearance correlating negatively with specific dimensions of the CSFQ. (3) The intensity of sexual thoughts and fantasies correlates positively with specific dimensions of the CSFQ. (4) The occurrence of painful sexual encounters correlates negatively with specific dimensions of the CSFQ. Additionally, we analyzed demographic and physical correlates of the sexual functioning of women with PCOS. This study was approved by the Ethics Committee of the Medical University of Silesia, No.: PCN/CBN/0022/KB1/77/21.

The inclusion criteria comprised women diagnosed with polycystic ovary syndrome (PCOS) according to the Rotterdam criteria, aged 18–40, with partners, and who gave written consent. The control group included women without PCOS, aged 18–40, with their partners, and who gave written consent.

The patients with PCOS were recruited through the Department of Gynecological Endocrinology of Medical University of Silesia in Katowice (Poland). The participants of the control group were recruited from the medical students of the Medical University of Silesia and the medical staff at the Upper Silesian Medical Centre in Katowice.

Patients with PCOS were recruited to the study group during their first diagnostic hospitalization at the Department of Gynecological Endocrinology. The diagnosis of PCOS was confirmed by gynecologists and endocrinologists according to the Rotterdam criteria and based on a physical examination and a set of laboratory tests tailored to each patient's symptoms. The topic of sexuality was not mentioned prior to the patients taking the survey. The information provided to the respondents included a brief description of the significance of the sexual function in women with PCOS for their further life satisfaction. Participating patients with a stable male partner gave written consent to the proposed study and completed a set of questionnaires for women (demographic, CSFQ-F-C, VAS) at the end of their stay in the hospital ward. The questionnaire intended for men (CSFQ-M-C) was taken home by the patients with PCOS and returned during their first follow-up visit at the Outpatient Clinic of Infertility Treatment. Of 147 women enrolled in our study, 91 provided CSFQ-M-C test results from their partners.

The control group included women without a diagnosis of PCOS or chronic diseases. They provided written consent to the study and completed our demographic questionnaire and the CSFQ-F-C. Their partners met the CSFQ-M-C criteria. All questionnaires were returned together. Of the 93 women included in the control group, 69 took the test.

All information about the physical condition of patients with PCOS came from medical records prepared during hospitalization by doctors of the Department of Gynecological Endocrinology. Information about the control group participants was obtained based on interviews with them.

2.1. Questionnaires and Scales

The demographic questionnaire included age, marital status, place of residence, education, employment, confirmation of having a permanent sexual partner, and confirmation of sexual activity in the last week or last month.

The Changes in Sexual Functioning Questionnaire 14 (CSFQ-14) was used to assess sexual dysfunction. The CSFQ-14 is well validated and contains sex-specific items and has proven useful in assessing changes in sexual function in various populations. The questionnaire measures overall sexual functioning (sum of 1 to 14 items), with 5 subdomains assessing pleasure (Item 1), desire/frequency (Items 2 + 3), desire/interest (Items 4 + 5 + 6), arousal (Items 7 + 8 + 9), and orgasm (Items 11 + 12 + 13). We defined sexual dysfunction on a standard basis (CSFQ—female clinical version global score ≤ 41 and CSFQ—male clinical version global score ≤ 47).

The Visual Analogue Scale (VAS) is a psychometric scale that can be used as a tool to measure subjective characteristics or attitudes. In our study, PCOS patients indicated their level of agreement with the question by indicating their position on a solid line between Points 1 and 10. Using the VAS scale used in several previous studies, we obtained 7 questions: (1) How important is a satisfying sex life to you? (2) How many sexual thoughts and fantasies have you had in the past? (3) Do you find yourself sexually attractive? (4) How does excessive body hair affect your sexuality? (5) Does your appearance make it difficult to establish social contacts? (6) In the last 4 weeks, how often have you experienced pain during intercourse? (7) How satisfied have you been with your sex life in the last 4 weeks [11]? The scale was not validated for the Polish version.

The Waist Hip Ratio (WHR) was calculated by dividing a waist measurement by a hip measurement. The Ferriman–Gallwey (m-F-G) score was used to evaluate terminal hair growth on a scale of 0–4 on eleven different body areas according to the authors' scoring system. A Ferriman–Gallwey score ≥ 8 was considered diagnostic of hirsutism. The presence and severity of acne was evaluated on a scale of 0–4.

2.2. Statistical Analyses

A mixed analysis of variance (ANOVA) model was used to examine the differences between women and their partners in PCOS and control groups. In each model, we included within subject effects (i.e., difference between women and their partners), between subject effects (i.e., difference between PCOS and control groups), and interaction between both effects (i.e., to answer the question if the differences between women and men are diverse in PCOS and control groups). We computed the ω^2 coefficient as a measure of the effect size due to its lower susceptibility in the cases of assumption violations [14]. In the case of statistically significant effects, Holm's post hoc tests (together with Cohen's ds as effect size measures) were computed.

To examine the correlation between CSFQ and VAS, we used Pearson's correlation coefficients. The same procedure was used to explore some demographic and physical correlates of the sexual functioning of women with PCOS. Yet, in this case, having in mind the ordinal (i.e., education) or nominal (i.e., residence, work, acne presence, and hirsutism), we also used Spearman's correlation (for ordinal variable) and the U Mann–Whitney test (for nominal variables) to explore possible correlates of sexual functioning of women with PCOS.

3. Results

3.1. Participants

The sample (n = 160) consisted of two subsamples: (1) women diagnosed with PCOS and their partners (n = 91) and (2) women without PCOS and their partners (control group; n = 69). The average age of the women participating in the study was 28.64 years (SD = 5.61) and was slightly higher in the PCOS group (M = 29.61, SD = 6.64) compared to the control group (M = 27, 91, SD = 4.57). However, the difference was not statistically significant (Mann–Whitney U test with rank-biserial correlation as a measure of effect size: W = 3532.00, p = 0.176, rbs = 0.09).

Most participants reported higher education (PCOS: n = 51, 56%; control: n = 44, 64%) or secondary education (PCOS: n = 33, 36%; control: n = 24, 35%). The majority also maintained stable work (PCOS: n = 69, 76%; control: n = 61, 88%). However, some of them remained unemployed (PCOS: n = 12, 13%; control: n = 7, 10%) or received a life pension (PCOS: n = 4, 4%; control: n = 1, 1%).

All respondents declared a stable heterosexual relationship. In both subsamples, the percentage of women in a formal relationship (PCOS: n = 42, 46%; control: n = 35, 51%) and an informal relationship (PCOS: n = 49, 54%; control: n = 29, 42%; n = 5, 7% of women in the control group declared they were divorced) remained similar. Most of the respondents lived with their family (PCOS: n = 76, 84%; control: n = 48, 70%; the rest declared living alone).

Regarding the PCOS group, the participants' average WHR was 0.86 (SD = 0.10), with the lowest value of 0.67 and the highest of 1.17. In the case of 32 (35%) women, the Ferriman–Gallwey test indicated a presence of hirsutism. Also, in the case of 55 (60%) women, the medical examination revealed acne.

3.2. Sexual Functioning—Descriptive Statistics

Table 1 presents descriptive statistics for the dimensions of the sexual functioning of women with PCOS and the control group and their partners.

Table 1. Sexual functioning of women with and without PCOS and their partners—descriptive statistics.

	M	SD	Min	Max	Skewness
PCOS group—women					
Pleasure	3.92	0.96	1.00	5.00	−0.78
Desire—frequency	6.95	1.37	3.00	10.00	−0.35
Desire—interest	8.75	2.06	3.00	12.00	−0.34
Arousal	10.56	2.05	5.00	14.00	−0.37
Orgasm	10.88	2.46	3.00	15.00	−0.40
Total CSFQ	49.59	7.47	27.00	63.00	−0.34
Control group—women					
Pleasure	3.93	0.99	1.00	5.00	−0.98
Desire—frequency	6.97	1.40	4.00	10.00	−0.28
Desire—interest	8.58	2.45	3.00	13.00	−0.29
Arousal	11.16	2.10	6.00	15.00	−0.83
Orgasm	11.15	2.94	3.00	15.00	−1.02
Total CSFQ	50.68	8.63	24.00	64.00	−1.31
PCOS group—men					
Pleasure	4.28	0.82	1.00	5.00	−1.55
Desire—frequency	7.42	1.39	4.00	10.00	−0.18
Desire—interest	9.77	2.19	4.00	15.00	−0.01
Arousal	12.88	1.46	9.00	15.00	−0.84
Orgasm	12.40	1.67	7.00	15.00	−0.71
Total CSFQ	56.12	5.55	40.00	70.00	−0.51

2.8.4. Interpretation of Results

Nonspecific Microbial Vaginitis (nMVitis)

All vaginal discharge smears that had a Nugent score between 4 and 10 and presented VIR (moderate or intense) were classified in this category. Vaginal microbiota with these characteristics were considered to present a proinflammatory state or acute inflammation.

Bacterial Vaginosis

Interpreted as a state of chronic inflammation of the vaginal microbiota, since an inflammatory reaction with the presence of PMN was not observed.

Definition of Altered and Normal Microbiota

For the preparation of the tables and statistical analysis of the group under study, all cases with intermediate microbiota, bacterial vaginosis, and cases with nMVitis were considered altered microbiota. According to Nugent's criteria, cases that scored between 0 and 3 were considered normal microbiota.

2.8.5. Identification of Neutrophil Extracellular Traps (NETs)

Immunofluorescence of vaginal discharge smears was performed to determine the presence of neutrophil extracellular DNA using a polyclonal primary antibody anti-rabbit IgG (reference no. ab68672 Abcam, Cambridge, UK) to identify NE elastase. The smears were incubated with polyclonal anti-NE antibody (reference no. ab68672 Abcam, Cambridge, UK) in PBS-BSA at a dilution of 1:300. They were then washed by manual shaking and incubated for 1 h with secondary antibody anti-Rabbit IgG conjugated with Alexa Fluor™ 488 (reference no. A11008, Life Technologies, Invitrogen, Thermo Fisher Scientific, Waltham, MA, USA). Subsequently, the samples were then washed by manual shaking with Sytox orange® (reference no. s11368, Invitrogen, Thermo Fisher Scientific, Waltham, MA, USA) (stain for DNA, 1:2000 in 1X PBS). The slides were covered with mounting medium (reference no. 00-4959-52, Invitrogen Thermo Fisher Scientific, Waltham, MA, USA) and a coverslip. The TissueFAXS i Plus Cytometry microscope (TissueGnostics, Vienna, Austria) was used to scan the smears. Then, the TissueFaxs-Viewer 7.0 software was used to obtain images of interest areas to observe fluorescence.

2.9. Statistical Analysis

The data obtained were entered in an Excel spreadsheet; they were analyzed with the SPSS program (IMB-SPSS, version 29.0 for Windows); descriptive statistics were used with the calculation of frequencies, percentages, measures of central tendency and dispersion, inferential statistics, and parametric and nonparametric tests according to each variable. For clinical and hormonal variables, OR values were calculated with their respective 95% CI. Values of $p \leq 0.005$ were considered statistically significant.

3. Results

The participants' age range was 18–36 (mean 23 years). Phenotype A was the most representative, with 60.6% (20/33), C and D both had 18.2% (6/33), and B was the least observed (1/33) 3.0%.

Vaginal microbiota status according to Bacova–Erige criteria were NM 30.3% (10/33), IM 33.3% (11/33), BV 15.2% (5/33), and nonspecific microbial vaginitis (nMVitis) 21.2% (7/33). A high number of patients, (23/33) 69.7%, presented an altered microbiota.

The variables age (≤ 23 years p-value = 0.07), phenotypes A and B (considered together), lifetime sexual partners, and oligomenorrhea represented the highest number of women with altered microbiota. Oral contraceptive use was the variable with the slightest variation among users and non-users of contraceptives. However, the most important and significant statistical association was observed with the variable active sexually transmitted infection at the time of sampling (p-value = 0.023) (Table 3).

Table 3. Clinical factors according to vaginal microbiota status in the study group (n = 33).

Variables	n	Normal	Altered	OR (IC)	p-Value
Phenotypes					
A and B	21(63.6)	5(23.8)	16(76.2)	2.29(0.50; 10.50)	0.283
C and D	12(36.4)	5(41.7)	7(58.3)		
Age of onset of sexual intercourse (years)					
≤18	20(60.6)	8(40.0)	12(60.0)	0.27(0.04; 1.57)	0.133
>18	13(39.4)	2(15.4)	11(84.6)		
Number of sexual partners					
None	6(18.18)	3(50.0)	3(50.0)	0.35(0.06; 2.15)	0.246
More than 1 sexual partner	27(81.82)	7(25.93)	20(74.07)		
Active STI					
Yes	25(75.8)	5(20.0)	20(80.0)	6.68(1.18; 37.78)	* 0.023
No	8(24.2)	5(62.5)	3(37.5)		
Oral contraceptives use					
Yes	19(57.6)	7(36.8)	12(63.2)	0.47(0.10; 2.27)	0.341
No	14(42.4)	3(21.4)	11(78.5)		
Oligomenorrhea					
Yes	27(81.8)	7(25.9)	20(74.1)	2.86(0.46; 17.58)	0.246
No	6(18.2)	3(50.0)	3(50.0)		

Number of sexual partners: in the last six months. **Active STI**: sexually transmitted infections detected in the laboratory by conventional PCR. **Statistical test:** Chi-squared, **OR**: Odds Ratio, **IC**: confidence interval, * p-value < 0.005.

About the hormonal variables, only insulin showed a significant p-value. More cases were observed in patients with normal insulin and altered microbiota. Glucose levels were also analyzed in association with the state of the microbiota, but no results could be obtained since the glucose levels of all the patients were reported as normal (Table 4).

Table 4. Hormonal variables according to vaginal microbiota status in the study group (n = 33).

Hormonal Variables	N	Normal	Altered	OR (IC)	p-Value
HOMA					
Normal	12(40.0)	5(25.0)	9(75.0)	0.52(0.10; 2.60)	0.429
Altered	18(60.0)	7(38.9)	7(61.1)		
Insulin					
Normal	26(86.7)	6(23.1)	20(76.9)	–	0.002
Altered	4(15.3)	4(100.0)	–		
Total Testosterone					
Normal	16(48.5)	7(43.8)	9(56.3)	0.28(0.06; 0.35)	0.103
Altered	17(51.5)	3(17.6)	14(82.4)		

Table 4. *Cont.*

		Vaginal Microbiota (%)			
Hormonal Variables	N	Normal	Altered	OR (IC)	*p*-Value
DHEAS					
Normal	26(89.7)	9(34.6)	17(65.4)	–	0.220
Altered	3(10.3)	-	3(100.0)		
17-OH progesterone					
Normal	15(53.6)	6(40.0)	9(60.0)	2.22(0.43; 11.6)	0.339
Altered	13(46.4)	3(23.1)	10(76.9)		
Androstenedione					
Normal	20(69.0)	7(35.0)	13(65.0)	1.07(0.2; 5.7)	0.930
Altered	9(31.0)	3(33.3)	6(66.7)		
LH					
Normal	17(54,8)	6(35.3)	11(64.7)	1.36(0.29; 6.28)	0.690
Altered	14(45.2)	4(28.6)	10(71.4)		
AMH					
Normal	2(7.7)	1(50.0)	1(50.0)	2.42(0.13; 44.50)	0.540
Altered	24(92.3)	7(29.2)	17(70.8)		
Vitamin D					
Normal	20(71.4)	7(35.0)	13(65.0)	0.23(0.03; 2.61)	0.234
Altered	8(28.6)	1(12.5)	7(87.5)		

DHEAS: dehydroepiandrosterone sulfate; **LH**: luteinizing hormone; **AMH**: Anti-Müllerian hormone. **Statistical test:** Chi-squared, **OR**: Odds Ratio, **IC**: confidence interval, *p*-value < 0.005.

The proinflammatory state assessed by cell destruction (debris) and naked nuclei was present in 72.7% (24/33) of cases with variable intensity (scarce 6/33, moderate 10/33, and intense 8/33), depending on whether they were found in some or all fields observed in Gram staining. A statistically significant difference was observed between the proinflammatory statuses present vs. absent concerning normal or altered vaginal microbiota *p*-value = 0.021. A higher percentage of proinflammatory status and altered vaginal microbiome was observed in 14 (60.9%) patients (Table 5).

Table 5. Proinflammatory state according to the states of the vaginal microbiota.

		Proinflammatory State (%)		
Vaginal Microbiota	n (%)	Absent	Present	*p*-Value
Normal	10(30.3)	0	10(100.0)	* 0.021
Altered	23(33.3)	9(39.1)	14(60.9)	
Total	33(100.0)	9(27.3)	24(72.7)	

The absence or presence of a proinflammatory state was defined by the amount of cell destruction and loose nuclei observed during Gram reading in 20 fields. Vaginal microbiota normal: a score between 0 and 3 was considered according to the Nugent criteria. Altered vaginal microbiota includes intermediate microbiota (IM), bacterial vaginosis (BV), and non-specific microbial vaginitis (nMVitis). **Statistical test:** Chi-squared, (*) corresponds to a statistically significant *p*-value (*p*< 0.05).

VIR was evaluated by the presence of PMN and Giemsa staining, and was present in 24.2% (8/33, 1 NM case and 7 IM cases).

The release of NETs was observed in the eight cases that presented VIR, and their characteristics are shown in Table 6. In cases with VIR, 62.5% (5/8) are of phenotype A, with no cases of phenotype B found. A total of 25% (2/8) of phenotype D and 12.5% (1/8) of phenotype C were also found. The proinflammatory status of the cases analyzed for

NETs were as follows: 50% (4/8) intense, 25% (2/8) moderate, 12.5% (1/8) scarce, and 12.5% (1/8) absent. Moreover, regarding the vaginal microbiota, 87.5% (7/8) of the cases presented nMVitis.

Table 6. Distribution of SOP phenotype, proinflammatory status, and vaginal microbiota in the eight cases examined for neutrophil extracellular traps (NETs).

Cases with VIR	Phenotypes	Proinflammatory State	Vaginal Microbiota
1	D	Scarce	MN
2	A	Intense	nMVitis
3	D	Intense	nMVitis
4	A	Moderate	nMVitis
5	A	Moderate	nMVitis
6	C	Intense	nMVitis
7	A	Absent	nMVitis
8	A	Intense	nMVitis

(VIR): vaginal inflammatory reaction; **(nMVitis):** non-specific microbial vaginitis.

By PCR, one-eighth of the samples were positive for *Candida albicans*, two-eighths were positive for *Atopobium vaginae*, and seven-eighths were positive for *Gardnerella vaginalis*. For *Trichomonas vaginalis* and *Chlamydia trachomatis*, all were negative.

As observed in (Figure 2) representative images of vaginal discharge smears from women with PCOS show anti-NE marking (Alexa fluor 488), sytox orange staining marking DNA, and Gram stain-marked structure suggestive of NETs (green arrow).

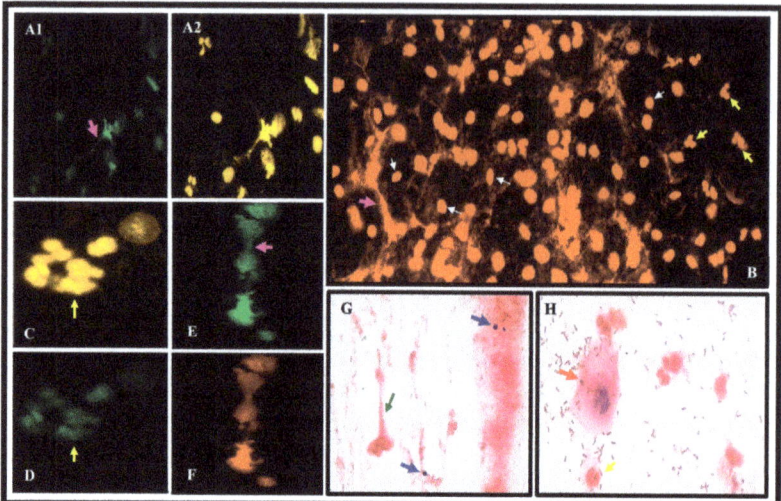

Figure 2. Representative images of vaginal discharge smears from women with PCOS. The Tissue-FAXS i Plus cytometry microscope was used to scan the smears at 20X magnification and TissueFaxs-Viewer software was used to obtain images at 100-450% zoom. Green staining in (**A1,D,E**) shows anti-NE labeling (Alexa fluor 488); Sytox orange staining marks DNA in images (**B,F**); Gram staining (**G**) shows structures suggestive of NET (green arrow), and presence of blastoconidia corresponding to Candida albicans diagnosed by PCR (blue arrows); Gram-stained image (**H**) indicates vaginal squamous cell (red arrow) showing different bacterial morphotypes corresponding to an intermediate microbiota; image (**F**) marks PMNs in the process of DNA release; yellow arrows indicate PMN nuclei (**B,C,D,H**); white arrows indicate squamous epithelial cell nuclei (**B**) and fuchsia arrows indicate NETs (**A1,E**) and (**A2,B**) channel merging. Images (**C,D,E,F**) (450% zoom), (**A1,A2,G,H**) (230% zoom), and (**B**) (100% zoom) were used.

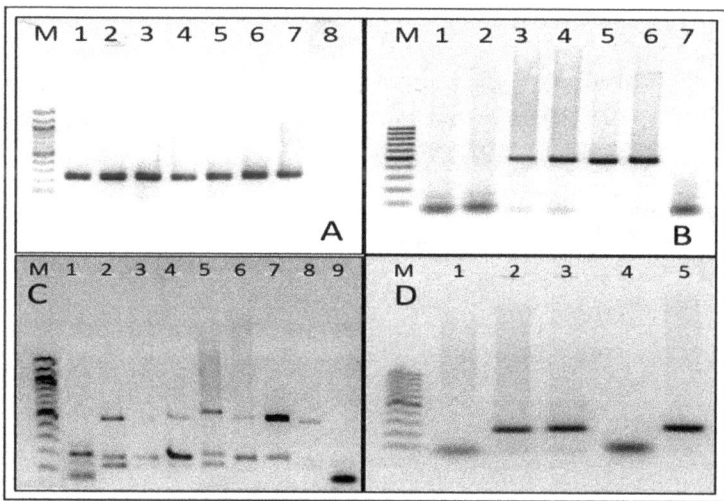

Figure 1. Representative images of PCR products from the conventional PCRs used in the study: (**M**) Molecular weight marker (100 bp) (**A**) PCR of the Beta-globin (268 bp) gene used as an internal control; (**B**) PCR of *Candida albicans* (496 bp), where lanes 1 and 2 are negative samples, lanes 3, 4, and 5 are positive samples, lane 6 is positive control, and lane 7 is blank control; (**C**) multiplex PCR for *Gardnerella vaginalis* (206 bp), *Atopobium vaginae* (558 bp) and *Megasphaera phylotype* 1 (144 bp), where lanes 1 and 2 are positive controls, lanes 3, 4, 5, 6, 7, and 8 are positive samples, and lane 9 is blank control; and (**D**) *Chlamydia trachomatis* PCR (241 bp), where lane 1 is negative sample, lanes 2 and 3 are positive samples, lane 4 is blank control, and lane 5 is positive control.

Table 2. Definition of basic vaginal states.

BVS in Women's Childbearing Age	NV	VIR
I Normal microbiota Predominance of *Lactobacilli*	0–3	No
II Normal microbiota + VIR Predominance of *Lactobacilli* with vaginal inflammatory reaction present.	0–3	Yes
III Intermediate microbiota Equilibrium of *Lactobacilli* and anaerobic Bacteria	4–6	No
IV Bacterial vaginosis Predominance of anaerobic bacteria	7–10	No
V Nonspecific Microbial Vaginitis Alteration of the ratio of *Lactobacilli* and anaerobic bacteria, or presence of foreign bacterial morphotypes with inflammatory reaction.	4–10	Yes

BVS: basic vaginal status; NV: Nugent's numerical value, VIR: vaginal inflammatory reaction.

2.8.3. Vaginal Inflammatory Reaction (VIR)

VIR was observed by Giemsa staining and counting leukocytes or PMN, applying criteria according to the Bacova–Erige manual [24]. Absent VIR: <5, moderate VIR: >5–<10, and intense VIR: >10 PMN per field. Reading was performed in 5 non-adjacent fields with a 100× objective and immersion oil.

2.7.2. Microorganism DNA Detection

Conventional one-step PCRs were used for *Chlamydia trachomatis*, *Candida albicans* [19], and *Trichomonas vaginalis* [20], using specific primers previously published. For the detection of *Gardnerella vaginalis* [21], *Atopobium vaginae*, and *Megasphaera phylotype* 1 [22], a conventional one-step multiplex PCR was used. Primer sequences and fragment sizes are shown in (Table 1). Positive controls: cultures or known clinical samples positive for each microorganism were used. Visualization: PCR products were confirmed relative to the positive control on 1.6% agarose gels stained with GelRed using a 100 bp marker (New England Biolabs, Ipswich, MA, USA).

Table 1. Primers used in PCR analysis.

Micro-Organism	Primers	Sequence 5′-3′	Fragment Base Pairs	Reference	GenBank
Chlamydia trachomatis	Forward Reverse	tccggagcgagttacgaaga aatcaatgcccgggattggt	241	Sánchez V. 2009 [23]	NZ_CP009926.1
Candida albicans	Forward Reverse	atgggtggtcaacatac tacatctatgtctaccacc	496	Burgener-kairuz 1994 [19]	X13296.1
Trichomonas vaginalis	Forward Reverse	attgtcgaacattggtcttaccctc tctgtgccgtcttcaagtatgc	262	Pačes J, 1992 [20]	L23861.1
Gardnerella vaginalis	Forward Reverse	gcgggctagagtgca acccgtggaatgggcc	206	Zariffard MR, 2002 [21]	GenBank: AY738665.1
Atopobium vaginae	Forward Reverse	gcagggacgaggccgcaa gtgtttccactgcttcacctaa	558	Fredricks D. 2007 [22]	AY738657.1
Megasphaera phylotype 1	Forward Reverse	gatgccaacagtatccgtccg Acagacttaccgaaccgcct	144	Fredricks D. 2007 [22]	AY738672.1

The result was determined by visualization of a band at the same height, as the positive control was interpreted as a positive sample for that micro-organism. Conversely, no band visualization was interpreted as a negative result (Figure 1).

2.8. Analysis of Vaginal Discharge Smears

The analysis of the smears was carried out according to the criteria stated in the BACOVA-ERIGE (Balance of Vaginal Contents-Study of the Genital Inflammatory Reaction) procedures manual, which classifies the vaginal microbiota into 5 basic vaginal states [24] (Table 2).

2.8.1. Gram Stain

Microscopic observation using a 100× objective and immersion oil allows differentiation between Gram-positive bacteria (violet color) and Gram-negative bacteria (reddish color). The reading was performed in 20 fields, counting Gram-positive bacilli (*Lactobacillus* spp.), pleomorphic Gram-variable bacilli (compatible with *Gardnerella vaginalis*), and Gram-variable curved bacilli (*Mobiluncus* spp.). A score was assigned to the number of morphotypes found, according to Nugent's criteria [25], allowing the microbiota to be classified with the following score: normal (NM) 0–3, intermediate (IM) 4–6, and bacterial vaginosis (BV) 7–10. In addition, the presence or absence of blastoconidia and pseudohyphae were recorded.

2.8.2. Proinflammatory State

Observed by Gram staining and defined by the amount of cellular damage (referred to as destroyed cells (detritus) and/or epithelial cell nuclei without cytoplasm), the following criteria were assigned: absent (0); present, grouping the cases that presented scarce (1+); moderate (2+); and intense (3+) cellular damage. The evaluation was performed in 20 fields at 1000× with immersion oil.

Committee (CEISH) 2023-006O-IE of the University of Cuenca, Ecuador, authorized the research protocol.

2.5. Survey Application

A survey was applied anonymously (using a code), which allowed the collection of clinical data of women with a diagnosis of PCOS. The items included in the survey were the following: age, age of onset of sexual intercourse, number of sexual partners in the last six months, use of oral contraceptives, oligomenorrhea. At the same time, blood tests for the following hormones were performed: HOMA (Homeostasis Model Assessment), insulin, total testosterone, DHEAS (dehydroepiandrosterone sulfate), 17—OH progesterone, androstenedione (A4), LH (luteinizing hormone), FSH (follicle stimulating hormone), AMH (Anti-Müllerian hormone), glucose, and vitamin D.

2.6. Patients

Thirty-three women over 18 years of age diagnosed with PCOS were included according to the recommendations of the 2018 international evidence-based guidelines [2], which allow for the classification of PCOS patients according to phenotypes A, B, C, and D. Exclusion criteria were as follows: menstruation on the day of sampling, having had sexual intercourse in the last 48 h, being a douche user, cognitive impairment, antimicrobial treatment in the last 30 days, immunosuppressive drugs or immunosuppression, chronic degenerative diseases (non-classical congenital adrenal hyperplasia, androgen-producing tumor, hyperprolactinemia, thyroid dysfunction, Cushing's syndrome, drugs with androgenic activity, etc.), and patients with ovarian cysts.

Four clinical phenotypes of the disease have been identified, each with clinical implications regarding severity. Phenotype A is known as "classic" or complete and consists of three criteria: hyperandrogenism, oligo-ovulation, and polycystic ovarian morphology. Phenotype B, also called "classic", has hyperandrogenism and oligo-ovulation. Both phenotypes A and B have a more severe clinical and metabolic impact. Phenotype C is called "ovulatory", characterized by hyperandrogenism and polycystic ovarian morphology, while phenotype D, "non-hyperandrogenic", is composed of oligo-ovulation and polycystic ovarian morphology, and being less severe [18].

2.7. Vaginal Discharge Samples

The samples were taken through speculoscopy by a professional gynecologist, using a cotton swab from the "vaginal fornix and vaginal walls". Subsequently, 5 smears were made on slides which were left to dry in the air and then stored in a transporting box. Each slide was used for the following purposes: DNA extraction, Gram staining, Giemsa, and immunofluorescence.

2.7.1. DNA Extraction

Vaginal material was scraped with a scalpel from each slide and placed in 1.5 mL tubes with lysis buffer (0.01 M Tris pH 7.8, 0.005 M EDTA pH 8, 0.5% SDS) and incubated at 85 °C for 15 min. Subsequently, 7.5 M ammonium acetate pH 7.5 was added, the tubes were cooled to -20 °C for 5 min, and the proteins were precipitated at 12,000 rpm for 5 min (min) at 4 °C. The supernatant was mixed with isopropanol and incubated overnight at -20 °C. DNA was precipitated at 12,000 rpm for 15 min at 4 °C, washed with 70% ethanol, and hydrated with TE buffer (10 mmol/L Tris-HCl, 1 mmol/L EDTA pH 8). Internal control: a conventional one-step polymerase chain reaction (PCR) was used as an internal control, which allowed us to discard samples with non-amplifiable inhibitory DNA. For this, primers PCO4 and GH20 were used: primers PCO4 5′-caacttcatccacgttcacc-3′ and GH20 5′-gaagagccaaggacaggacaggacaggtac-3′, which amplify a fragment of 268 base pairs (bp) of the Beta-Globin gene.

factors [4]. There is a close association between microbial dysbiosis and pathological changes in PCOS [3].

In this association, the release of proinflammatory and inflammatory factors, the primary mechanism driven by altered microbiota, could be associated with the clinical characteristics of polycystic ovary syndrome, predominantly obesity, insulin resistance, and vitamin D deficiency in the different phenotypes of patients with PCOS [5,6]. Likewise, there is an imbalance in the vaginal microbiota, generated mainly by irregular menses and hormonal changes associated with hyperandrogenism and hyperinsulinemia with anovulation and oligo- or amenorrhea. This maintains an estrogenic tone not counteracted by postovulatory progesterone, so that estrogen stimulates the accumulation of glycogen in the cells of the vaginal epithelium. This glycogen is used by Lactobacillus within vagina to produce lactic acid, keeping the vaginal pH under 4.5 and thus preventing the growth of pathogenic or opportunistic micro-organisms such as *Candida* spp. or *Gardnerella* spp. [4]. However, this estrogenic tone, which should be a protective factor in patients with PCOS, is only basal, and the necessary increases associated with the normal menstrual cycle do not occur [5]; thereby leadings to increased destruction of epithelial cells and local inflammation [7]. These conditions create a favorable environment for microorganisms to colonize the lower genital tract. *Gardnerella vaginalis*, *Prevotella* spp., and *Mycoplasma hominis* have been described with a higher prevalence in the vaginal microbiota of patients with PCOS [8]. This disruption of the vaginal microbiome would potentially lead to an increase in local inflammatory factors, such as interleukin-8 and tumor necrosis factor-α, which, together with other metabolites, trigger chronic systemic inflammation that can affect the hypothalamic–pituitary–ovarian axis. At the vaginal level, the increase in polymorphonuclear neutrophils (PMN), and their activation induces the formation and release of neutrophil extracellular traps (NETs), which allow PMN to perform a process of cell death (NETosis) through which the release of nuclear chromatin, peptides, and antimicrobial enzymes, including defensins, catalysins, neutrophil elastase (NE) and myeloperoxidase (MPO) occurs, controlling and helping the organism to defend itself from inflammatory and infectious processes [9–12].

The effect of sex steroid hormones as well as the intestinal microbiome have been extensively investigated [13–15], but inflammatory states and the vaginal microbiota require further evaluation [16,17]. This study explores the diversity of the vaginal microbiota in patients with PCOS, as well as the vaginal inflammatory reaction (VIR) and PMN activation with the production of neutrophil extracellular traps.

2. Materials and Methods

2.1. Study Design

Cross-sectional study.

2.2. Sample

The sample corresponded to the first 33 patients who attended the consultation at the Hospital UTPL-Santa Inés de Loja, Ecuador, from May to August 2023 and diagnosed with PCOS. This study was considered random due to the characteristics of the sampling.

2.3. Location

Conducted in 2022–2023 at the Hospital Santa Inés, Loja, Ecuador, and the Center of Excellence in Translational Medicine and Scientific and Technological Bioresource Nucleus (CEMT-BIOREN), Universidad de La Frontera, Temuco, Chile.

2.4. Ethical Aspects

The women participating in the study participated voluntarily and without monetary reward. They were given a written informed consent form that was read and explained to them, and a copy was provided and signed by each of them. The Human Research Ethics

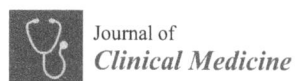 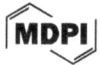

Article

Vaginal Microbiota and Proinflammatory Status in Patients with Polycystic Ovary Syndrome: An Exploratory Study

María Elena Espinosa [1,2], Angélica Melo [3], Marion Leon [3], Estefanía Bautista-Valarezo [2], Fabiola Zambrano [3,4], Pamela Uribe [3,5], Anita Bravo [3], Anja Taubert [6], Carlos Hermosilla [6], Virginia Iturrieta [3] and Raul Sánchez [3,4],*

[1] Ph.D. Program in Medical Sciences, Faculty of Medicine, Universidad de La Frontera, Temuco 4780000, Chile; meespinosax@utpl.edu.ec
[2] Department of Health Sciences, Faculty of Health Sciences, Universidad Técnica Particular de Loja, UTPL, San Cayetano Alto s/n, Loja 1101608, Ecuador; mebautista@utpl.edu.ec
[3] Center of Excellence in Translational Medicine-Scientific and Technological Bioresource (CEMT-BIOREN), Temuco 4780000, Chile; angelica.melo@ufrontera.cl (A.M.); m.leon06@ufromail.cl (M.L.); fabiola.zambrano@ufrontera.cl (F.Z.); pamela.uribe@ufrontera.cl (P.U.); a.bravo02@ufromail.cl (A.B.); v.iturrieta01@ufrontera.cl (V.I.)
[4] Department of Preclinical Sciences, Faculty of Medicine, Universidad de La Frontera, Temuco 4780000, Chile
[5] Department of Internal Medicine, Faculty of Medicine, Universidad de La Frontera, Temuco 4780000, Chile
[6] Institute of Parasitology, Justus Liebig University Giessen, 35392 Giessen, Germany; anja.taubert@vetmed.uni-giessen.de (A.T.); carlos.r.hermosilla@vetmed.uni-giessen.de (C.H.)
* Correspondence: raul.sanchez@ufrontera.cl

Abstract: Background/Purpose: Polycystic ovary syndrome (PCOS) is an endocrine-metabolic disease most common in patients of childbearing age. This pathology is associated with clinical, metabolic, and reproductive complications. We evaluated the diversity of the vaginal microbiota (VM), the vaginal inflammatory reaction (VIR), the proinflammatory state, and the activation of polymorphonuclear neutrophils (PMN) with the production of neutrophil extracellular traps (NETs). **Methods**: Thirty-three patients who attended a consultation at the Hospital UTPL-Santa Inés, Loja, Ecuador, from May to August 2023 who were diagnosed with PCOS participated in this study. Blood samples, vaginal discharge, and a survey were obtained. **Results**: A high number of patients, 23/33 (69.7%), presented altered microbiota in clinical variables associated with PCOS phenotypes A and B, sexual partners (>2), and oligomenorrhoea. A significant statistical association was only observed for sexually transmitted infections at sampling ($p = 0.023$) and insulin ($p = 0.002$). All eight cases studied with VIR had PMN/NETotic activity. A high frequency of proinflammatory states was observed in all vaginal microbiota states. **Conclusions**: These results suggest that the PCOS could trigger a proinflammatory state in the vaginal epithelium independently of the state of the vaginal microbiota. Furthermore, the presence of NETs observed in the cases studied could decrease fertility in these PCOS patients.

Keywords: polycystic ovary syndrome; phenotypes; vaginal inflammatory reaction; vaginal microbiota; neutrophil extracellular traps (NETs)

1. Introduction

Polycystic ovary syndrome (PCOS) is a neuroendocrine, metabolic, and reproductive disorder that can affect up to 20% of women in their reproductive age. It is characterized by oligo-anovulation, clinical and/or biochemical hyperandrogenism, and ultrasonography with diagnosis of polycystic ovaries [1]. Applying the recommendations of the 2019 international evidence-based guideline for diagnosing PCOS, the diagnosis of the different phenotypes of PCOS (A, B, C, and D) can be made, allowing its categorization and type of treatment [2,3]. Its etiopathogenesis is complex, multifactorial, and heterogeneous in its presentation, including the interaction of genetic, epigenetic, and environmental

29. Dewailly, D.; Andersen, C.Y.; Balen, A.; Broekmans, F.; Dilaver, N.; Fanchin, R.; Griesinger, G.; Kelsey, T.W.; La Marca, A.; Lambalk, C.; et al. The physiology and clinical utility of anti-Mullerian hormone in women. *Hum. Reprod. Update* **2014**, *20*, 370–385. [CrossRef] [PubMed]
30. Robin, G.; Gallo, C.; Catteau-Jonard, S.; Lefebvre-Maunoury, C.; Pigny, P.; Duhamel, A.; Dewailly, D. Polycystic Ovary-Like Abnormalities (PCO-L) in women with functional hypothalamic amenorrhea. *J. Clin. Endocrinol. Metab.* **2012**, *97*, 4236–4243. [CrossRef] [PubMed]
31. Carmina, E.; Fruzzetti, F.; Lobo, R.A. Features of polycystic ovary syndrome (PCOS) in women with functional hypothalamic amenorrhea (FHA) may be reversible with recovery of menstrual function. *Gynecol. Endocrinol.* **2018**, *34*, 301–304. [CrossRef]
32. Alvero, R.; Kimzey, L.; Sebring, N.; Reynolds, J.; Loughran, M.; Nieman, L.; Olson, B.R. Effects of fasting on neuroendocrine function and follicle development in lean women. *J. Clin. Endocrinol. Metab.* **1998**, *83*, 76–80. [CrossRef]
33. Stamatiades, G.A.; Kaiser, U.B. Gonadotropin regulation by pulsatile GnRH: Signaling and gene expression. *Mol. Cell Endocrinol.* **2018**, *463*, 131–141. [CrossRef]
34. Burger, H.G. Androgen production in women. *Fertil. Steril.* **2002**, *77* (Suppl. S4), S3–S5. [CrossRef]
35. Dewailly, D.; Robin, G.; Peigne, M.; Decanter, C.; Pigny, P.; Catteau-Jonard, S. Interactions between androgens, FSH, anti-Mullerian hormone and estradiol during folliculogenesis in the human normal and polycystic ovary. *Hum. Reprod. Update* **2016**, *22*, 709–724. [CrossRef]
36. Belda, X.; Fuentes, S.; Daviu, N.; Nadal, R.; Armario, A. Stress-induced sensitization: The hypothalamic-pituitary-adrenal axis and beyond. *Stress* **2015**, *18*, 269–279. [CrossRef]
37. Selzer, C.; Ott, J.; Dewailly, D.; Marculescu, R.; Steininger, J.; Hager, M. Prolactin levels in Functional hypothalamic amenorrhea: A retrospective case-control study. *Arch. Gynecol. Obstet.* **2023**, *309*, 651–658. [CrossRef]
38. Macotela, Y.; Triebel, J.; Clapp, C. Time for a New Perspective on Prolactin in Metabolism. *Trends Endocrinol. Metab.* **2020**, *31*, 276–286. [CrossRef]
39. Melmed, S.; Casanueva, F.F.; Hoffman, A.R.; Kleinberg, D.L.; Montori, V.M.; Schlechte, J.A.; Wass, J.A.; Endocrine, S. Diagnosis and treatment of hyperprolactinemia: An Endocrine Society clinical practice guideline. *J. Clin. Endocrinol. Metab.* **2011**, *96*, 273–288. [CrossRef] [PubMed]
40. Rosenfield, R.L.; Ehrmann, D.A. The Pathogenesis of Polycystic Ovary Syndrome (PCOS): The Hypothesis of PCOS as Functional Ovarian Hyperandrogenism Revisited. *Endocr. Rev.* **2016**, *37*, 467–520. [CrossRef] [PubMed]
41. He, Y.; Tian, J.; Blizzard, L.; Oddy, W.H.; Dwyer, T.; Bazzano, L.A.; Hickey, M.; Harville, E.W.; Venn, A.J. Associations of childhood adiposity with menstrual irregularity and polycystic ovary syndrome in adulthood: The Childhood Determinants of Adult Health Study and the Bogalusa Heart Study. *Hum. Reprod.* **2020**, *35*, 1185–1198. [CrossRef]
42. Ezeh, U.; Pisarska, M.D.; Azziz, R. Association of severity of menstrual dysfunction with hyperinsulinemia and dysglycemia in polycystic ovary syndrome. *Hum. Reprod.* **2022**, *37*, 553–564. [CrossRef]
43. La Marca, A.; Pati, M.; Orvieto, R.; Stabile, G.; Carducci Artenisio, A.; Volpe, A. Serum anti-mullerian hormone levels in women with secondary amenorrhea. *Fertil. Steril.* **2006**, *85*, 1547–1549. [CrossRef] [PubMed]
44. Lie Fong, S.; Schipper, I.; Valkenburg, O.; de Jong, F.H.; Visser, J.A.; Laven, J.S. The role of anti-Mullerian hormone in the classification of anovulatory infertility. *Eur. J. Obstet. Gynecol. Reprod. Biol.* **2015**, *186*, 75–79. [CrossRef]
45. Luisi, S.; Ciani, V.; Podfigurna-Stopa, A.; Lazzeri, L.; De Pascalis, F.; Meczekalski, B.; Petraglia, F. Serum anti-Mullerian hormone, inhibin B, and total inhibin levels in women with hypothalamic amenorrhea and anorexia nervosa. *Gynecol. Endocrinol.* **2012**, *28*, 34–38. [CrossRef]
46. Qu, X.; Donnelly, R. Sex Hormone-Binding Globulin (SHBG) as an Early Biomarker and Therapeutic Target in Polycystic Ovary Syndrome. *Int. J. Mol. Sci.* **2020**, *21*, 8191. [CrossRef]

Disclaimer/Publisher's Note: The statements, opinions and data contained in all publications are solely those of the individual author(s) and contributor(s) and not of MDPI and/or the editor(s). MDPI and/or the editor(s) disclaim responsibility for any injury to people or property resulting from any ideas, methods, instructions or products referred to in the content.

4. Hager, M.; Dewailly, D.; Marculescu, R.; Ghobrial, S.; Parry, J.P.; Ott, J. Stress and polycystic ovarian morphology in functional hypothalamic amenorrhea: A retrospective cohort study. *Reprod. Biol. Endocrinol.* **2023**, *21*, 42. [CrossRef] [PubMed]
5. Bonazza, F.; Politi, G.; Leone, D.; Vegni, E.; Borghi, L. Psychological factors in functional hypothalamic amenorrhea: A systematic review and meta-analysis. *Front. Endocrinol.* **2023**, *14*, 981491. [CrossRef] [PubMed]
6. Shufelt, C.L.; Torbati, T.; Dutra, E. Hypothalamic Amenorrhea and the Long-Term Health Consequences. *Semin. Reprod. Med.* **2017**, *35*, 256–262. [CrossRef] [PubMed]
7. Blenck, C.L.; Harvey, P.A.; Reckelhoff, J.F.; Leinwand, L.A. The Importance of Biological Sex and Estrogen in Rodent Models of Cardiovascular Health and Disease. *Circ. Res.* **2016**, *118*, 1294–1312. [CrossRef] [PubMed]
8. Barbagallo, F.; Pedrielli, G.; Bosoni, D.; Tiranini, L.; Cucinella, L.; Calogero, A.E.; Facchinetti, F.; Nappi, R.E. Sexual functioning in women with functional hypothalamic amenorrhea: Exploring the relevance of an underlying polycystic ovary syndrome (PCOS)-phenotype. *J. Endocrinol. Investig.* **2023**, *46*, 1623–1632. [CrossRef]
9. Fontana, L.; Garzia, E.; Marfia, G.; Galiano, V.; Miozzo, M. Epigenetics of functional hypothalamic amenorrhea. *Front. Endocrinol.* **2022**, *13*, 953431. [CrossRef]
10. Gordon, C.M.; Ackerman, K.E.; Berga, S.L.; Kaplan, J.R.; Mastorakos, G.; Misra, M.; Murad, M.H.; Santoro, N.F.; Warren, M.P. Functional Hypothalamic Amenorrhea: An Endocrine Society Clinical Practice Guideline. *J. Clin. Endocrinol. Metab.* **2017**, *102*, 1413–1439. [CrossRef]
11. Phylactou, M.; Clarke, S.A.; Patel, B.; Baggaley, C.; Jayasena, C.N.; Kelsey, T.W.; Comninos, A.N.; Dhillo, W.S.; Abbara, A. Clinical and biochemical discriminants between functional hypothalamic amenorrhoea (FHA) and polycystic ovary syndrome (PCOS). *Clin. Endocrinol.* **2021**, *95*, 239–252. [CrossRef]
12. Teede, H.J.; Misso, M.L.; Costello, M.F.; Dokras, A.; Laven, J.; Moran, L.; Piltonen, T.; Norman, R.J.; on behalf of the International PCOS Network. Recommendations from the international evidence-based guideline for the assessment and management of polycystic ovary syndrome. *Fertil. Steril.* **2018**, *110*, 364–379. [CrossRef]
13. The Rotterdam ESHRE/ASRM-Sponsored PCOS Consensus Workshop Group. Revised 2003 consensus on diagnostic criteria and long-term health risks related to polycystic ovary syndrome (PCOS). *Hum. Reprod.* **2004**, *19*, 41–47. [CrossRef]
14. Teede, H.J.; Tay, C.T.; Laven, J.; Dokras, A.; Moran, L.J.; Piltonen, T.T.; Costello, M.F.; Boivin, J.; Redman, L.M.; Boyle, J.A.; et al. Recommendations from the 2023 International Evidence-based Guideline for the Assessment and Management of Polycystic Ovary Syndrome. *Fertil. Steril.* **2023**, *120*, 767–793. [CrossRef]
15. Makolle, S.; Catteau-Jonard, S.; Robin, G.; Dewailly, D. Revisiting the serum level of anti-Mullerian hormone in patients with functional hypothalamic anovulation. *Hum. Reprod.* **2021**, *36*, 1043–1051. [CrossRef]
16. Beitl, K.; Dewailly, D.; Seemann, R.; Hager, M.; Bunker, J.; Mayrhofer, D.; Holzer, I.; Ott, J. Polycystic Ovary Syndrome Phenotype D versus Functional Hypothalamic Amenorrhea with Polycystic Ovarian Morphology: A Retrospective Study about a Frequent Differential Diagnosis. *Front. Endocrinol.* **2022**, *13*, 904706. [CrossRef] [PubMed]
17. Piltonen, T.T.; Komsi, E.; Morin-Papunen, L.C.; Korhonen, E.; Franks, S.; Järvelin, M.-R.; Arffman, R.K.; Ollila, M.-M. AMH as part of the diagnostic PCOS workup in large epidemiological studies. *Eur. J. Endocrinol.* **2023**, *188*, 547–554. [CrossRef]
18. Berga, S.L.; Mortola, J.F.; Girton, L.; Suh, B.; Laughlin, G.; Pham, P.; Yen, S.S. Neuroendocrine aberrations in women with functional hypothalamic amenorrhea. *J. Clin. Endocrinol. Metab.* **1989**, *68*, 301–308. [CrossRef]
19. Morrison, A.E.; Fleming, S.; Levy, M.J. A review of the pathophysiology of functional hypothalamic amenorrhoea in women subject to psychological stress, disordered eating, excessive exercise or a combination of these factors. *Clin. Endocrinol.* **2021**, *95*, 229–238. [CrossRef] [PubMed]
20. Jonard, S.; Pigny, P.; Jacquesson, L.; Demerle-Roux, C.; Robert, Y.; Dewailly, D. The ovarian markers of the FSH insufficiency in functional hypothalamic amenorrhoea. *Hum. Reprod.* **2005**, *20*, 101–107. [CrossRef] [PubMed]
21. Genazzani, A.D.; Meczekalski, B.; Podfigurna-Stopa, A.; Santagni, S.; Rattighieri, E.; Ricchieri, F.; Chierchia, E.; Simoncini, T. Estriol administration modulates luteinizing hormone secretion in women with functional hypothalamic amenorrhea. *Fertil. Steril.* **2012**, *97*, 483–488. [CrossRef]
22. Marshall, J.C.; Dalkin, A.C.; Haisenleder, D.J.; Griffin, M.L.; Kelch, R.P. GnRH pulses—The regulators of human reproduction. *Trans. Am. Clin. Climatol. Assoc.* **1993**, *104*, 31–46.
23. Tsutsumi, R.; Webster, N.J. GnRH pulsatility, the pituitary response and reproductive dysfunction. *Endocr. J.* **2009**, *56*, 729–737. [CrossRef]
24. Herpertz, S.; Hagenah, U.; Vocks, S.; von Wietersheim, J.; Cuntz, U.; Zeeck, A. The diagnosis and treatment of eating disorders. *Dtsch. Arztebl. Int.* **2011**, *108*, 678–685. [CrossRef]
25. Schneider, L.F.; Warren, M.P. Functional hypothalamic amenorrhea is associated with elevated ghrelin and disordered eating. *Fertil. Steril.* **2006**, *86*, 1744–1749. [CrossRef]
26. Tinahones, F.J.; Martinez-Alfaro, B.; Gonzalo-Marin, M.; Garcia-Almeida, J.M.; Garrido-Sanchez, L.; Cardona, F. Recovery of menstrual cycle after therapy for anorexia nervosa. *Eat. Weight. Disord.* **2005**, *10*, e52–e55. [CrossRef]
27. Hager, M.; Ott, J.; Marschalek, J.; Marschalek, M.L.; Kinsky, C.; Marculescu, R.; Dewailly, D. Basal and dynamic relationships between serum anti-Mullerian hormone and gonadotropins in patients with functional hypothalamic amenorrhea, with or without polycystic ovarian morphology. *Reprod. Biol. Endocrinol.* **2022**, *20*, 98. [CrossRef] [PubMed]
28. Mayrhofer, D.; Dewailly, D.; Hager, M.; Marculescu, R.; Beitl, K.; Ott, J. Functional hypothalamic amenorrhea with or without polycystic ovarian morphology: A retrospective cohort study about insulin resistance. *Fertil. Steril.* **2022**, *118*, 1183–1185. [CrossRef] [PubMed]

been suggested as a possible cause for the high PCOM prevalence [4], the exact mechanism remains unknown. FHA women with PCOM revealed higher AMH levels (Table 4), which has been found previously and seems plausible [15,27], as well as lower SHBG levels, which is a new finding in patients with FHA. SHBG production is lower in PCOS women with insulin resistance [46]. Although FHA patients with PCOM revealed higher HOMA index levels for insulin resistance [28], this might not completely explain the difference in SHBG levels. However, the clinical relevance is questionable, since both groups revealed median SHBG levels within the normal range (with PCOM: 67.0 nmol/L, without PCOM: 79.4 nmol/L). However, and this seems of importance, there was no difference in the main outcome parameter LH:FSH ratio between FHA women with and without PCOM (median 0.8 versus 0.7, respectively; $p = 0.728$; Table 4). Although it has been proposed that some FHA women with PCOM initially had simple PCOS before [4,15,27,28] and that they reveal a hyper-responsiveness of LH to a GnRH bolus similar to PCOS patients [27], the data suggest that in both groups, the demise in GnRH pulsatility was comparable. It is still unclear how many FHA patients with PCOM have underlying PCOS. It would be reasonable if this would apply only to a minority of patients. However, the question of why so many women with FHA reveal PCOM remains open. When talking to other experts, some suggest that PCOM would reflect a different state of ovarian stimulation in these women. However, the data presented herein do not support this hypothesis.

Concerning limitations, the retrospective study design must be taken into account in addition to the above-mentioned difficulties to completely separate FHA from PCOS patients. However, the large sample size with well-defined FHA (negative progestogen challenge test, normal pituitary MRI, clear cause for FHA) might be considered a study strength.

5. Conclusions

Our data show that an LH:FSH ratio ≤ 1 is found in >80% of women with FHA, whereas most of these patients revealed FSH levels >2 mIU/mL. Thus, physicians should not rely on normal FSH levels to rule out FHA. Notably, this decrease in the LH:FSH ratio seems to be relevantly associated with dysfunction of the hypothalamic GnRH pulsatility. The LH:FSH ratio might also be a promising parameter for the differential diagnosis between FHA and PCOS in the future.

Author Contributions: M.B., M.H., D.D., R.M. and J.O. conceived the study design. M.B. wrote the original draft of the manuscript. M.H. participated in article writing. M.B., M.H. and J.O. performed the statistical analysis. M.H., J.O., J.S. and M.B. collected, analyzed, and interpreted the data. D.D., R.M. and J.S. provided useful comments for data interpretation. D.D. implemented valuable aspects to the discussion. All authors have read and agreed to the published version of the manuscript.

Funding: This research received no external funding.

Institutional Review Board Statement: The study was approved by the Ethics Committee of the Medical University of Vienna (Institutional Review Board number 2436/2020) and conducted in accordance with the principles of the Declaration of Helsinki. Oral and written informed consent was obtained from all study participants before study-related activities began.

Informed Consent Statement: Not applicable.

Data Availability Statement: Data will be made available upon reasonable request.

Conflicts of Interest: The authors declare no conflicts of interest.

References

1. Klein, D.A.; Paradise, S.L.; Reeder, R.M. Amenorrhea: A Systematic Approach to Diagnosis and Management. *Am. Fam. Physician* **2019**, *100*, 39–48.
2. Munster, K.; Helm, P.; Schmidt, L. Secondary amenorrhoea: Prevalence and medical contact--a cross-sectional study from a Danish county. *Br. J. Obstet. Gynaecol.* **1992**, *99*, 430–433. [CrossRef] [PubMed]
3. Gordon, C.M. Clinical practice. Functional hypothalamic amenorrhea. *N. Engl. J. Med.* **2010**, *363*, 365–371. [CrossRef] [PubMed]

was of influence. Therefore, a lower LH:FSH ratio may be considered as a specific reflection of the GnRH dysregulation of FHA, i.e., greater suppression of LH than FSH, presumably due to slow GnRH pulsatility [23]. Thus, one might consider the LH:FSH ratio better than LH itself, for which we have no consensual threshold [11], since the ratio also integrates FSH. Moreover, based on the fact that it seems to be influenced by GnRH dysregulation alone rather than other factors, the LH:FSH ratio could help clinical decision making in the future, especially concerning the above-mentioned differential diagnosis to PCOS. Thus, comparative studies, especially challenging FHA vs. PCOS in large populations, are needed in the future. Indeed, although the LH:FSH ratio is not a definition criterion for PCOS [13], an elevated LH:FSH ratio is commonly associated with the presence of PCOS.

Concerning the correlation analyses (Table 2), the positive correlation between the LH:FSH ratio and LH and between the LH:FSH ratio and estradiol seem to confirm the above-mentioned results and considerations. A higher GnRH pulse frequency also leads to a higher LH pulse frequency [33]. Accordingly, a higher LH level could reflect a better overall GnRH pulse generator function and, thus, better ovarian function reflected by higher estradiol levels would be logical. This is somehow also supported by the positive correlation between LH and testosterone, since a relevant amount of androstenedione, the most important precursor of testosterone, is produced by the theca cells in the ovary [34], under the influence of LH [35]. The positive correlation between estradiol and testosterone is in line with these observations. In addition, the LH:FSH ratio revealed a positive correlation with the serum prolactin level. It has been mentioned that the prolactin level could be considered a "sensor" of the hypothalamic–pituitary dysregulation even when it is within the normal range [36]. As shown previously by our study group, eating disorders and excessive exercise tended to lower prolactin levels in FHA women [37]. Therefore, the lower the LH:FSH ratio, the lower the prolactin level. The relevance of the prolactin level, which also affects metabolism, osmoregulation, immune function, behavior, and many more [38,39], needs to be elucidated in women with FHA in the future. However, despite the fact that prolactin levels do not differ between FHA patients and normally cycling controls, it has been mentioned that prolactin levels might be some kind of "sensor" of the hypothalamic activity as mentioned above. However, since increased prolactin levels are usually an exclusion criterion for FHA and since prolactin also exerts metabolic effects, further studies are needed to elucidate the relevance of prolactin FHA women [36]. It seems noteworthy that in the previous analysis, the presence of PCOM in ultrasound was associated with higher prolactin levels [36], which was not the case in the analysis presented herein.

The lack of data on adrenal androgens must also be considered as a minor limitation. Several factors are associated with insulin resistance in PCOS, including genetic mutations, lipodystrophy [40], and childhood obesity according to the Bogalusa Heart Study's findings [41]. In addition, it has been shown that anovulatory patients with PCOS have a higher risk of dysglycemia and hyperinsulinemia compared to oligo-amenorrheic or eumenorrheic patients [42]. Whether the inclusion of data about insulin resistance in FHA would be of relevance remains open for discussion. At least it was shown recently that the majority of women with FHA did not reveal abnormal levels according to the "Homeostasis Model Assessment of Insulin Resistance" (ZITAT EINFÜGEN).

It seems reasonable that higher FSH levels were positively correlated with higher estradiol levels (Table 2). Estradiol is synthetized by granulosa cells through the action of aromatase, which is also present in small growing follicles and is FSH-dependent [35]. Moreover, higher FSH levels were associated with higher AMH levels. This phenomenon has been reported previously [27], which lends support to the hypothesis that the relative FSH deficiency, which is typical for FHA, leads to a decrease in the pool of growing follicles and therefore to a decrease in ovarian AMH production [15,27]. This relationship between FSH and AMH had no impact whatsoever on the LH:FSH ratio.

Once again, a high rate of PCOM in women with FHA was found (43.0%), which is in accordance with previous case series [4,15,20,30,43–45]. Although stress sensitivity has

In a last step, we compared the 77 FHA women without (57.0%) to the 58 FHA women with PCOM (43.0%) (Table 4). The latter revealed higher AMH values (6.3 ng/mL, IQR 4.9–7.6 versus 2.0 ng/mL, IQR 1.1–2.7; $p < 0.001$) as well as lower SHGB values (67.0 nmol/L, IQR 39.7–94.1 versus 79.4 nmol/L, IQR 63.3–104.0; $p = 0.008$). The ranges of the LH:FSH ratio were similar between the two groups.

Table 4. Comparison of FHA with and without PCOM.

	PCOM (n = 58)	Non-PCOM (n = 77)	p
Age (years)	26 (22;28)	26 (22;30)	0.299
BMI (kg/m^2)	20.4 (18.8;22.5)	20.0 (18.4;21.4)	0.190
Prolactin (ng/mL)	9.6 (6.6;13.0)	8.8 (6.7;12.8)	0.964
FSH (mIU/mL)	4.8 (3.5;6.5)	4.7 (3.2;6.2)	0.426
LH (mIU/mL)	2.8 (1.5;5.5)	2.6 (1.3;4.6)	0.290
LH:FSH ratio	0.8 (0.3;1.0)	0.7 (0.4;1.0)	0.728
Estradiol (pg/mL)	24 (11;34)	22 (12;29)	0.719
Testosterone (ng/mL)	0.20 (0.14;0.29)	0.19 (0.13;0.29)	0.881
SHBG (nmol/L)	67.0 (39.7;94.1)	79.4 (63.3;104.0)	0.008
AMH (ng/mL)	6.3 (4.9;7.6)	2.0 (1.1;2.7)	< 0.001

Data are provided as median (interquartile range). Please find hormones described in Table 1. A p-value < 0.05 was considered significant.

4. Discussion

In this retrospective analysis, about 13% of FHA patients revealed FSH levels < 2.0 mIU/mL, whereas decreased LH levels < 2 mIU/mL were found in about 39% of patients. Importantly, over 80% of women revealed an LH:FSH ratio ≤ 1. In addition, an LH:FSH ratio >1 was associated with higher LH levels only. Last but not least, FHA women with PCOM did not reveal an altered LH:FSH ratio.

Before discussing these findings in detail, the focus should be on basic patient characteristics. We consider the fact that only women with well-defined FHA were included a study strength. Notably, excessive exercise was the most common cause for FHA (40.7%) followed by stress (32.6%). A low median BMI of 20.3 kg/m^2 [10] as well as the low median FSH, LH, and testosterone levels (Table 1) seem typical for FHA patients and are comparable to previous studies [10,15,30,31]. Notably, a negative progestogen challenge test and clear causes for FHA were mandatory definition criteria in our study population. However, since PCOS is an important and difficult differential diagnosis and since there is a lack of clear diagnostic criteria [15], we cannot completely rule out that very few PCOS patients might have been included. Nonetheless, we consider this circumstance only a minor study limitation.

The main finding was that a relevant proportion of our FHA patients revealed normal FSH and LH levels even though this was more often the case for FSH than for LH. From a pathophysiological perspective, this seems reasonable since reduced GnRH pulsatility has been reported to favor FSH secretion [23]. Notably, FSH levels in FHA patients have been reported to vary from study to study, leading to ambiguity in clinical practice [32]. Given the mentioned pathophysiologic considerations, where a decrease in GnRH pulsatility will likely result in substantially decreased LH levels, but only a modest decline in FSH levels, it seems comprehensible that so many FHA women in our study population revealed an LH:FSH ratio ≤ 1.0 (81.5%). It is noteworthy that, to the best of our knowledge, this parameter has not been reported previously in FHA patients [15]. Our data show that women with an LH:FSH ratio >1 revealed higher LH levels in both the univariable and multivariable analysis, whereas the association with higher estradiol levels was only found in the univariable model (Table 3). It seems of particular interest that no other parameter

The results showed statistically significant positive correlations between the WHR ratio, social struggles related to appearance (VAS5; $r = 0.23$, $p = 0.031$), and level of last month's sexual satisfaction (VAS7; $r = 0.30$, $p = 0.004$). In both cases, the higher the WHR was, the higher both the social struggles related to appearance and the declared sexual satisfaction were. Both statistical effects were small.

Also, the Ferriman–Gallwey score was positively correlated with the level of perceived impact of excessive hair on personal sexuality (VAS4; $r = 0.41$, $p < 0.001$). It suggested that women diagnosed with PCOS with higher Ferriman–Gallwey scores declared higher levels of perceived impact of excessive hair on personal sexuality. In this case, the effect size was medium.

To analyze the associations between VAS scores and other physical characteristics (i.e., presence of hirsutism and acne), we performed a Mann–Whitney U test, with the same rationale as in the previous paragraph.

Overall, the results showed no statistically significant differences in VAS scores between groups of women diagnosed with PCOS with and without acne. The only difference that turned out to be statistically significant concerned the number of painful sexual contacts (VAS6), which was higher in women with PCOS and acne (median = 2.00, IQR = 4.00) compared to women without acne (median = 1.00, IQR = 1.00). However, the effect size of this difference was rather small. As a result, the results showed no statistically significant differences in VAS results between groups of women diagnosed with PCOS with and without hirsutism. In this case, the only difference that turned out to be statistically significant was the perceived impact of excessive hair on personal sexuality (VAS4), which was higher in women with PCOS and hirsutism (median = 7.00, IQR = 6.00) compared to people without hirsutism (median = 2.00, IQR = 4.00). The effect size of this difference was medium.

3.7. Association between Sexual Activity in Last Week and Sexual Functioning in Women Diagnosed with PCOS

We examined the association between sexual activity and sexual functioning in women diagnosed with PCOS using the Mann–Whitney U test. We decided on this procedure due to (1) the dichotomous nature of the variable related to sexual activity (possible answers: yes or no) and (2) differences in n groups (in the case of sexual activity in the last week—for "no": n = 56; for "yes": n = 35). Also, taking into account a small n (i.e. the variable indicating sexual activity in the last month—for "no": n = 8; for "yes": n = 83) or the lack of cases in one group (i.e. the variable indicating sexual activity during the last three months) in the case of other variables related to sexual activity, we decided to conduct this test only for the variable related to sexual activity during the last week.

The results showed no statistically significant differences in sexual functioning between the group of women with PCOS who declared sexual activity within the last week and those who did not perform any sexual activity in that time.

4. Discussion

The impact of PCOS on sexual function in women is still a matter of debate. Although reviews and meta-analyses devoted to the topic of sexual dysfunction in women with PCOS [11–13] do not lead to one consistent conclusion, they do indicate that there is a possible relationship between PCOS and FSD in these women. Pastor et al. showed that women with PCOS experienced FSD in terms of arousal, lubrication, sexual satisfaction, orgasm, and overall scores compared to controls [11]. However, Zhao et al. showed that there are no statistically significant differences in FSD between women with PCOS and women without this diagnosis [12]. Loh et al. conducted the most extensive meta-analysis and found that women with PCOS have a 30% higher risk of developing FSD compared to women without PCOS [13]. They confirmed that total scores on the Female Sexual Function Index (FSFI) did not differ significantly between the study and control groups, while women with PCOS obtained significantly lower scores on the pain and satisfaction subscales than the control groups [13]. In their opinion, this indicated limitations in the use of this scale to assess sexual desire [13] and the overlap between desire and arousal [15]. Regardless of the limitations of FSFI, it is important to remember that both men and women may have difficulty distinguishing between desire and arousal because sexual stimuli trigger both desire and arousal simultaneously [16,17].

Stovall et al. are the only ones in the past who have used the CSFQ questionnaire to assess sexual functions in women with PCOS [18]. Although they described decreased sexual function in most domains, they showed statistically significant differences between the study and control groups only in the orgasm/fulfillment domain. In our study, we did not obtain statistically significant differences between women with PCOS and the control group in terms of domains and the total score on the CSFQ scale confirming the occurrence of FSD in the study group. However, a detailed analysis of the CSFQ subscales showed that in both groups of women the average values of the subscales of pleasure (3.92 vs. 3.93), desire/interest (8.75 vs. 8.58) and arousal (10.56 vs. 11, 16) were below the cut-off limit—points excluded (Table 1). Additionally, the mean values in the orgasm domain (10.88) were also below the threshold for sexual dysfunction in women with PCOS (Table 1). The results presented are like those reported by Stovall et al. and generally support mild FSD in women; we would like to note, however, that our study provides insight into the sexuality of women with PCOS in the context of their sexual partners. In terms of all domains and general functioning on the CSFQ scale, we obtained a pattern of statistically significant differences between women and men in favor of men (Table 2). This effect ranged from small to medium on the pleasure, desire/interest, orgasm, and total score subscales, but from medium to large on the desire/frequency and arousal subscales.

To explain the above results, it is necessary to refer to sexual response models. The linear model supplemented by Kaplan included four phases: desire, arousal, orgasm, and decisiveness, and assumed that male desire is stable and high [19]. The latest research focuses on assessing the short-term variability of the desires of women and men in the context of their emotional state and closeness in a partnership and does not confirm significant differences between women and men [20]. This is consistent with Basson's later model assuming that the motivations for sexual activity are numerous, sexual desire does not have to be present at the beginning of the sexual response, but it is achieved after the brain processes sexual signals that combine desire with arousal [21]. It has been suggested that women with different levels of sexual function identify with different models of the sexual response cycle [22], and women identifying with Basson's model had significantly lower levels of sexual function [23]. Clinical observations confirm that the dominant reasons for initiating and partnering in sexual activity in women are emotional, and in men, physical [21]. The central role of attention processes in stimulating the subjective and physiological components of sexual arousal has been proven [24]. Conscious evaluation of sexual stimuli and contextual cues can lead to subjective sexual arousal (SSA). The latter may be increased by awareness of genital congestion, which is more typical of the male experience [25].

(SSA) has been defined as positive cognitive [26] or emotional engagement [27] in response to a sexual stimulus, suggesting that one must be directly or indirectly aware of the sexual stimulus, which may be internal (sexual thoughts) or external (partner's), to experience SSA [28]. SSA reduces sexual restraint [29] and motivates individuals to engage in sexual activity [30]. It is also believed that increased SSA may increase pleasure and satisfaction during sexual activity, which are associated with engagement in future sexual activity [31]. This knowledge may lead us to another result in our study, that the intensity of sexual thoughts and fantasies was associated with higher levels of desire/frequency, desire/interest, but also arousal and orgasm (Table 3). Attempts to enhance SSA by administering drugs did not produce consistent results, which is most likely related to the excessive heterogeneity of the studied women and the drug dose [32–34]. Cognitive interventions are more effective (91% of studies) than pharmacological ones (31% of studies) [35]. This may be partially explained by psychological variables (mood, attention, relationship satisfaction), which may have a stronger impact on women's experience of SSA than pharmacological agents [35]. Velten et al. showed that women with clinical and subclinical sexual dysfunctions engage in sexual stimuli to a lesser extent [36]. This finding suggests that therapeutic efforts should focus on increasing attention to sexual cues and simultaneously analyzing women's emotional and cognitive evaluation of these cues [36].

Empirical research indicates that the motivation to engage in sexual activity is related to sexual thoughts and fantasies, which influence the level of sexual well-being [21]. Gender differences in the way women and men respond to sexual situations highlight the importance of the potential for sexual arousal to decline or disappear "if everything goes wrong" [21]. In this context, the most interesting result concerns the domain of arousal in women with PCOS. They declare only slightly lower arousal compared to women from the control group, but there is a large discrepancy between them and their partners in this respect (Table 2). This may be complemented by the dual control model, which states that sexual arousal is influenced by excitatory and inhibitory mechanisms, with women generally exhibiting greater inhibition and men greater arousal [37,38]. The central neuroendocrine mechanisms regulating the sexual response in women are today described as dynamic, creating a balance between stimulating and inhibiting factors [39,40]. Several studies have confirmed the occurrence of arousal disorders in women with PCOS [12,41–44]. Bazarganipour et al. noticed a possible relationship between arousal and hirsutism, acne, and obesity [42]. Bahadori et al. showed that arousal dysfunction was associated with phenotype B characterized by hyperandrogenism, hirsutism, and anovulation [43]. Gniew et al. suggested that this may be due to the degree of personal distress observed within the team [44]. In this context, our results require further research due to the lack of an objective assessment of the affective state and the relationship with specific phenotypic characteristics of PCOS patients.

The assessment of individual sexual domains leads to the conclusion that women with PCOS derive significantly less satisfaction from their sexual life than women without this syndrome [11,41,45,46]. It may be the result of specific symptoms such as hyperandrogenism, hirsutism, and oligoanovulation or anovulation, characteristic of both phenotype A and B [47]. These symptoms had a negative impact on physical appearance, resulting in a decreased perception of "feminine identity" and a feeling of "unattractiveness" [48], as well as a deterioration of "self-image" and lowered "self-esteem" [49]. Indeed, higher levels of subjective attractiveness (VAS3) in our patients were associated with higher scores in almost all domains and the CSFQ total score, except for the desire/frequency subscale (Table 3). This finding indicates the importance of a positive attitude towards oneself, which can strengthen individual psychological mechanisms that eliminate frustration caused by the diagnosis and course of PCOS.

Eftenkhar et al. found lower scores in all FSFI domains if the Ferriman–Gallwey scale scores were 6–8 [50]. Elsenbruch et al. described concerns about excessive hair growth among women with PCOS, who confirmed that it had a detrimental effect on their sexual life [45]. Our study shows two conclusions on this subject: firstly, the greater the impact of excessive hair on sexuality (VAS4) and the greater social problems resulting from appearance (VAS5), the lower the level of pleasure was (Table 3), and secondly, the higher results on the Ferriman–Gallwey scale worsened the subjectively perceived impact of excessive hair on sexuality (VAS4) (Table 6). Ercan et al. reported a significant negative correlation between the results of total FSFI and the levels of total and free testosterone [51]. Veras et al. showed a negative correlation between sexual functions and the levels of total testosterone and dehydroepiandrosterone sulfate [52]. On the contrary, Mansson et al. and Stovall et al. proved the inverse relationship [18,41]. Rellini et al. confirmed that clinical symptoms suggesting sensitivity to androgen levels, but not biological androgen levels per se, predicted levels of sexual desire [53]. In this context, the role of testosterone in modulating female sexual desire and sexual function in general is still poorly understood. Although there is evidence of benefits from short-term transdermal testosterone administration in postmenopausal women with low sexual drive, there is no specific serum level or lower limit for androgens or androgen precursors to recognize decreased female sexual function [54,55]. Our findings confirm that physical characteristics associated with hyperandrogenism have a negative impact on women's sexuality.

There are various research results describing the association of sexual functions with obesity, BMI, and WHR in women with PCOS, namely that obesity and hirsutism correlate with reduced sexual satisfaction [56], an increase in BMI has a negative relationship with satisfaction with sexual life [41], with lower results in FSFI [57], an increase in body weight and abdominal circumference negatively correlated with sexual satisfaction in women [58,59], and a progressive increase in sexual dysfunctions correlated with a constant increase in the WHR index [60]. De Frene et al. concluded that an increase in BMI in women leads to a decrease in sexual satisfaction and in their relationships, but this was inconsistent with the feelings of their partners, which increased in proportion to their body weight [61]. Benetti-Pinto et al. noticed that BMI correlates with quality of life, i.e., the higher the BMI, the lower the quality of life [62]. The studies by Elsenbruch et al. and Stovall et al. showed that BMI changes did not correlate with the level of satisfaction in women with PCOS [18,45]. In the case of our study, it was shown that the higher the WHR index, the greater the social problems resulting from appearance and the greater the sexual satisfaction reported by women with PCOS in the last month (Table 6). It cannot be concluded that a higher WHR had a negative impact on perceived sexual satisfaction, but it did cause greater social struggles.

The more frequent occurrence of painful sexual intercourse in our patients is associated with a lower quality of orgasm, as well as a lower level of pleasure, arousal, and overall functioning (Table 3). Loh et al. showed a lower pain score in women with PCOS, which they interpreted as the possibility of dyspareunia caused by relatively low FSH levels preventing the growth of ovarian follicles and resulting in estrogen deficiency with possible vaginal atrophy [13]. It is worth mentioning the results of the study by Nohr EA et al., who found that dyspareunia occurs more often in the group of patients with a history of PCOS [63]. The authors interpreted this finding in the context of decreased thirst and reduced ability to relax due to chronic pain and medical conditions. This observation is limited by the fact that the mean age of the patients was over 40 years. In this context, our results call for deeper research into the somatic causes of intercourse pain.

Research on sexual functions poses many methodological difficulties, which are also visible in our study. The described discrepancy in results—the presence vs. absence of FSD and statistical difference vs. absence of this difference compared to the control group—can be explained by the multifactorial nature of women's sexual functions, the severity of PCOS, and the nature of sexual relationships, as well as different populations of research groups, inclusion criteria, and assessment methods [64]. Additionally, the limited number of participants in the study group did not allow for the analysis of sexual functions in terms of specific PCOS phenotypes and sex hormone levels.

5. Conclusions

We confirmed that there are no statistically significant differences in sexual function between women with PCOS and women without this diagnosis. This finding concerns young cisgender women who reported living in stable heterosexual relationships. Our attempt to compare the sexual function of women and their partners in the study group showed significant differences in all sexual areas and total sexual functioning, but the difference in arousal was particularly important. The intensity of sexual thoughts and fantasies especially increased desire. We have proven that self-esteem has a huge impact on women's sexuality. Our results concern young cisgender women who reported living in stable heterosexual relationships.

Our findings should be translated into a model of care for women with PCOS. Multidisciplinary care models should offer integrated care with tailored therapies, education, and lifestyle support, as well as treatment. A wide range of health care for this group of patients should include not only gynecologists, endocrinologists, primary care physicians, dietitians, and exercise physiologists, but open access to psychologists and sexologists should be ensured. The involvement of various specialists should facilitate the preparation of a question list, a structured list of patient-generated and applied health questions that can be integrated with evidence-based information and answers. This facilitates patient–caregiver interaction and may contribute to improving patient knowledge and support [1].

Author Contributions: Conceptualization, A.W. and M.K. (Marek Krzystanek); methodology, A.W. and P.M.; software, A.W. and M.K. (Marek Krzystanek); validation, M.K. (Marek Krzystanek), P.M. and M.K. (Marta Kochanowicz); formal analysis, A.W. and P.M.; investigation, M.K. (Marta Kochanowicz) and P.M.; resources, P.M. and M.K. (Marta Kochanowicz); data curation, A.W.; writing—original draft preparation, A.W.; writing—review and editing, M.K. (Marek Krzystanek); visualization, M.K. (Marek Krzystanek); supervision, M.K. (Marek Krzystanek) and P.M.; project administration, A.W. and P.M.; funding acquisition, M.K. (Marek Krzystanek). All authors have read and agreed to the published version of the manuscript.

Funding: This research received no external funding.

Institutional Review Board Statement: The study was approved by the Ethics Committee of Medical University of Silesia No PCN/CBN/0022/KB1/77/21 (21 September 2021).

Informed Consent Statement: Informed consent was obtained from all subjects involved in the study.

Data Availability Statement: Patient medical records are available in patient medical records and are available upon request from the authors: Paweł Madej and Marta Kochanowicz.

Conflicts of Interest: The authors declare no conflicts of interest.

References

1. Joham, A.E.; Norman, R.J.; Stener-Victorin, E.; Legro, R.S.; Franks, S.; Moran, L.J.; Boyle, J.; Teede, H.J. Polycystic ovary syndrome. *Lancet Diabetes Endocrinol.* **2022**, *10*, 668–680, Erratum in *Lancet Diabetes Endocrinol.* **2022**, *10*, e11. [CrossRef] [PubMed]
2. Rotterdam ESHRE/ASRM-Sponsored PCOS Consensus Workshop Group. Revised 2003 consensus on diagnostic criteria and long-term health risks related to polycystic ovary syndrome (PCOS). *Hum. Reprod.* **2004**, *19*, 41–47. [CrossRef]
3. Lizneva, D.; Suturina, L.; Walker, W.; Brakta, S.; Gavrilova-Jordan, L.; Azziz, R. Criteria, prevalence, and phenotypes of polycystic ovary syndrome. *Fertil. Steril.* **2016**, *106*, 6–15. [CrossRef] [PubMed]
4. Hamilton-Fairley, D.; Taylor, A. Anovulation. *BMJ* **2003**, *327*, 546–549. [CrossRef]
5. Kakoly, N.S.; Earnest, A.; Teede, H.J.; Moran, L.J.; Joham, A.E. The Impact of Obesity on the Incidence of Type 2 Diabetes Among Women With Polycystic Ovary Syndrome. *Diabetes Care* **2019**, *42*, 560–567. [CrossRef] [PubMed]
6. Dokras, A.; Stener-Victorin, E.; Yildiz, B.O.; Li, R.; Ottey, S.; Shah, D.; Epperson, N.; Teede, H. Androgen Excess-Polycystic Ovary Syndrome Society: Position statement on depression, anxiety, quality of life, and eating disorders in polycystic ovary syndrome. *Fertil. Steril.* **2018**, *109*, 888–899. [CrossRef] [PubMed]
7. Coffey, S.; Mason, H. The effect of polycystic ovary syndrome on health-related quality of life. *Gynecol. Endocrinol.* **2003**, *17*, 379–386. [CrossRef] [PubMed]
8. Deeks, A.A.; Gibson-Helm, M.E.; Teede, H.J. Anxiety and depression in polycystic ovary syndrome: A comprehensive investigation. *Fertil. Steril.* **2010**, *93*, 2421–2423. [CrossRef] [PubMed]
9. Tay, C.T.; Teede, H.J.; Hill, B.; Loxton, D.; Joham, A.E. Increased prevalence of eating disorders, low self-esteem, and psychological distress in women with polycystic ovary syndrome: A community-based cohort study. *Fertil. Steril.* **2019**, *112*, 353–361. [CrossRef]
10. American Psychiatric Association. *Diagnostic and Statistical Manual of Mental Disorders*, 5th ed.; APA: Arlington, VA, USA, 2013.
11. Pastoor, H.; Timman, R.; de Klerk, C.; Bramer, W.M.; Laan, E.T.; Laven, J.S. Sexual function in women with polycystic ovary syndrome: A systematic review and meta-analysis. *Reprod. Biomed. Online* **2018**, *37*, 750–760. [CrossRef]
12. Zhao, S.; Wang, J.; Xie, Q.; Luo, L.; Zhu, Z.; Liu, Y.; Luo, J.; Zhao, Z. Is polycystic ovary syndrome associated with risk of female sexual dysfunction? A systematic review and meta-analysis. *Reprod. Biomed. Online* **2019**, *38*, 979–989. [CrossRef] [PubMed]
13. Loh, H.H.; Yee, A.; Loh, H.S.; Kanagasundram, S.; Francis, B.; Lim, L.L. Sexual dysfunction in polycystic ovary syndrome: A systematic review and meta-analysis. *Hormones* **2020**, *19*, 413–423. [CrossRef]
14. Albers, C.; Lakens, D. 2018 When power analyses based on pilot data are biased: Inaccurate effect size estimators and follow-up bias. *J. Exp. Soc. Psychol.* **2018**, *74*, 187–195. [CrossRef]
15. Forbes, M.K.; Baillie, A.J.; Schniering, C.A. Critical flaws in the Female Sexual Function Index and the international index of Erectile Function. *J. Sex Res.* **2014**, *51*, 485–491. [CrossRef] [PubMed]
16. Janssen, E.; McBride, K.R.; Yarber, W.; Hill, B.J.; Butler, S.M. Factors that influence sexual arousal in men: A focus group study. *Arch. Sex Behav.* **2008**, *37*, 252–265. [CrossRef]
17. Brotto, L.A.; Heiman, J.R.; Tolman, D.L. Narratives of desire in mid-age women with and without arousal difficulties. *J. Sex Res.* **2009**, *46*, 387–398. [CrossRef]

18. Stovall, D.W.; Scriver, J.L.; Clayton, A.H.; Williams, C.D.; Pastore, L.M. Sexual function in women with polycystic ovary syndrome. *J. Sex Med.* **2012**, *9*, 224–230. [CrossRef]
19. Regan, P.C.; Berscheid, E. Gender differences in beliefs about the cause of male and female sexual desire. *Pers. Relatsh.* **1995**, *2*, 345–358. [CrossRef]
20. Harris, E.A.; Hornsey, M.J.; Hofmann, W.; Jern, P.; Murphy, S.C.; Hedenborg, F.; Barlow, F.K. Does Sexual Desire Fluctuate More Among Women than Men? *Arch. Sex Behav.* **2023**, *52*, 1461–1478. [CrossRef] [PubMed]
21. Basson, R. Human sexual response. *Handb. Clin. Neurol.* **2015**, *130*, 11–18. [CrossRef] [PubMed]
22. Sand, M.; Fisher, W.A. Women's endorsement of models of female sexual response: The nurses' sexuality study. *J. Sex Med.* **2007**, *4*, 708–719. [CrossRef] [PubMed]
23. Basson, R. The female sexual response: A different model. *J. Sex Marital Ther.* **2000**, *26*, 51–65. [CrossRef] [PubMed]
24. de Jong, D.C. The role of attention in sexual arousal: Implications for treatment of sexual dysfunction. *J. Sex Res.* **2009**, *46*, 237–248. [CrossRef]
25. Basson, R. Human sex-response cycles. *J. Sex Marital Ther.* **2001**, *27*, 33–43. [CrossRef]
26. Spiering, M.; Everaerd, W.; Janssen, E. Priming the sexual system: Implicit versus explicit activation. *J. Sex Res.* **2003**, *40*, 134–145. [CrossRef]
27. Parish, S.J.; Meston, C.M.; Althof, S.E.; Clayton, A.H.; Goldstein, I.; Goldstein, S.W.; Heiman, J.R.; McCabe, M.P.; Segraves, R.T.; Simon, J.A. Toward a More Evidence-Based Nosology and Nomenclature for Female Sexual Dysfunctions-Part III. *J. Sex Med.* **2019**, *16*, 452–462. [CrossRef]
28. Althof, S.E.; Meston, C.M.; Perelman, M.A.; Handy, A.B.; Kilimnik, C.D.; Stanton, A.M. Opinion Paper: On the Diagnosis/Classification of Sexual Arousal Concerns in Women. *J. Sex Med.* **2017**, *14*, 1365–1371. [CrossRef] [PubMed]
29. Skakoon-Sparling, S.; Cramer, K.M.; Shuper, P.A. The Impact of Sexual Arousal on Sexual Risk-Taking and Decision-Making in Men and Women. *Arch. Sex Behav.* **2016**, *45*, 33–42. [CrossRef]
30. Meston, C.M.; Buss, D.M. Why humans have sex. *Arch. Sex Behav.* **2007**, *36*, 477–507. [CrossRef] [PubMed]
31. McNulty, J.K.; Wenner, C.A.; Fisher, T.D. Longitudinal Associations Among Relationship Satisfaction, Sexual Satisfaction, and Frequency of Sex in Early Marriage. *Arch. Sex Behav.* **2016**, *45*, 85–97. [CrossRef]
32. Hackbert, L.; Heiman, J.R. Acute dehydroepiandrosterone (DHEA) effects on sexual arousal in postmenopausal women. *J. Womens Health Gend.-Based Med.* **2002**, *11*, 155–162. [CrossRef] [PubMed]
33. Schmid, Y.; Hysek, C.M.; Preller, K.H.; Bosch, O.G.; Bilderbeck, A.C.; Rogers, R.D.; Quednow, B.B.; Liechti, M.E. Effects of methylphenidate and MDMA on appraisal of erotic stimuli and intimate relationships. *Eur. Neuropsychopharmacol.* **2015**, *25*, 17–25. [CrossRef]
34. Sipski, M.L.; Rosen, R.C.; Alexander, C.J.; Hamer, R.M. Sildenafil effects on sexual and cardiovascular responses in women with spinal cord injury. *Urology* **2000**, *55*, 812–815. [CrossRef] [PubMed]
35. Handy, A.B.; Stanton, A.M.; Meston, C.M. Understanding Women's Subjective Sexual Arousal Within the Laboratory: Definition, Measurement, and Manipulation. *Sex Med. Rev.* **2018**, *6*, 201–216. [CrossRef] [PubMed]
36. Velten, J.; Milani, S.; Margraf, J.; Brotto, L.A. Visual attention and sexual arousal in women with and without sexual dysfunction. *Behav. Res. Ther.* **2021**, *144*, 103915. [CrossRef] [PubMed]
37. Bancroft, J.; Graham, C.A.; Janssen, E.; Sanders, S.A. The dual control model: Current status and future directions. *J. Sex Res.* **2009**, *46*, 121–142. [CrossRef] [PubMed]
38. Janssen, E.; Bancroft, J. The Dual Control Model of Sexual Response: A Scoping Review, 2009–2022. *J. Sex Res.* **2023**, *60*, 948–968. [CrossRef]
39. Davis, S.R.; Guay, A.T.; Shifren, J.L.; Mazer, N.A. Endocrine aspects of female sexual dysfunction. *J. Sex Med.* **2004**, *1*, 82–86. [CrossRef]
40. Kingsberg, S.A.; Clayton, A.H.; Pfaus, J.G. The Female Sexual Response: Current Models, Neurobiological Underpinnings and Agents Currently Approved or Under Investigation for the Treatment of Hypoactive Sexual Desire Disorder. *CNS Drugs* **2015**, *29*, 915–933. [CrossRef]
41. Månsson, M.; Norström, K.; Holte, J.; Landin-Wilhelmsen, K.; Dahlgren, E.; Landén, M. Sexuality and psychological wellbeing in women with polycystic ovary syndrome compared with healthy controls. *Eur. J. Obstet. Gynecol. Reprod. Biol.* **2011**, *155*, 161–165. [CrossRef] [PubMed]
42. Bazarganipour, F.; Ziaei, S.; Montazeri, A.; Foroozanfard, F.; Kazemnejad, A.; Faghihzadeh, S. Sexual Functioning among Married Iranian Women with Polycystic Ovary Syndrome. *Int. J. Fertil. Steril.* **2014**, *8*, 273–280. [PubMed]
43. Bahadori, F.; Jahanian Sadatmahalleh, S.; Montazeri, A.; Nasiri, M. Sexuality and psychological well-being in different polycystic ovary syndrome phenotypes compared with healthy controls: A cross-sectional study. *BMC Womens Health* **2022**, *22*, 390. [CrossRef]
44. Anger, J.T.; Brown, A.J.; Amundsen, C.L. Sexual Dysfunction in Women With Polycystic Ovary Syndrome: The Effects of Testosterone, Obesity, and Depression. *J. Pelvic Med. Surg.* **2007**, *13*, 119–124. [CrossRef]
45. Elsenbruch, S.; Hahn, S.; Kowalsky, D.; Offner, A.H.; Schedlowski, M.; Mann, K.; Janssen, O.E. Quality of life, psychosocial well-being, and sexual satisfaction in women with polycystic ovary syndrome. *J. Clin. Endocrinol. Metab.* **2003**, *88*, 5801–5807. [CrossRef] [PubMed]

46. Stapinska-Syniec, A.; Grabowska, K.; Szpotanska-Sikorska, M.; Pietrzak, B. Depression, sexual satisfaction, and other psychological issues in women with polycystic ovary syndrome. *Gynecol. Endocrinol.* **2018**, *34*, 597–600. [CrossRef] [PubMed]
47. Tian, X.; Ruan, X.; Du, J.; Cheng, J.; Ju, R.; Mueck, A.O. Sexual function in Chinese women with different clinical phenotypes of polycystic ovary syndrome. *Gynecol. Endocrinol.* **2023**, *39*, 2221736. [CrossRef] [PubMed]
48. Morotti, E.; Persico, N.; Battaglia, B.; Fabbri, R.; Meriggiola, M.C.; Venturoli, S.; Battaglia, C. Body imaging and sexual behavior in lean women with polycystic ovary syndrome. *J. Sex Med.* **2013**, *10*, 2752–2760. [CrossRef]
49. Sills, E.S.; Perloe, M.; Tucker, M.J.; Kaplan, C.R.; Genton, M.G.; Schattman, G.L. Diagnostic and treatment characteristics of polycystic ovary syndrome: Descriptive measurements of patient perception and awareness from 657 confidential self-reports. *BMC Womens Health* **2001**, *1*, 3. [CrossRef] [PubMed]
50. Eftekhar, T.; Sohrabvand, F.; Zabandan, N.; Shariat, M.; Haghollahi, F.; Ghaghaei-Nezamabadi, A. Sexual dysfunction in patients with polycystic ovary syndrome and its affected domains. *Iran. J. Reprod. Med.* **2014**, *12*, 539–546. [PubMed]
51. Ercan, C.M.; Coksuer, H.; Aydogan, U.; Alanbay, I.; Keskin, U.; Karasahin, K.E.; Baser, I. Sexual dysfunction assessment and hormonal correlations in patients with polycystic ovary syndrome. *Int. J. Impot. Res.* **2013**, *25*, 127–132. [CrossRef]
52. Veras, A.B.; Bruno, R.V.; de Avila, M.A.; Nardi, A.E. Sexual dysfunction in patients with polycystic ovary syndrome: Clinical and hormonal correlations. *Compr. Psychiatry* **2011**, *52*, 486–489. [CrossRef]
53. Rellini, A.H.; Stratton, N.; Tonani, S.; Santamaria, V.; Brambilla, E.; Nappi, R.E. Differences in sexual desire between women with clinical versus biochemical signs of hyperandrogenism in polycystic ovarian syndrome. *Horm. Behav.* **2013**, *63*, 65–71. [CrossRef] [PubMed]
54. Davis, S.R.; Davison, S.L.; Donath, S.; Bell, R.J. Circulating androgen levels and self-reported sexual function in women. *JAMA* **2005**, *294*, 91–96. [CrossRef]
55. Wierman, M.E.; Arlt, W.; Basson, R.; Davis, S.R.; Miller, K.K.; Murad, M.H.; Rosner, W.; Santoro, N. Androgen therapy in women: A reappraisal: An Endocrine Society clinical practice guideline. *J. Clin. Endocrinol. Metab.* **2014**, *99*, 3489–3510. [CrossRef] [PubMed]
56. Hahn, S.; Janssen, O.E.; Tan, S.; Pleger, K.; Mann, K.; Schedlowski, M.; Kimmig, R.; Benson, S.; Balamitsa, E.; Elsenbruch, S. Clinical and psychological correlates of quality-of-life in polycystic ovary syndrome. *Eur. J. Endocrinol.* **2005**, *153*, 853–860. [CrossRef] [PubMed]
57. Ferraresi, S.R.; Lara, L.A.; Reis, R.M.; Rosa e Silva, A.C. Changes in sexual function among women with polycystic ovary syndrome: A pilot study. *J. Sex Med.* **2013**, *10*, 467–473. [CrossRef]
58. Yaylali, G.F.; Tekekoglu, S.; Akin, F. Sexual dysfunction in obese and overweight women. *Int. J. Impot. Res.* **2010**, *22*, 220–226. [CrossRef] [PubMed]
59. Brody, S.; Weiss, P. Slimmer women's waist is associated with better erectile function in men independent of age. *Arch. Sex Behav.* **2013**, *42*, 1191–1198. [CrossRef]
60. Zueff, L.N.; Lara, L.A.; Vieira, C.S.; Martins, W.P.; Ferriani, R.A. Body composition characteristics predict sexual functioning in obese women with or without PCOS. *J. Sex Marital Ther.* **2015**, *41*, 227–237. [CrossRef]
61. De Frène, V.; Verhofstadt, L.; Loeys, T.; Stuyver, I.; Buysse, A.; De Sutter, P. Sexual and relational satisfaction in couples where the woman has polycystic ovary syndrome: A dyadic analysis. *Hum. Reprod.* **2015**, *30*, 625–631. [CrossRef] [PubMed]
62. Benetti-Pinto, C.L.; Ferreira, S.R.; Antunes, A., Jr.; Yela, D.A. The influence of body weight on sexual function and quality of life in women with polycystic ovary syndrome. *Arch. Gynecol. Obstet.* **2015**, *291*, 451–455. [CrossRef] [PubMed]
63. Nohr, E.A.; Hansen, A.B.; Andersen, M.S.; Hjorth, S. Sexual health in parous women with a history of polycystic ovary syndrome: A national cross-sectional study in Denmark. *Int. J. Gynaecol. Obstet.* **2022**, *157*, 702–709. [CrossRef] [PubMed]
64. March, W.A.; Moore, V.M.; Willson, K.J.; Phillips, D.I.; Norman, R.J.; Davies, M.J. The prevalence of polycystic ovary syndrome in a community sample assessed under contrasting diagnostic criteria. *Hum. Reprod.* **2010**, *25*, 544–551. [CrossRef] [PubMed]

Disclaimer/Publisher's Note: The statements, opinions and data contained in all publications are solely those of the individual author(s) and contributor(s) and not of MDPI and/or the editor(s). MDPI and/or the editor(s) disclaim responsibility for any injury to people or property resulting from any ideas, methods, instructions or products referred to in the content.

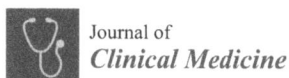 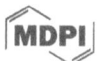

Article

Translation of the Modified Polycystic Ovary Syndrome Questionnaire (mPCOSQ) and the Polycystic Ovary Syndrome Quality of Life Tool (PCOSQOL) in Dutch and Flemish Women with PCOS

Geranne Jiskoot [1,*,†], Sara Somers [2,*,†], Chloë De Roo [2], Dominic Stoop [2] and Joop Laven [1]

[1] Division of Reproductive Endocrinology and Infertility, Department of Obstetrics and Gynaecology, Erasmus Medical Centre, P.O. Box 2040, 3000 CA Rotterdam, The Netherlands
[2] Department of Reproductive Medicine, Ghent University Hospital, Corneel Heymanslaan 10, 9000 Ghent, Belgium
* Correspondence: l.jiskoot@erasmusmc.nl (G.J.); sara.somers@uzgent.be (S.S.)
† These authors contribute equally to this work.

Abstract: This study aims to determine the test–retest reliability and to confirm the domain structures of the Dutch version of the modified polycystic ovary syndrome questionnaire (mPCOSQ) and the Polycystic Ovary Syndrome Quality of Life Scale (PCOSQOL) in Dutch and Flemish women with Polycystic Ovary Syndrome (PCOS). PCOS patients were contacted with a request to complete both questionnaires (including additional demographic questions) online in their home environment on T0 and on T1. The study was approved by the Ethics Committee of Erasmus Medical Centre and of Ghent University Hospital. In this study, 245 participants were included between January and December 2021. The mPCOSQ has excellent internal consistency (α: 0.95) and a high to excellent Intraclass Correlation Coefficient (ICC) for all six domains (ICC: 0.88–0.96). The PCOSQOL demonstrates excellent internal consistency (α: 0.96) and ICC (ICC: 0.91–0.96) for all four domains. The original six-factor structure of the mPCOSQ is partly confirmed. An extra domain is added to the PCOSQOL which included coping items. Most women have no preference for one of the two questionnaires (55.9%). In conclusion, The Dutch mPCOSQ and PCOSQOL are reliable and disease-specific QoL measures for women with PCOS. Both questionnaires are recommended for clinical practice.

Keywords: polycystic ovary syndrome; PCOS; health-related quality of life; QoL; questionnaire; modified PCOSQ; PCOSQOL

Citation: Jiskoot, G.; Somers, S.; De Roo, C.; Stoop, D.; Laven, J. Translation of the Modified Polycystic Ovary Syndrome Questionnaire (mPCOSQ) and the Polycystic Ovary Syndrome Quality of Life Tool (PCOSQOL) in Dutch and Flemish Women with PCOS. *J. Clin. Med.* **2023**, *12*, 3927. https://doi.org/10.3390/jcm12123927

Academic Editor: Enrico Carmina

Received: 5 May 2023
Revised: 27 May 2023
Accepted: 2 June 2023
Published: 8 June 2023

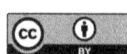

Copyright: © 2023 by the authors. Licensee MDPI, Basel, Switzerland. This article is an open access article distributed under the terms and conditions of the Creative Commons Attribution (CC BY) license (https://creativecommons.org/licenses/by/4.0/).

1. Introduction

Polycystic Ovary Syndrome (PCOS) is the most common endocrine condition in women of reproductive age and affects 8–15% of that age group [1–3]. The diagnosis of PCOS requires at least two out of three of the following criteria: (1) oligo-ovulation or anovulation (irregular or no menstrual cycle), (2) clinical hyperandrogenism (e.g., hirsutism) and/or biochemical signs of hyperandrogenism (elevated free androgen index or elevated testosterone levels), and (3) polycystic ovarian morphology (PCOM) (by transvaginal ultrasound), and the exclusion of other etiologies that might cause hyperandrogenism or cycle irregularity [4]. Most women with PCOS experience one or more of the following symptoms: psychological (anxiety, depression, and body image dissatisfaction), physical (hirsutism and acne), reproductive (irregular menstrual cycles, and infertility), and metabolic (insulin resistance, metabolic syndrome, prediabetes, and type 2 diabetes) disorders [5]. In general, women with PCOS encounter more depressive and anxiety complaints, they have lower self-esteem, and they experience a more negative body image than women without PCOS [6,7]. The prevalence of clinically significant symptoms associated with depression among women diagnosed with PCOS is reported to be 37%, which is notably higher compared to the rate of 14.2% observed in healthy women. Furthermore, the prevalence of symptoms related to anxiety is found to be 42% in women with PCOS, whereas it is only 8.5% among healthy women [8]. Additionally, these women report lower quality of life (QoL) due to their PCOS symptoms [9,10]. Most women with PCOS report that weight concerns have the largest impact on QoL. Other PCOS symptoms, such as menstrual problems, infertility, hirsutism, and acne, impact their QoL less [11]. According to the latest PCOS guideline of the European Society of Human Reproduction and Embryology (ESHRE), healthcare professionals should be more aware of the negative impact of PCOS on quality of life [12].

Implementing QoL questionnaires in research and routine practice provides significant added value in understanding the impact of a particular condition or treatment on an individual's well-being and overall quality of life. QoL questionnaires are standardized instruments that assess various aspects of an individual's physical, psychological, and social functioning, and their overall satisfaction with life. For women with PCOS, the polycystic ovary syndrome questionnaire (PCOSQ) [13] was developed to complement generic health-related QoL instruments, such as the Standard short-form health survey questionnaire (SF-36) [14]. The PCOSQ has already been translated into English [15,16], Arabic [17], German [18], Chinese [19], Swedish [20], and Iranian [21]. Recent research suggested that psychological, social, or environmental aspects are less represented than the physical impact of PCOS measured by the PCOSQ. Others suggested that more QoL measures should be developed [22] to obtain a more sensitive measure of QoL in all PCOS phenotypes [23]. Therefore, the Polycystic Ovary Syndrome Quality of Life Scale (PCOSQOL) was developed in 2018 based on these recommendations [24].

Globally, women have reported insufficient access to information, delayed diagnosis, and inconsistent care for PCOS [12]. The provision of comprehensive and accurate information has been shown to enhance satisfaction with care and improve the overall patient experience [25]. Language barriers further exacerbate the issue, as the majority of consumer information is predominantly available in English. This poses challenges for immigrant populations and women residing in countries where English is not their primary language, such as the Netherlands and Belgium. Therefore, this study aims to determine the test–retest reliability and to confirm the domain structure of the Dutch version of the mPCOSQ and the PCOSQOL in Dutch-speaking samples. Additionally, we want to examine which questionnaire is preferred by women with PCOS.

2. Materials and Methods

2.1. Study Design

Two independent translators performed a forward and backward translation of the original English mPCOSQ and PCOSQOL. Between January and December 2021, patients with PCOS were contacted with a request to complete the mPCOSQ and PCOSQOL questionnaires (and some additional demographic questions) online in their home environment (T0). A test–retest design was applied to demonstrate stability over time by having all women complete the same questionnaires a second time after two to four weeks (T1). At both points in time, participants were asked if they had a preference for one of the two questionnaires. We also performed a factor analysis. All materials, including the information sheet, the consent form, and the questionnaires, were completed using Gemstracker (www.gemstracker.org). The study was approved by the Ethics Committee of the Erasmus Medical Centre (The Netherlands) (MEC-2019-0628) and Ghent University Hospital (Belgium) (B6702020000388).

2.2. Questionnaires

The original PCOSQ [13] was developed in 1998 by Cronin et al. It consisted of 26 items and took 10 to 15 min to complete. The questionnaire included five subscales: emotions, body hair, infertility, weight, and menstrual problems [13]. Based on a validation study by Jones and colleagues [15], an acne domain was added to improve the validity of the

PCOSQ. This resulted in a 30-item mPCOSQ with 6 subscales: emotions (8 items), body hair (5 items), weight concerns (5 items), infertility concerns (4 items), menstrual problems (4 items), and acne (4 items). Each item is answered based on a 7-point Likert scale, where one represents the poorest function, and seven represents an optimal function. A higher score on the mPCOSQ denotes a higher quality of life [26]. The PCOSQOL is developed by Williams et al. and is a 35-item self-administered questionnaire with four domains: impact of PCOS (16 items), infertility (7 items), hirsutism (6 items), and mood (6 items). Each item is answered based on a 7-point Likert scale, ranging from 1 (usually) to 7 (does not apply). A higher score on the PCOSQOL denotes a higher quality of life [24].

2.3. Population

Women of at least 18 years old, who were able to speak and write Dutch, and who were diagnosed with PCOS according to the Rotterdam criteria [4] or according to the international evidence-based guideline for the assessment and management of PCOS [12] were eligible for the study. Women who were pregnant at T0 or T1 were excluded from the study. The definition of PCOM varies according to the PCOS criteria that are used. According to the Rotterdam criteria, PCOM is defined as $\geq$12 follicles (measuring 2–10 mm) and/or ovarian volume > 10 cm^3 in at least one ovary [27]. According to the international evidence-based guideline for the assessment and management of PCOS, PCOM is defined as a follicle number per ovary of $\geq$20 (on either ovary) and/or an ovarian volume $\geq$ 10 mL, ensuring no corpora lutea, cysts, or dominant follicles [12]. Both definitions are used to define PCOS in this study.

2.4. Recruitment

Participants were recruited via Erasmus MC (the Netherlands) and Ghent University Hospital (Belgium). At the Erasmus MC, all patients were recruited via a PCOS database of the Division of Reproductive Endocrinology and Infertility. This database includes all women with menstrual cycle disorders that are systematically screened using a standardized protocol. They were all contacted via email and received a link to the online questionnaires. At Ghent University Hospital, Belgian PCOS patients were recruited in several ways: (1) PCOS patients who were included in a previous study and who agreed to be contacted for future research received an email with the link to the questionnaires, (2) the gynecologists working at the Women's Clinic and in a later stage the endocrinologists working at the Endocrinology Department of the hospital were informed about the study and recruited patients in their daily practice, (3) the treating gynecologists of the Department of Reproductive Medicine (RM) emailed PCOS patients that were eligible for the study with a request to reply in case of interest in the study, (4) a flyer was distributed in the waiting room of the Department of RM and later in the waiting room of the Endocrinology Department of the hospital, (5) a message was put on the website of the Department of RM. In May 2022, it was decided to stop recruitment. At that time, 64 Belgian PCOS patients had completed the questionnaires at both points in time.

2.5. Statistical Considerations

Applying the procedure described by Bonett [28] for a Pearson correlation of at least 0.80 and a 95% confidence interval width of 0.10, requires a sample size of 240 patients. Therefore, 120 Dutch patients and 120 Flemish patients need to be enrolled.

The Cronbach alpha was used together with the Intraclass Correlation Coefficient (ICC) for the test–retest of the mPCOSQ and the PCOSQOL. To assess the reliability within the mPCOSQ and the PCOSQOL domains, the one-way random-effects analysis of variance technique was used to estimate the Mean Square values required for subsequent calculation of the ICC. The ICC ranges from 0 to 1. Values near 0 indicate unreliable test–retest structure, and values above 0.90 indicate excellent reliability. Factor analysis (using principal components analysis with varimax rotation) was used to measure which questions belong to each domain. The factor indicates the relationship between a set of items and is defined by the items that load on it or the factor loadings. Loadings > 0.5 were considered satisfactory. The data were analyzed using SPSS Software version 28 (IBM). Data not normally distributed were presented as medians, including the interquartile range (IQR) for continuous data and n (%) for categorical data. Mann–Whitney U-tests were used to determine significant differences between continuous variables. For categorical variables, Fisher's exact and χ2 tests were used. p-values of ≤ 0.05 defined statistical significance.

3. Results

A total of 245 women participated in the study and completed the test–retest of both questionnaires; 64 women were included in Belgium and 181 in the Netherlands. The median age of the women who completed the mPCOSQ and the PCOSQOL assessments was 31 (IQR 27.0–34.0) years. The median weight was 79 (IQR 65.0–98.0) kg. The median BMI was 32.1 (IQR 27.7–39.2) kg/m^2. Most women received their PCOS diagnosis one to five years ago (44.1%) and were not actively trying to become pregnant (63.7%). Most women were married (40.8%) and worked on a full-time basis (45.3%). They did not smoke (91.4%), drank alcohol (58.4%), and the majority did not use drugs (98.0%). Most women were Caucasian and were born in the Netherlands or in Belgium (89.0%). Seven women in total were born in Suriname (3.3%), Turkey (0.8%), and Morocco (0.4%), and fourteen women were born elsewhere (5.7%), see Table 1. At baseline, women in Belgium had a significantly lower BMI ($p = 0.003$) and were more likely to work on a full-time basis ($p < 0.001$). There were no significant differences in age ($p = 0.966$), marital status ($p = 0.141$), smoking status ($p = 0.298$), alcohol use ($p = 0.464$), and the proportion of women that were trying to conceive ($p = 0.291$).

Table 1. Patient characteristics.

Characteristics	Belgium (IQR)	The Netherlands (IQR)
	N = 64	N = 181
Median age (years)	31.0 (28.0–33.8)	30.0 (27.0–34.0)
Median weight (kg)	69.0 (58–80.8)	82.0 (70.0–100.0)
Median body mass index (BMI) (kg/m^2)	30.0 (25.3–35.5)	34.3 (28.7–40.5)
	N (%)	N (%)
Time since PCOS diagnosis:		
<1 year	16 (25.0)	27 (14.9)
1 to 5 years	31 (48.4)	77 (42.5)
5 to 10 years	9 (14.1)	43 (23.8)
>10 years	8 (12.5)	34 (18.8)
Trying to conceive (yes)	27 (42.2)	62 (34.3)
Marital status (married)	21 (32.8)	79 (43.6)
Education:		
Low	12 (18.8)	6 (3.3)
Intermediate	2 (3.1)	84 (46.4)
High	50 (78.1)	91 (50.3)
Working status (full time)	46 (71.9)	65 (35.9)
Smoking (yes)	3 (4.7)	18 (9.9)
Alcohol use (yes)	40 (62.5)	103 (56.9)
Drug use (yes)	1 (1.6)	4 (2.2)

Note: "Low" refers to the International Standard Classification of Education (ISCED) levels 0–2 (early childhood education, primary education, and lower secondary education), "intermediate" refers to ISCED levels 3–4 (upper secondary education, and post-secondary non-tertiary education), and "high" refers to ISCED levels 5–8 (tertiary education, including bachelor's, master's, and doctoral degrees). IQR = interquartile range.

3.1. Test–Retest Reliability

For the 30-item mPCOSQ, the overall Cronbach's alpha (α) was 0.95, which is considered excellent internal consistency. The ICC for the six domains ranged from 0.88 to 0.96, which is high to excellent. For the 35-item PCOSQOL, the overall Cronbach's α was

0.96. The ICC for the four domains ranged from 0.91 to 0.96. These values are considered excellent (Table 2).

Table 2. mPCOSQ and PCOSQOL subscales at T0 and T1.

Questionnaire	Domain	Median Score T0 (Min–Max)	Median Score T1 (Min–Max)	Cronbach's Alpha (α)	ICC (95% CI)
mPCOSQ	Emotions	3.8 (1–7)	4.1 (1–7)	0.919	0.92 (0.90–0.94)
	Body hair	3.8 (1–7)	3.8 (1–7)	0.959	0.96 (0.95–0.97)
	Weight	3.0 (1–7)	2.8 (1–7)	0.955	0.96 (0.94–0.97)
	Infertility	3.8 (1–7)	4.0 (1–7)	0.932	0.93 (0.90–0.95)
	Menstrual problems	3.3 (1–7)	3.3 (1–7)	0.879	0.88 (0.84–0.90)
	Acne	5.8 (1–7)	5.8 (1–7)	0.916	0.92 (0.89–0.94)
PCOSQOL	Impact of PCOS	3.9 (1–7)	3.9 (1–7)	0.952	0.95 (0.94–0.96)
	Infertility	4.6 (1–7)	4.6 (1–7)	0.951	0.95 (0.94–0.96)
	Hirsutism	4.5 (1–7)	4.3 (1–7)	0.961	0.96 (0.95–0.97)
	Mood	4.2 (1–7)	4.2 (1–7)	0.914	0.91 (0.89–0.93)

Note: CI = confidence interval.

3.2. Factor Analysis

For the mPCOSQ, we found that the original six-factor structure was partly confirmed (Supplemental Tables S1 and S2). Two items ("How much of the time during the last two weeks did you feel a lack of control over the situation with PCOS?" (item 23) and "In relation to your last menstruation, how much was a late menstrual period a problem for you?" (item 20)) did not load on their original domain. Therefore, item 23 was moved from the domain "infertility" to "emotions", and item 20 was moved from the domain "emotions" to "menstrual problems".

For the PCOSQOL, the original four-factor structure was changed into a five-factor structure: impact of PCOS (11 items), infertility (7 items), hirsutism (7 items), coping with PCOS (6 items), and mood (4 items). The domain "coping with PCOS" was added, which includes items from the original domain "impact of PCOS": 19, 27, 28, 29, 32, and 33. Item 19 ("Felt like your PCOS is in control of your life") loaded on two domains which are "impact of PCOS" and "coping with PCOS". We decided to include item 19 in the new domain, "coping with PCOS". Item 20 ("Felt embarrassed about the way you look"), originally in the domain "hirsutism", failed to obtain a value of 0.50.

3.3. Baseline Differences

The overall total score on the mPCOSQ was 3.97 (SD = 1.20). The difference between the overall score in Belgium and in the Netherlands was significant (4.74 vs. 3.70; $p < 0.001$). On the PCOSQOL, women recruited in Belgium had an overall total score of 4.90 (SD = 1.23), and women recruited in the Netherlands had a total score of 3.86 (SD = 1.23) ($p < 0.001$). This suggests that women in Belgium had better QoL compared to women in the Netherlands. The mean scale scores of the mPCOSQ showed that "menstrual problems" and "weight" scored the lowest, indicating the worst health in these two dimensions. For the PCOSQOL, the scales "mood" and "impact of PCOS" scored the lowest (Table 3). Additional analyses were performed to examine the difference between overall scores for Belgium and the Netherlands.

Assuming that BMI performed an important role in the difference between mPCOSQ and PCOSQOL scores in both countries, we performed additional analyses based on BMI and if women were trying to conceive. Women with a BMI below 30 had better QoL compared to women with a BMI above 30 on the mPCOSQ (4.48 vs. 3.93, $p < 0.002$) and on the PCOSQOL (4.64 vs. 3.60, $p < 0.001$). Additionally, women who were not trying to conceive had better QoL compared to women who were trying to conceive based on the mPCOSQ (4.38 vs. 3.68, $p < 0.001$) and the PCOSQOL (4.14 vs. 3.68, $p = 0.002$).

Table 3. Baseline mPCOSQ and PCOSQOL subscales for Belgium and the Netherlands.

Questionnaire	Domain	Overall Score (SD)	Score for Belgium (SD)	Score for The Netherlands (SD)	p Value
mPCOSQ	Emotions	3.99 (1.36)	4.93 (1.37)	3.65 (1.19)	<0.001
	Body hair	4.00 (2.03)	4.92 (2.01)	3.67 (1.95)	<0.001
	Weight	3.59 (2.19)	4.61 (2.10)	3.22 (2.11)	<0.001
	Infertility	3.73 (1.94)	4.37 (2.08)	3.50 (1.84)	0.002
	Menstrual problems	3.41 (1.40)	3.96 (1.67)	3.22 (1.24)	0.003
	Acne	5.17 (1.75)	5.43 (1.65)	5.09 (1.78)	0.167
	Total score (with acne)	3.97 (1.20)	4.74 (1.24)	3.70 (1.07)	<0.001
	Total score (without acne)	3.78 (1.28)	4.63 (1.28)	3.48 (1.14)	<0.001
PCOSQOL	Impact of PCOS	4.00 (1.47)	4.88 (1.47)	3.70 (1.35)	<0.001
	Infertility	4.38 (1.92)	4.74 (1.89)	4.26 (1.92)	0.094
	Hirsutism	4.29 (1.88)	5.13 (1.74)	3.99 (1.84)	<0.001
	Mood	3.99 (1.42)	4.91 (1.17)	3.67 (1.36)	<0.001
	Total score	4.13 (1.31)	4.90 (1.23)	3.86 (1.23)	<0.001

3.4. Acceptability

Most women (70.6%) completed the questionnaires in approximately 15 min. They found the time spent on the questionnaires to be good (93.9%). Most women experienced the questionnaires as medium relevant (36.3%), while 23.5% found the questionnaires highly relevant, and 24.1% found them not relevant. Most women had no preference for one of the two questionnaires (55.9%).

4. Discussion

The results of this study showed that the Dutch mPCOSQ and PCOSQOL are reliable and disease-specific QoL measures for Dutch and Flemish women with PCOS. Both questionnaires had excellent internal consistency and high to excellent ICC for all domains. For the mPCOSQ, the original six-factor structure was partly confirmed. Based on the factor analysis of the PCOSQOL, an extra domain was added, which included coping items. Most women had no preference for one of the two questionnaires. We found that Belgian women with PCOS had better QoL compared to women in the Netherlands. This might be related to the significantly lower BMI in Belgian patients.

4.1. mPCOSQ

The original PCOSQ was translated into many languages [15–20] but not yet for Dutch-speaking women. Therefore, we have translated the 30-item Dutch version of the modified PCOSQ, including a sixth subscale for acne [21,26]. The acne domain was added because acne is related to a worse quality of life in women with PCOS [15] and because previous validation studies have shown that adding acne questions improved the validity of the original PCOSQ [15,26]. Others have introduced a version of the mPCOSQ with seven domains; the domain "menstrual factor" of the PCOSQ was divided into "menstrual symptoms" and "menstrual predictability" [26]. This change was installed because Guyatt et al. had found that two questions on the menstrual period (item 8 on irregular menstrual period and item 20 on last (late) menstrual period) loaded on a new—at that time undefined—factor of the PCOSQ [15,17]. Other authors suggested a change of item 20 from the emotional domain to the menstrual domain [20,21]. Another possible explanation for the low internal consistency in the menstrual domain of the PCOSQ was the fact that the question on headaches did not fit in that domain [16]. Due to the inconsistency in the literature, we decided to use the mPCOSQ with six domains. Although some earlier studies found a lower internal consistency for the menstrual domain compared to the other PCOSQ domains [15–18], our data showed an excellent Cronbach's α [21]. However, we also found that item 20 did not load on the original emotional domain and suggested it be moved to the menstrual domain, which is in line with the findings of other research groups [20,21]. Our results showed that item 23 (lack of control over the situation with PCOS) should be moved from the domain "infertility" to the emotional domain. This finding is in line with the results of previous studies [15,20].

In our study, the time interval between the completion of the questionnaires was two to four weeks. Previous PCOSQ/mPCOSQ studies have used intervals of three to six days [15], seven days [20], five days to two weeks [17], two weeks [21], four weeks [18], and 44 weeks [16]. Jedel and colleagues suggested an interval of three days to limit the impact on health status [20]. Our belief is that a longer time between T0 and T1 would be preferable to prevent participants from recalling their previous answers and reproducing them at T1. However, we acknowledge that a four-week timeframe may be more prone to changes in health compared to shorter intervals [16]. However, our data showed high to excellent test–retest reliability.

4.2. PCOSQOL

Our results with regard to internal consistency and test–retest reliability of the PCOSQOL were in line with the development and preliminary validation study [24]. Contrary to that study, we found that six items of the domain "impact of PCOS" loaded on a new domain "coping with PCOS". Moreover, it can be debated to exclude items 19 and 20 because of very low loadings to the original domain. This, too, is in contrast with the findings of Williams et al. [24].

4.3. Strengths, Limitations, and Future Research

The strengths of our study are worth mentioning. In contrast to some previous studies [17,20], we strived for identical settings (the home environment) at the two points in time of completing the questionnaires [15,21,24]. Furthermore, we questioned the same participants twice [16,18]) and not a subgroup of the first cohort [21] or a different cohort [24]. Additionally, it was a strength that two fertility centers in different countries were involved because most studies were monocentric [15,17–20] or performed within one country [21,24]. Additionally, we included both PCOS patients with and without a wish for a child and patients with and without a recent PCOS diagnosis which improves the generalizability of the results. Nonetheless, the proportion of participants with irregular cycles and infertility might be larger and the proportion of participants with hirsutism and acne might be smaller compared to the general population since we mainly recruited via fertility centers [15,18,21].

Some limitations could be identified. Although much effort was put into recruitment at Ghent University Hospital, the target of 120 Belgian inclusions could not be reached within a reasonable time. However, a predominance of Dutch patients led to the intended sample size of 240 patients. Yet, this might have influenced the results of the study as significant differences between Belgian and Dutch participants were present at baseline, with Belgians having a lower BMI and being more likely to work on a full-time basis. Additionally, the sample is prone to self-selection bias: it is possible that participants were more eager to take part in the study because of more severe symptoms related to PCOS or because of an impaired quality of life [18]. A small cohort of Belgian participants presented themselves to take part in the study (e.g., after reading a message on the hospital website). For these patients, it was not possible to verify the diagnosis of PCOS [21].

More translations of the PCOSQOL in different ethnic populations are necessary to evaluate if adjustments to the original questionnaire are necessary. Future research should also focus on whether differences in quality of life in PCOS patients could be correlated with different PCOS phenotypes.

5. Conclusions

The Dutch mPCOSQ and PCOSQOL are reliable and disease-specific QoL measures for Dutch and Flemish women with PCOS. For the mPCOSQ, the original six-factor structure was partly confirmed. Based on the factor analysis of the PCOSQOL, an extra domain was added, which included coping items. Most women had no preference for one of the two questionnaires.

Supplementary Materials: The following supporting information can be downloaded at: https://www.mdpi.com/article/10.3390/jcm12123927/s1. Table S1: mPCOSQ factor analysis; Table S2: PCOSQOL factor analysis; File S1: Dutch version of the mPCOSQ; File S2: Dutch version of the PCOSQOL.

Author Contributions: Conceptualization, G.J.; methodology, G.J.; software, G.J.; validation, G.J.; formal analysis, G.J.; investigation, G.J. and S.S.; resources, G.J.; data curation, G.J.; writing—original draft preparation, G.J. and S.S.; writing—review and editing, G.J., S.S., C.D.R., D.S. and J.L.; visualization, G.J. and S.S.; supervision, C.D.R., D.S. and J.L.; project administration, G.J. and S.S. All authors have read and agreed to the published version of the manuscript.

Funding: This research received no external funding.

Institutional Review Board Statement: The study was conducted in accordance with the Declaration of Helsinki, and approved by the Ethics Committee of Erasmus Medical Centre (The Netherlands) (protocol code MEC-2019-0628; 10 February 2020) and Ghent University Hospital (Belgium) (protocol code B6702020000388; 6 August 2020).

Informed Consent Statement: Informed consent was obtained from all subjects involved in the study.

Data Availability Statement: The data presented in this study are available on request from the corresponding authors.

Acknowledgments: We thank all the women for participating in this study. Our Flemish colleagues are acknowledged for their efforts in recruitment.

Conflicts of Interest: G.J. received an unrestricted research grant from the Waterloo Foundation and she received consultancy fees from Ferring®. D.S. received unrestricted research grants from Ferring®, Organon®, Gedeon Richter®, and Vitrolife®. He also received consultancy fees from Ferring®, Organon®, Gedeon Richter®, and Merck Serono®. J.L. received unrestricted research grants from Ferring®, Merck Serono®, Roche Diagnostics®, and Anshlabs®. He also received consultancy fees from Ferring®, Anshlabs®, Roche Diagnostics®, and Titus healthcare®. The other authors declare no conflict of interest.

References

1. March, W.A.; Moore, V.M.; Willson, K.J.; Phillips, D.I.; Norman, R.J.; Davies, M.J. The prevalence of polycystic ovary syndrome in a community sample assessed under contrasting diagnostic criteria. *J. Hum. Reprod.* **2010**, *25*, 544–551. [CrossRef]
2. Bozdag, G.; Mumusoglu, S.; Zengin, D.; Karabulut, E.; Yildiz, B.O. The prevalence and phenotypic features of polycystic ovary syndrome: A systematic review and meta-analysis. *Hum. Reprod.* **2016**, *31*, 2841–2855. [CrossRef] [PubMed]
3. Azziz, R.; Carmina, E.; Chen, Z.; Dunaif, A.; Laven, J.S.; Legro, R.S.; Lizneva, D.; Natterson-Horowtiz, B.; Teede, H.J.; Yildiz, B.O. Polycystic ovary syndrome. *Nat. Rev. Dis. Primers* **2016**, *2*, 16057. [CrossRef] [PubMed]
4. ESHRE, R. ASRM-Sponsored PCOS Consensus Workshop Group Revised 2003 consensus on diagnostic criteria and long-term health risks related to polycystic ovary syndrome. *Fertil. Steril.* **2004**, *81*, 19–25.
5. Laven, J.S.; Imani, B.; Eijkemans, M.J.; Fauser, B.C. New approach to polycystic ovary syndrome and other forms of anovulatory infertility. *Obstet. Gynecol. Surv.* **2002**, *57*, 755–767. [CrossRef]
6. Veltman-Verhulst, S.M.; Boivin, J.; Eijkemans, M.J.; Fauser, B.J. Emotional distress is a common risk in women with polycystic ovary syndrome: A systematic review and meta-analysis of 28 studies. *Hum. Reprod. Update* **2012**, *18*, 638–651. [CrossRef] [PubMed]
7. Teede; Deeks, A.; Moran, L. Polycystic ovary syndrome: A complex condition with psychological, reproductive and metabolic manifestations that impacts on health across the lifespan. *BMC Med.* **2010**, *8*, 41. [CrossRef] [PubMed]
8. Cooney, L.G.; Lee, I.; Sammel, M.D.; Dokras, A. High prevalence of moderate and severe depressive and anxiety symptoms in polycystic ovary syndrome: A systematic review and meta-analysis. *Hum. Reprod.* **2017**, *32*, 1075–1091. [CrossRef]
9. Kitzinger, C.; Willmott, J. 'The thief of womanhood': Women's experience of polycystic ovarian syndrome. *Soc. Sci. Med.* **2002**, *54*, 349–361. [CrossRef]
10. McCook, J.G.; Reame, N.E.; Thatcher, S.S. Health-related quality of life issues in women with polycystic ovary syndrome. *J. Obstet. Gynecol. Neonatal Nurses* **2005**, *34*, 12–20. [CrossRef]
11. Jones, G.L.; Hall, J.M.; Balen, A.H.; Ledger, W.L. Health-related quality of life measurement in women with polycystic ovary syndrome: A systematic review. *Hum. Reprod. Update* **2008**, *14*, 15–25. [CrossRef] [PubMed]

12. Teede; Misso, M.L.; Costello, M.F.; Dokras, A.; Laven, J.; Moran, L.; Piltonen, T.; Norman, R.J.; International PCOS Network. Recommendations from the international evidence-based guideline for the assessment and management of polycystic ovary syndrome. *Fertil. Steril.* **2018**, *110*, 364–379. [CrossRef] [PubMed]
13. Cronin, L.; Guyatt, G.; Griffith, L.; Wong, E.; Azziz, R.; Futterweit, W.; Cook, D.; Dunaif, A. Development of a health-related quality-of-life questionnaire (PCOSQ) for women with polycystic ovary syndrome (PCOS). *J. Clin. Endocrinol. Metab.* **1998**, *83*, 1976–1987. [CrossRef] [PubMed]
14. Aaronson, N.K.; Muller, M.; Cohen, P.D.; Essink-Bot, M.L.; Fekkes, M.; Sanderman, R.; Sprangers, M.A.; te Velde, A.; Verrips, E. Translation, validation, and norming of the Dutch language version of the SF-36 Health Survey in community and chronic disease populations. *J. Clin. Epidemiol.* **1998**, *51*, 1055–1068. [CrossRef] [PubMed]
15. Jones, G.L.; Benes, K.; Clark, T.L.; Denham, R.; Holder, M.G.; Haynes, T.J.; Mulgrew, N.C.; Shepherd, K.E.; Wilkinson, V.H.; Singh, M.; et al. The Polycystic Ovary Syndrome Health-Related Quality of Life Questionnaire (PCOSQ): A validation. *Hum. Reprod.* **2004**, *19*, 371–377. [CrossRef] [PubMed]
16. Guyatt, G.; Weaver, B.; Cronin, L.; Dooley, J.A.; Azziz, R. Health-related quality of life in women with polycystic ovary syndrome, a self-administered questionnaire, was validated. *J. Clin. Epidemiol.* **2004**, *57*, 1279–1287. [CrossRef]
17. Alghadeer, S.; Algarawi, A.; Abu-Rkybah, F.; Alshebly, M.M.; Alruthia, Y. The translation and validation of the Arabic Version of the Polycystic Ovary Syndrome Health-Related Quality of Life Questionnaire (AR-PCOSQ). *BMC Womens Health* **2020**, *20*, 244. [CrossRef]
18. Bottcher, B.; Fessler, S.; Friedl, F.; Toth, B.; Walter, M.H.; Wildt, L.; Riedl, D. Health-related quality of life in patients with polycystic ovary syndrome: Validation of the German PCOSQ-G. *Arch. Gynecol. Obs.* **2018**, *297*, 1027–1035. [CrossRef]
19. Ou, H.T.; Wu, M.H.; Lin, C.Y.; Chen, P.C. Development of Chinese Version of Polycystic Ovary Syndrome Health-Related Quality of Life Questionnaire (Chi-PCOSQ). *PLoS ONE* **2015**, *10*, e0137772. [CrossRef]
20. Jedel, E.; Kowalski, J.; Stener-Victorin, E. Assessment of health-related quality of life: Swedish version of polycystic ovary syndrome questionnaire. *Acta Obs. Gynecol. Scand.* **2008**, *87*, 1329–1335. [CrossRef]
21. Bazarganipour, F.; Ziaei, S.; Montazeri, A.; Faghihzadeh, S.; Frozanfard, F. Psychometric properties of the Iranian version of modified polycystic ovary syndrome health-related quality-of-life questionnaire. *Hum. Reprod.* **2012**, *27*, 2729–2736. [CrossRef] [PubMed]
22. Malik-Aslam, A.; Reaney, M.D.; Speight, J. The suitability of polycystic ovary syndrome-specific questionnaires for measuring the impact of PCOS on quality of life in clinical trials. *Value Health* **2010**, *13*, 440–446. [CrossRef] [PubMed]
23. Barry, J.A.; Leite, N.; Sivarajah, N.; Keevil, B.; Owen, L.; Miranda, L.C.; Qu, F.; Hardiman, P. Relaxation and guided imagery significantly reduces androgen levels and distress in Polycystic Ovary Syndrome: Pilot study. *Contemp. Hypn. Integr. Ther.* **2017**, *32*, 21–29.
24. Williams, S.; Sheffield, D.; Knibb, R.C. The Polycystic Ovary Syndrome Quality of Life scale (PCOSQOL): Development and preliminary validation. *Health Psychol. Open* **2018**, *5*, 2055102918788195. [CrossRef]
25. Gibson-Helm, M.; Teede, H.; Dunaif, A.; Dokras, A. Delayed diagnosis and a lack of information associated with dissatisfaction in women with polycystic ovary syndrome. *J. Clin. Endocrinol. Metab.* **2017**, *102*, 604–612. [CrossRef]
26. Barnard, L.; Ferriday, D.; Guenther, N.; Strauss, B.; Balen, A.H.; Dye, L. Quality of life and psychological well being in polycystic ovary syndrome. *Hum. Reprod.* **2007**, *22*, 2279–2286. [CrossRef]
27. Balen, A.H.; Laven, J.S.E.; Tan, S.L.; Dewailly, D. Ultrasound assessment of the polycystic ovary: International consensus definitions. *Hum. Reprod. Update* **2003**, *9*, 505–514. [CrossRef]
28. Bonett, D.G.; Wright, T.A. Sample size requirements for estimating Pearson, Kendall and Spearman correlations. *Psychometrika* **2000**, *65*, 23–28. [CrossRef]

Disclaimer/Publisher's Note: The statements, opinions and data contained in all publications are solely those of the individual author(s) and contributor(s) and not of MDPI and/or the editor(s). MDPI and/or the editor(s) disclaim responsibility for any injury to people or property resulting from any ideas, methods, instructions or products referred to in the content.

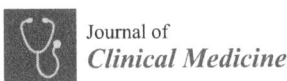

Article

The Effect of Tailored Short Message Service (SMS) on Physical Activity: Results from a Three-Component Randomized Controlled Lifestyle Intervention in Women with PCOS

Alexandra Dietz de Loos [1,*], Geranne Jiskoot [1,2], Rita van den Berg-Emons [3], Yvonne Louwers [1], Annemerle Beerthuizen [2], Jan van Busschbach [2] and Joop Laven [1]

1. Division of Reproductive Endocrinology and Infertility, Department of Obstetrics and Gynaecology, Erasmus University Medical Center, 3015 GD Rotterdam, The Netherlands
2. Department of Psychiatry, Section Medical Psychology and Psychotherapy, Erasmus University Medical Center, 3015 GD Rotterdam, The Netherlands
3. Department of Rehabilitation Medicine, Erasmus University Medical Center, 3015 GD Rotterdam, The Netherlands
* Correspondence: a.dietzdeloos@erasmusmc.nl; Tel.: +31-622-666-365

Abstract: This analysis of secondary outcome measures of a randomized controlled trial was conducted to study the effect of a one-year three-component (cognitive behavioural therapy, diet, exercise) lifestyle intervention (LSI), with or without additional Short Message Service (SMS) support, on physical activity and aerobic capacity in overweight or obese women with polycystic ovary syndrome (PCOS). Women diagnosed with PCOS and a BMI > 25 kg/m^2 were randomly assigned to LSI with SMS support (SMS+, n = 60), LSI without SMS support (SMS−, n = 63) or care as usual (CAU, n = 60) in order to lose weight. Based on results from the International Physical Activity Questionnaire (IPAQ), we found a significant within-group increase after one year for SMS+ in the high physical activity category (+31%, p < 0.01) and sitting behaviour decreased (Δ −871 min/week, p < 0.01). Moreover, the peak cycle ergometer workload increased within SMS+ (Δ +10 watts, p < 0.01). The SMS+ group also demonstrated a significantly different increase in walking metabolic equivalent of task minutes (METmin)/week compared with CAU after one year (Δ 1106 METmin/week, p < 0.05). Apart from this increase in walking activity, no other between-group differences were found in this trial. Overall, based on within-group results, SMS support seemed to help with improving physical activity and aerobic capacity and decreasing sedentary behaviour.

Keywords: PCOS; lifestyle intervention; three-component; Short Message Service; exercise; physical activity; aerobic capacity

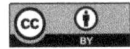

1. Introduction

Polycystic ovary syndrome (PCOS), characterized by ovulatory dysfunction, hyperandrogenism and polycystic ovarian morphology, is currently the most common endocrine disorder in reproductive-aged women [1]. This endocrine disorder is often associated with overweightness and obesity [2]. Furthermore, other clinical problems in women with PCOS may include derangements in reproductive, mental or metabolic parameters. The severity of the clinically expressed PCOS phenotype in these women is in turn negatively associated with increasing body mass index [3,4], which indicates that treatment strategies should focus on weight management.

Physical activity (any bodily movement produced by skeletal muscles that requires energy expenditure) and structured exercise (activity requiring physical effort, carried out to sustain or improve health and fitness), deliver metabolic, cardiovascular and psychological health benefits in the general population [1,5–8]. Additionally, isometric strength training (placing tension on particular muscles without moving the surrounding joints) demonstrated positive effects on dynamic strength and sport-related performance [9]. By contrast, sedentary behaviour (activities during waking hours in a seated or reclined position with energy expenditure less than 1.5 times resting metabolic rate [10]) has a negative impact on health and is linked to all-cause mortality [11,12]. Improving physical activity is a common element in the process of weight management. There are contradictory results on physical activity levels in women with PCOS. One study found these to be lower in women with than without PCOS. In particular, overweight or obese women with PCOS were less prone to be aligned with physical activity recommendations for weight maintenance or weight loss [13,14]. On top of this, high sedentary behaviour was extremely prevalent in this particular group. Additionally, women with PCOS were found to have an impaired aerobic capacity [15,16]. However, another study concluded that physical activity levels did not differ between obese women with and without PCOS [17]. Nonetheless, physical activity has a positive effect on overall health. Therefore, with the knowledge that obese women with PCOS suffer from poor metabolic, reproductive and mental health, this population should be motivated to be more physically active, achieve weight loss and maintain a healthy lifestyle [13].

The PCOS guidelines recommend a multi-component lifestyle intervention, including diet, behavioural strategies and physical activity, to achieve and maintain healthy weight [1]. However, health care providers are still searching for strategies to motivate this particular population and improve adherence to healthy lifestyle choices [18]. For example, one could promote physical activity by focusing on daily activities such as movement during transportation, work, leisure time or household and gardening chores when considering women's individual and family routines as well as cultural preferences [1]. Furthermore, eHealth, the use of information and communication technology to improve health, has demonstrated to have the potential to effectively promote physical activity in adults with obesity [19]. Mobile health options such as text messages through the Short Message Service (SMS) may be used for this purpose [20]. Where SMS support is given, tailored text messages appear to be more effective than generic ones in the general population [21,22]. However, the evidence on changes in physical activity resulting from motivational strategies such as SMS support in addition to a lifestyle intervention is still limited in women with PCOS.

We previously performed a randomized controlled one-year multidisciplinary lifestyle intervention aimed at changing cognitions and dietary habits and encouraging and promoting physical activity [23]. Half of the participants allocated to this three-component lifestyle intervention also received additional SMS support. The control group received care as usual, which consisted of advice to lose weight through methods of their own choosing. The primary outcome measure, weight loss, was achieved more in the lifestyle intervention groups and especially in the group with SMS support. Moreover, the chance of achieving a 5% weights loss was 7.0 times greater in the lifestyle intervention groups than the care as usual group [24]. The current study in the same cohort focused on the effect of the lifestyle intervention, with or without SMS support, on weekly physical activity levels when compared with care as usual. We hypothesized that physical activity levels increased in those women who received the three-component lifestyle intervention and that tailored SMS support might have amplified these results. Additionally, changes in aerobic capacity were also evaluated within the lifestyle intervention groups.

2. Materials and Methods
2.1. Trial Design

The PCOS lifestyle study was a randomized controlled trial (RCT) performed between August 2010 and March 2016. Women were included within the division of Reproductive Endocrinology and Infertility of the Department of Obstetrics and Gynaecology, at the Erasmus University Medical Centre, the Netherlands. The following three groups were compared: (1) one-year three-component lifestyle intervention with SMS support (SMS+), (2) one-year three-component lifestyle intervention without SMS support (SMS−) and (3) one-year care as usual (CAU). Data were collected every three months from baseline up to and including one year. The study protocol was published previously [23]. This RCT was approved by the Medical Research Ethics Committee of the Erasmus MC in Rotterdam (MEC2008-337) and registered with the clinical trial number NTR2450 (www.trialsearch.who.int (accessed on 1 February 2023)).

2.2. Participants

Women were included who were actively trying to become pregnant, had a body mass index (BMI) > 25 kg/m^2, were between 18 and 38 years of age and had a diagnosis of PCOS according to the Rotterdam 2003 consensus criteria [25]. Exclusion criteria comprised inadequate command of the Dutch language, severe mental illness, obesity due to another somatic cause, androgen excess caused by adrenal diseases or ovarian tumours and other malformations of the internal genitalia. All participants provided written informed consent. The sample size calculation was based on a notable difference in weight as the primary outcome measure of this RCT. A minimum of 60 participants was needed in each group, when accounting for an expected dropout proportion of 40%. Randomisation of participants was in a 1:1:1 ratio to one of the three groups with the use of a computer-generated random numbers table, which was executed by a research nurse who was not involved in the study.

2.3. Three-Component Lifestyle Intervention (LSI) and Control Group (CAU)

The three-component lifestyle intervention for both the SMS+ and SMS− groups consisted of twenty 2.5 h group meetings over the one-year period that covered the following topics: (1) cognitive behavioural therapy (CBT), (2) normo-caloric diet and (3) physical activity. The first 1.5 h of each group meeting was supervised by a mental health professional and a dietician. CBT techniques were used to create awareness and to restructure dysfunctional thoughts about, e.g., self-esteem and weight (loss). Furthermore, dietary advice was discussed as recommended by the 'Dutch Food Guide' [26]. The last hour of each session focused on physical activity and was supervised by two physical therapists. During each session, different sports and exercises were performed to encourage participants to try new forms of physical exercise. Furthermore, participants were also encouraged to increase their general physical activity during their daily routine. Recommendations were based on the Global Recommendations for Physical Activity by the World Health Organization [27]. These recommendations included: (1) five days of moderate physical activity for thirty min each day, (2) vigorous exercise one to three days a week (at least twenty min per session) and (3) perform eight to ten muscle-strengthening activities involving major muscle groups twice a week. Every 3 months, participants discussed their improvements and pitfalls with the psychologist, dietician and physical therapist.

After three months, the SMS+ group received SMS support in addition to the lifestyle intervention program. This group sent weekly self-monitored information regarding their diet, physical activity and emotions by SMS. A semi-automated software program returned patient-tailored SMS feedback to encourage positive behaviour. Additionally, two messages per week were sent addressing eating behaviour and physical activity; see Table 1.

In order to get acquainted with the program, we tested the lifestyle intervention in a pilot group (*n* = 26), of which the data were not included in the final analyses.

The control group received care as usual (CAU) as provided by health care professionals of our department for any woman with PCOS, excess weight and a wish to become pregnant. Their treating physician discussed the risk of excess weight for both mother and child and the relationship between overweightness and infertility. Subsequently, weight loss was encouraged by publicly available services such as visiting a dietician or gym.

Table 1. Examples of text messages focused on physical activity.

- Did you know that cleaning the house is also a moment of exercise? You can burn up to 140 calories in an hour!
- Nordic walking is a fun form of walking that burns extra calories. Maybe it's something for you?
- Take the stairs one extra time every day this week. Your goal doesn't have to be big, think of something small that you can change.
- Vacuuming is also a form of exercise! Start cleaning this weekend!
- Challenge: if you encounter an elevator this week, take the stairs!
- Go for a walk during your break from work!
- Household chores are also a form of exercise! While scrubbing the floor you can burn about 140 calories (per 60 min).
- Try to go swimming with a friend this week. That will be fun!
- Did you stick to the exercise standard of 30 min a day this week?
- Did you know that exercise helps against fatigue and negative feelings?

2.4. Clinical and Endocrine Assessments

Participants of all three groups (SMS+, SMS− and CAU) received five standardized assessments every three months from baseline up to and including one year. These included general medical, obstetric and family history, physical measurements (height, weight, BMI (kg/m^2), waist and hip circumference, blood pressure), transvaginal ultrasound (probe < 8 MHz) and an extensive endocrine assessment on fasting blood samples. Additionally, in order to monitor physical activity behaviour, all participants filled in the International Physical Activity Questionnaire (IPAQ) Long Form [28] at the above-mentioned three-monthly evaluation moments. Furthermore, a maximal cycle ergometer test was performed in the SMS+ and SMS− groups to evaluate changes in aerobic capacity. The CAU group did not perform the maximal cycle ergometer test intentionally, in order not to perform any form of intervention in this control group.

2.5. Outcome Measures

The primary outcome measure included the change in physical activity category (low, moderate, high) between and within all three groups over the course of the study period from baseline up to and including one year. These data were retrieved from the international physical activity questionnaires. Secondary outcome measures included changes in total weekly physical activity (metabolic equivalent of task minutes (METmin)/week), further subdivided per domain (work, transportation, household activities, leisure time (METmin/week)) and intensity (walking, moderate, vigorous (METmin/week)). Changes in sedentary behaviour (minutes/week) were also analysed. Furthermore, aerobic capacity within (only) the lifestyle intervention groups were evaluated and expressed as the achieved peak load (watt) resulting from the maximal cycle ergometer test.

2.5.1. International Physical Activity Questionnaire (IPAQ)

The IPAQ assesses the frequency, duration and intensity of physical activity in the course of the previous week and covers the following four domains: (1) at work, (2) during transportation, (3) during household activities and (4) during leisure time. The intensity of these various activities can be represented in metabolic equivalents (METs), which express energy expenditure in multiples of resting energy cost [29]. According to standardized procedures, time and days per activity and intensity were converted to MET minute/week scores by calculating METs x days x daily time. One minute of moderate household activities comprises 3.0 METs, walking 3.3 METs, general moderate intensity activities 4.0 METs, vigorous yard work 5.5 METs, cycling 6.0 METs and vigorous intensity activities 8.0 METS. Sedentary behaviour is also evaluated as an extra domain, which is expressed in minutes/week. Subsequently, subjects can be divided into three different physical activity categories:

1. Low: no activity is reported or some activity is reported but not enough to meet categories 'moderate or high'. These women reported activity equivalent to less than 600 METmin/week.
2. Moderate: These women reported 3 or more days of vigorous activity of at least 20 min per day, 5 or more days of moderate-intensity activity and/or walking of at least 30 min per day, or 5 or more days of any combination of walking, moderate-intensity or vigorous-intensity activities equivalent to at least 600 METmin/week.
3. High: These women reported vigorous-intensity activity on at least 3 days equivalent to at least 1500 METmin/week or 7 or more days of any combination of walking, moderate- or vigorous-intensity activities equivalent to at least 3000 METmin/week [28,29].

2.5.2. Maximal Cycle Ergometer Test

Before the start of every test we screened participants for cardiac and/or pulmonary contraindications with the Physical Activity Readiness Questionnaire (PAR-Q) [30]. Participants performed a standard ramp protocol on a cycle ergometer starting with a 5 min warm-up (20 watt) followed by an increase in load with 10, 15 or 20 watt every minute, based on the level of the participant. Participants must keep up a speed of 60 to 80 revolutions per minute. The test endpoint was a decrease of 15 revolutions per minute; at this point the peak load (watt), peak heart rate (beats per minute (BPM)) and modified Borg scale were evaluated. A maximum effort was defined as achieving an arbitrary 85% of the predicted maximum heart rate [31]. The predicted maximum heart rate was calculated with the use of Tanaka's equation (maximum heart rate: $(208 - (0.7 \times age))$) [32]. The modified Borg scale provides insight into the subjectively perceived effort level and ranges from 0 (no effort at all) to 10 (maximum exhaustion) [33]. A measurement in which the participant did not perform a maximum effort was excluded from the analyses.

2.6. Statistical Methods

Physical activity category, weekly METs and sedentary behaviour minutes from the IPAQ responses were calculated according to standardized procedures [29]. Data distribution was evaluated using the Kolmogorov–Smirnov test. Baseline primary and secondary outcome measures were displayed as mean (standard deviation) in case of a normal distribution or as median (interquartile range (IQR)) in case of a non-normal distribution for continuous variables and as n (%) for categorical variables. Within-group and between-group differences over time were analysed with multilevel linear or logistic regression analyses for continuous and categorical variables, respectively. The reason being that mixed modelling is a preferred method when datasets have missing data and unbalanced time-points [34]. The model contained two levels comprising the participants and their repeated measures. Furthermore, the study group, logarithmic time and interactions were included as independent variables. In case of a non-normal distribution, we performed a bootstrap procedure with 10,000 samples in order to fulfil the assumption of normality for the multilevel regression analyses. The estimates of the models were displayed as means for multilevel linear regression analyses and as percentages for multilevel logistic regression analyses. Statistical significance was defined as $p < 0.05$. IBM SPSS statistics version 27.0 was used for multilevel linear analyses including the bootstrap procedure. SAS version 9.4 (SAS Institute Inc., Cary, NC, USA) was used for multilevel logistic regression analyses.

3. Results

For this RCT, we identified 561 eligible women between August 2010 and March 2016. Of these women, 352 were excluded for reasons further specified in Figure 1, and 26 women participated in the pilot study, which was not included in the final analysis. Eventually, 183 women were allocated to SMS+ ($n = 60$), SMS− ($n = 63$) or CAU ($n = 60$) and had a median age of 29 years (IQR 26–32) and median BMI of 32.8 kg/m^2 (IQR 30.1–36.1). At baseline, only a small proportion of the participants were classified into the low physical activity category, ranging between 4.4 and 12.2% for all groups. The proportions of participants in the moderate and high physical activity categories ranged from 24.4 to 35.6% and from 60.9 to 63.4%, respectively; differences were all non-significant. Walking METmin/week was significantly different at baseline between the SMS+ (792 METmin/week) and CAU groups (1931 METmin/week) ($p = 0.027$) but not when compared with the SMS− group (1148 METmin/week). However, total physical activity METmin/week was similar between the groups, with 3834 (2007–5567), 3911 (2084–6555) and 3960 (1973–8573) for SMS+, SMS− and CAU, respectively; see Table 2.

Table 2. Baseline characteristics.

	Lifestyle Intervention				Care as Usual	
	SMS+ $n = 60$	Missing Values	SMS− $n = 63$	Missing Values	$n = 60$	Missing Values
	n (%)	n	n (%)	n	n (%)	n
Nulliparous	47 (79.7)	1	47 (75.8)	1	44 (75.9)	2
Caucasian	30 (50.0)	-	21 (35.0)	3	25 (42.4)	1
Smoking	13 (21.7)	-	11 (17.7)	1	14 (23.7)	1
Alcohol consumption	12 (20.0)	-	15 (24.2)	1	19 (32.2)	1
Education						
Low	5 (8.3)	-	5 (8.2)	2	8 (14.3)	4
Intermediate	33 (55.0)	-	34 (55.7)	2	35 (62.5)	4
High	22 (36.7)	-	22 (36.1)	2	13 (23.2)	4
IPAQ physical activity category	$n = 45$		$n = 46$		$n = 41$	
Low	2 (4.4)		3 (6.5)		5 (12.2)	
Moderate	16 (35.6)		15 (32.6)		10 (24.4)	
High	27 (61.4)		28 (60.9)		26 (63.4)	
	Median (IQR)	Missing values n	Median (IQR)	Missing values n	Median (IQR)	Missing values n
Age (year)	28 (26–32)	-	30 (27–33)	1	28 (26–32)	-
Weight (kg)	95 (85–105)	-	89 (80–104)	1	84 (79–97)	-
BMI (kg/m^2)	33.5 (30.9–37.1)	-	33.6 (30.4–36.0)	1	30.6 (29.3–34.3)	-
Waist (cm)	102 (94–110)	4	100 (93–107)	4	96 (89–109)	1
IPAQ	$n = 46$		$n = 47$		$n = 43$	
Walking (METmin/week)	792 (330–2112)		1148 (446–2153)		1931 (512–4158)	
Moderate (METmin/week)	1935 (686–4447)		2160 (1050–4187)		1350 (720–3300)	
Vigorous (METmin/week)	960 (240–3840)		1096 (380–3540)		1440 (520–5280)	
Total physical activity (METmin/week)	3834 (2007–5567)		3911 (2084–6555)		3960 (1973–8573)	
Sitting (min/week)	2520 (1710–3630)		2730 (1725–3240)		2865 (1725–3360)	
Maximum cycle ergometer test	$n = 31$		$n = 23$			
Peak load	179 (148–210)		166 (134–208)		-	
Peak heart rate	173 (170–181)		168 (162–178)		-	
mBorg	7 (4–7)		6 (5–8)		-	

Note: Values are displayed as numbers (percentages) or as medians (interquartile range). Abbreviations: SMS+, lifestyle intervention with SMS support; SMS−, lifestyle intervention without SMS support; IQR, interquartile range; IPAQ, international physical activity questionnaire; BMI, body mass index; MET, metabolic equivalent of task; mBorg, modified Borg (rating of perceived exertion scale).

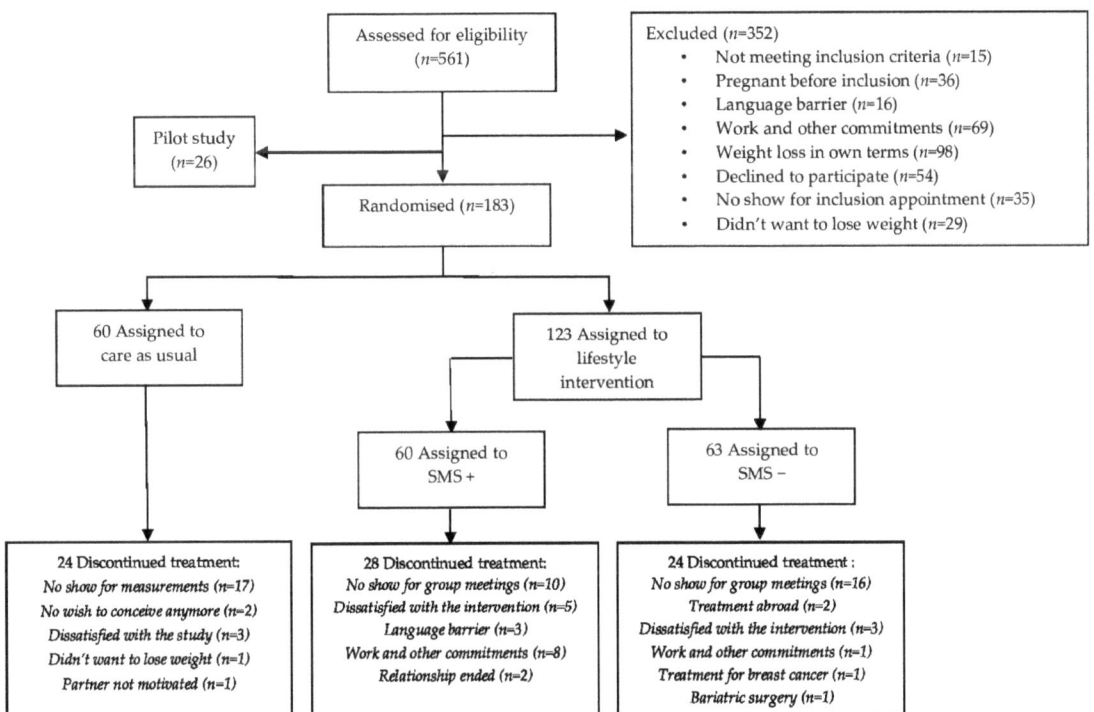

Figure 1. CONSORT flowchart.

3.1. Changes in Low, Moderate and High Physical Activity Categories Estimates

Remarkably, the biggest and statistically significant changes within the high, moderate and low physical activity categories were observed within the SMS+ group. There was a within-group increase of 31.0% (from 60.0% to 91.1%) in the high physical activity category over 12 months ($p = 0.007$) and a within-group decrease in moderate physical activity category (from 35.8% to 9.6%, Δ −26.1% within 12 months, $p = 0.018$). The low physical activity category within SMS+ did not change significantly (from 5.4% to 2.4%, Δ −3.0% within 12 months, $p = 0.358$). Within the SMS− group these differences were less prominent, with changes from 6.5% to 10.7% (Δ 4.2% within 12 months, $p = 0.443$) within the low category, 31.6% to 20.4% (Δ −11.3%, $p = 0.251$) within the moderate category and 62.6% to 69.6% (Δ 7.0% within 12 months, $p = 0.515$) within the high category. Moreover, for the CAU group there were changes from 9.5% to 8.7% (Δ −0.7% within 12 months, $p = 0.917$) in the low category, 25.6% to 18.4% (Δ −7.3%, $p = 0.453$) within the moderate category and 64.8% to 73.3% (Δ 8.4% within 12 months, $p = 0.442$) within the high category; see Figure 2. We did not observe any statistically significant between-group differences for changes in physical activity categories; see Table 3.

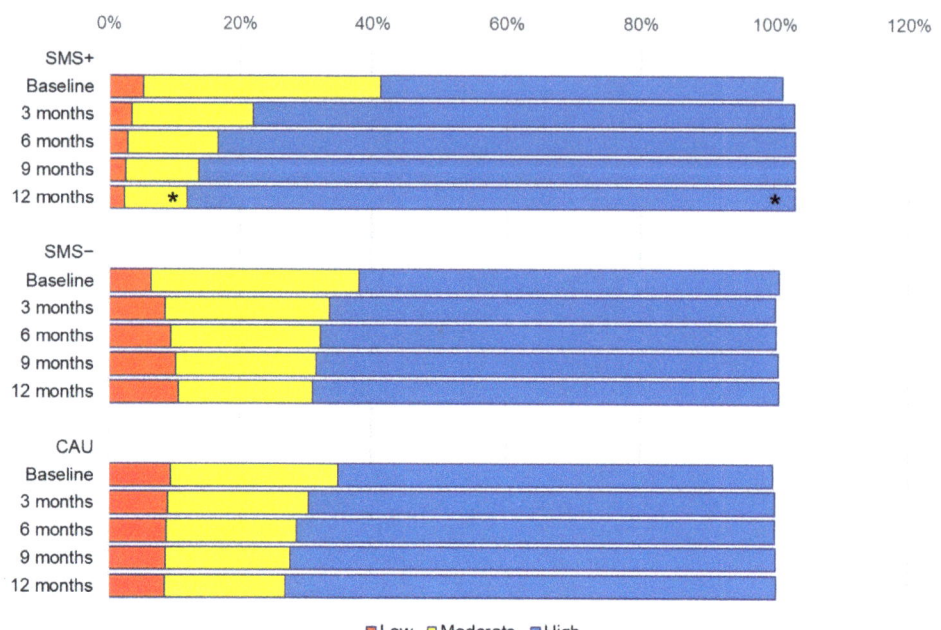

Figure 2. Changes in physical activity category estimates over time. Note: differences were tested with multilevel logistic regression analyses. * indicates significant within-group differences compared with baseline ($p < 0.05$). SMS+, lifestyle intervention with SMS support; SMS−, lifestyle intervention without SMS support; CAU, care as usual.

Table 3. Differences in physical activity categories and METmin/week between study groups at 12 months.

	SMS+ vs. CAU Difference	p Value	SMS− vs. CAU Difference	p Value	SMS+ vs. SMS− Difference	p Value
Category %						
Low	−2.2	0.312	4.9	0.543	−7.1	0.232
Moderate	−18.9	0.182	−4.0	0.823	−14.9	0.220
High	22.6	0.079	−1.5	0.922	24.0	0.060
Domains METmin/week						
Work	1574	0.293	1615	0.318	−42	0.981
Transport	−7	0.952	259	0.635	−266	0.479
Domestic and garden	−776	0.145	−264	0.665	−512	0.330
Leisure	547	0.502	−103	0.883	650	0.298
Intensity METmin/week						
Walking	1106	**0.047**	403	0.421	703	0.134
Moderate	−645	0.351	−508	0.417	−138	0.833
Vigorous	622	0.634	293	0.824	329	0.797
Total physical activity	2095	0.195	530	0.195	1565	0.243
Sedentary behaviour min/week						
Total sitting	−510	0.172	55	0.858	−565	0.141

Note: Differences were tested with multilevel logistic regression analyses for categorical variables, and with multilevel linear regression analyses for continuous variables, combined with a bootstrap procedure in case of a non-normal distribution. Boldface indicates significant difference ($p < 0.05$). Abbreviations: MET, metabolic equivalent of task; SMS+, lifestyle intervention with SMS support; SMS−, lifestyle intervention without SMS support; CAU, care as usual.

3.2. Physical Activity METminutes Estimates after 12 Months

Total physical activity METmin increased significantly within the SMS+ group, with 2175 METmin/week ($p = 0.043$), and non-significantly within the SMS− and CAU groups, with 610 METmin/week ($p = 0.460$) and 80 METmin/week ($p = 0.944$), respectively; see Figure 3. Between-group differences for total physical activity were non-significant. With regard to the different physical activity intensities, we observed a statistically significant higher increase in walking METmin/week within the timeframe of 12 months in the SMS+ group (from 1404 METmin/week to 2057 METmin/week) compared with the CAU group (from 2131 METmin/week to 1677 METmin/week) ($p = 0.047$, Δ 1106 METmin/week). Further details on estimated within-group and between-group physical activity changes within the different domains and for the different intensities are presented in Tables 3 and 4.

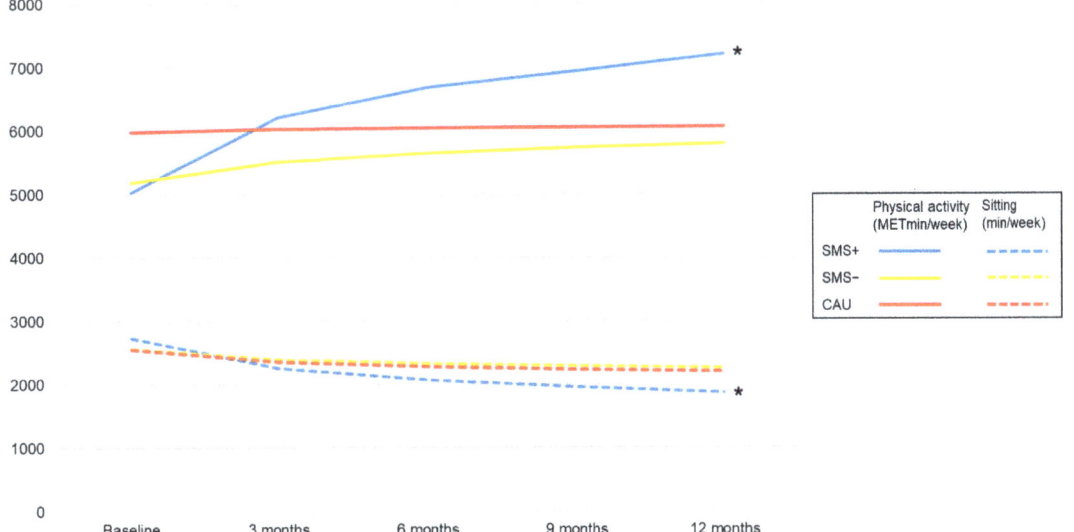

Figure 3. Changes in total physical activity METminutes and sitting behaviour minutes over time. Note: differences were tested with multilevel linear regression analyses, combined with a bootstrap procedure in case of a non-normal distribution. * indicates significant within-group differences ($p < 0.05$). MET, metabolic equivalent of task; min, minutes; SMS+, lifestyle intervention with SMS support; SMS−, lifestyle intervention without SMS support; CAU, care as usual.

3.3. Sedentary Behaviour Estimates after 12 Months

Sedentary behaviour decreased significantly within SMS+ from 2735 min/week at baseline to 1864 min/week at 12 months (Δ −871 min/week, $p = 0.005$). Additionally, a non-significant decrease was observed within SMS−, from 2563 min/week at baseline to 2257 min/week at 12 months (Δ −306 min/week, $p = 0.183$), and within CAU, from 2559 min/week at baseline to 2198 min/week at 12 months (Δ −361 min/week, $p = 0.157$); see Table 4. Between-group differences with regard to sitting minutes were non-significant; see Table 3.

Table 4. Within-group changes in METmin/week from baseline to 12 months.

IPAQ Responses	Group	Baseline	3 Months	6 Months	9 Months	12 Months		
n	SMS+	46	21	10	8	5		
n	SMS−	47	29	22	17	14		
n	CAU	43	21	28	21	11		
Domains METmin/week	Group	Baseline	3 months	6 months	9 months	12 months	Change	p value within
Work	SMS+	3704	3845	3902	3938	3964	260	0.858
	SMS−	3428	3591	3656	3698	3729	302	0.823
	CAU	5047	4337	4050	3867	3733	−1313	0.200
Transport	SMS+	1203	1169	1155	1147	1140	−63	0.826
	SMS−	987	1097	1141	1169	1190	203	0.421
	CAU	1217	1187	1174	1167	1161	−56	0.904
Domestic and garden	SMS+	1633	1392	1295	1233	1187	−446	0.251
	SMS−	1531	1567	1581	1590	1597	66	0.853
	CAU	1446	1624	1697	1743	1776	331	0.220
Leisure	SMS+	1348	1783	1959	2071	2153	805	0.132
	SMS−	1393	1477	1510	1532	1548	155	0.639
	CAU	1481	1620	1677	1713	1739	258	0.661
Intensity METmin/week	Group	Baseline	3 months	6 months	9 months	12 months	Change	p value within
Walking	SMS+	1404	1757	1899	1990	2057	652	0.063
	SMS−	1483	1455	1444	1437	1432	−51	0.879
	CAU	2131	1886	1787	1724	1677	−453	0.245
Moderate	SMS+	2505	2563	2587	2602	2613	107	0.833
	SMS−	2446	2579	2632	2666	2691	245	0.590
	CAU	2094	2500	2665	2769	2846	753	0.066
Vigorous	SMS+	2366	2415	2435	2448	2457	91	0.927
	SMS−	2609	2481	2429	2396	2371	−238	0.835
	CAU	3203	2916	2800	2726	2672	−531	0.660
Total physical activity	SMS+	5031	6207	6681	6984	7206	2175	**0.043**
	SMS−	5186	5516	5649	5734	5796	610	0.460
	CAU	5986	6029	6046	6057	6065	80	0.944
Sedentary min/week	Group	Baseline	3 months	6 months	9 months	12 months	Change	p value within
Total sitting	SMS+	2735	2265	2074	1953	1864	−871	**0.005**
	SMS−	2563	2397	2331	2288	2257	−306	0.183
	CAU	2559	2364	2285	2235	2198	−361	0.157

Note: Differences were tested with multilevel linear regression analyses combined with a bootstrap procedure in case of a non-normal distribution. Boldface indicates significant differences ($p < 0.05$). Abbreviations: IPAQ, international physical activity questionnaire; n, number; MET, metabolic equivalent of task; SMS+, lifestyle intervention with SMS support; SMS−, lifestyle intervention without SMS support; CAU, care as usual.

3.4. Aerobic Capacity Estimates after 12 Months within SMS+ and SMS−

We observed a significant increase in peak load resulting from the maximal cycle ergometer test within SMS+ from 177 watts at baseline to 187 watts at 12 months (Δ 10 watts (+5.5%) within 12 months, $p = 0.005$). For SMS−, this was 168 watts at baseline and 170 watts at 12 months (Δ 3 watts (+1.6%) within 12 months, $p = 0.102$). This was non-significant between the two groups ($p = 0.222$). Participants achieved on average 92–93% of the predicted maximum heart rate, which remained stable over the course of the study. The number of participants who delivered a maximum performance according to the pre-specified cut-off of ≥85% of the predicted maximum heart rate is further specified in Table 5.

Table 5. Within-group changes in maximal cycle ergometer test outcomes from baseline to 12 months.

	Group	Baseline	3 Months	6 Months	9 Months	12 Months	Change	p Value within	p Value between
Max performance n (total)	SMS+	31 (46)	22 (25)	13 (15)	11 (12)	9 (11)	-	-	-
	SMS−	23 (40)	25 (29)	19 (22)	14 (18)	16 (19)	-	-	-
Peak load (watts)	SMS+	177	182	184	186	187	10	**0.016**	0.222
	SMS−	168	169	170	170	170	3	0.516	
% of achieved maximum HR *	SMS+	93	93	93	93	93	0	0.557	0.195
	SMS−	92	93	93	93	93	1	0.228	
Peak HR (BPM)	SMS+	175	174	173	173	173	−2	0.226	0.173
	SMS−	172	172	173	173	173	1	0.442	
mBorg	SMS+	6	6	6	6	6	0	0.688	0.552
	SMS−	6	6	6	6	6	0	0.647	

Note: Differences were tested with multilevel linear regression analyses for continuous variables, combined with a bootstrap procedure in case of a non-normal distribution. Boldface indicates significant differences ($p < 0.05$). * Achieved maximum HR was calculated with the Tanaka equation. Abbreviations: SMS+, lifestyle intervention with SMS support; SMS−, lifestyle intervention without SMS support; HR, heart rate; BPM, beats per minute; mBorg, modified Borg (rating of perceived exertion scale).

4. Discussion

This randomized controlled study reports on physical activity outcomes following a three-component lifestyle intervention with or without additional SMS support. Apart from an increase in walking METmin/week in the SMS+ group compared with the CAU group after one year, we did not observe any other statistically significant between-group differences. However, the SMS+ group was successful at improving categories of self-reported physical activity and also demonstrated a statistically significant positive within-group effect on aerobic capacity and decreased weekly sitting minutes.

Other lifestyle interventions have described positive health benefits as a result of increased physical activity behaviour. Modest increases in step count were associated with reduced levels of inflammatory markers in women with PCOS [35]. Both high-intensity interval training (HIIT) and continuous aerobic exercise training have shown to improve reproductive function [36], anthropometrics and some cardiometabolic health markers [37,38]. However, HIIT has shown to offer greater improvements in aerobic capacity, insulin sensitivity and menstrual cyclicity and larger reductions in hyperandrogenism compared with moderate intensity training [39]. In the end, a recent meta-analysis concluded that improvements in health outcomes were more dependent on exercise intensity rather than dose [40]. However, especially with regard to adherence to a lifestyle intervention in this population, one should keep in mind an individual's personal and cultural preferences when composing an exercise program in order to make it a sustainable lifestyle change. This may sometimes mean that health care providers should focus more on increasing general daily physical activity rather that promoting vigorous exercise.

Weekly sitting minutes decreased significantly within the SMS+ group during our one-year lifestyle intervention. Sedentary behaviour is extremely prevalent in the PCOS population [13], and positive associations were found between increased sitting time and weight gain [14,41], as well as PCOS symptom severity [42]. In the general population, sedentary behaviour is linked to all-cause mortality and adverse health impacts [11,12]. Therefore, one of the most important aspects should be to diminish sedentary behaviour in women with PCOS who struggle with weight loss or weight maintenance.

The lifestyle intervention with SMS support demonstrated a statistically significant within-group increase in peak workload over the course of the study. However, the clinical relevance of the magnitude of this finding can be questioned. Notable improvements in aerobic capacity are generally to be expected following an increase in moderate and, especially, vigorous exercise [39,43]. An explanation for the modest improvements could be that one of the main goals of our lifestyle program was to encourage the implementation of a combination of moderate, vigorous and muscle-strengthening activities in the participant's daily routine [23,27] and was therefore not designed as an intense, solely high-intensity exercise intervention. There are no studies that clearly define the clinical relevance of changes in peak workload or IPAQ responses in women with PCOS and excess weight. However, evidence does exists on the effect of weight loss and favourable changes in aerobic capacity [44]. Around 85.7% of the women in the SMS+ group achieved >5% weight loss [24], suggesting that the improvements in body weight might have positively impacted the results on peak workload. Furthermore, the observed positive changes to the high category at least indicates an increase in general weekly physical activity. Walking METmin/week improved more in the SMS+ group, corresponding to an increase of almost 30 min daily walking activity. Taking more steps per day has been found to be associated with a progressively lower risk of all-cause mortality in the general population [45]. Moreover, the decrease in sitting behaviour minutes, which in the SMS+ group amounted to several hours a day, may also be seen as a significant improvement. One could hypothesize that the above-mentioned findings do count as clinically relevant in this population of women with PCOS in which lifestyle habits are known to be difficult to improve [46].

A strength of our study was the use of tailored SMS in order to encourage and reinforce positive behavioural changes and increase physical activity. Although the PCOS guidelines recommend considering the use of mobile health applications for this purpose, limited evidence is available on the effectiveness of this method. In general, studies have suggested that the use of mobile technology for health promotion might be effective in improving long-term health-related outcomes [47,48]. Recently, a study concluded that a mobile health application, in addition to a lifestyle modification program, could decrease BMI, waist circumference, anxiety and depression and improve exercise and diet adherence in patients with PCOS in the long term [49]. Furthermore, another mobile health application called 'AskPCOS' has been recently developed in response to the specific needs of women with PCOS [50,51]. These are all indications that the use of supporting mobile health technology has a positive effect on behavioural changes and should be used to motivate adherence to a healthy lifestyle in the PCOS population.

A limitation of the study is recall bias for weekly physical activity measured with IPAQ, which is a common problem in retrospective assessment with questionnaires. Self-reporting can cause over- and underestimation of weekly physical activity that may bias the results [52]. However, the IPAQ is an internationally used questionnaire with acceptable measurement properties and is at least as good as other established self-reporting methods [28]. In order to address the above-mentioned limitations, specific rules for processing data were applied according to the IPAQ protocol [29]. Nonetheless, the IPAQ data provide a good reflection of the participant's weekly activities. Future studies should consider using devices such as an accelerometer or pedometer in order to objectively measure physical activity. Furthermore, when interpreting the results, one should keep in mind that this randomized controlled trial was powered on weight loss (primary outcome) and not on physical activity [23]. Additionally, the preferred assessment of aerobic capacity is measuring the maximum amount of oxygen uptake during exercise (VO_2max) [53], which can be conducted using an open-circuit spirometry method. By measuring the gas exchange, the oxygen demands of the skeletal muscles during maximal physical exercise give a reflection of the peak capacity of the participant's cardiovascular and pulmonary systems [54]. Open-circuit spirometry was not performed in our study population. However, VO_2max is closely related to exercise workload. Therefore, the interpretation of the results of these two outcomes are comparable, although conclusions should be interpreted with caution. Finally, one could also interpret the absence of maximum cycle ergometer tests in the CAU group as a limitation. However, this was implemented intentionally because any form of interference could have influenced the control group's actions. A recurrent maximal cycle ergometer test is not in line with care as usual and therefore could have impaired the results from the control group.

5. Conclusions

Apart from an increase in walking activity in SMS+, no other between-group differences were found in this one-year three-component lifestyle intervention. However, based on within-group results, additional SMS support seemed superior in improving physical activity and aerobic capacity and decreasing sedentary behaviour in overweight and obese women with PCOS and a wish to become pregnant. Future adequately powered studies should be performed in order to confirm this positive tendency for eHealth options in the promotion of a physically active lifestyle.

Author Contributions: Conceptualization, A.D.d.L., G.J., R.v.d.B.-E., Y.L., A.B., J.v.B. and J.L.; data curation, A.D.d.L. and G.J.; formal analysis, A.D.d.L.; investigation, A.D.d.L. and G.J.; methodology, A.D.d.L., G.J., R.v.d.B.-E., Y.L., A.B., J.v.B. and J.L.; project administration, A.D.d.L., G.J. and J.L.; supervision, J.L.; writing—original draft, A.D.d.L.; writing—review and editing, A.D.d.L., G.J., R.v.d.B.-E., Y.L., A.B., J.v.B. and J.L. All authors have read and agreed to the published version of the manuscript.

Funding: This research received no external funding.

Institutional Review Board Statement: The study was conducted according to the guidelines of the Declaration of Helsinki and approved by the Medical Research Ethics Committee of the Erasmus MC in Rotterdam (MEC-2008-337, date of approval: 4 December 2008).

Informed Consent Statement: Informed consent was obtained from all subjects involved in the study.

Data Availability Statement: The data presented in this study are available on request from the corresponding author. The data are not publicly available due to privacy restrictions.

Acknowledgments: We thank the entire PCOS team of the Erasmus MC.

Conflicts of Interest: A.D., G.J., R.B., Y.L., A.B. and J.B. have nothing to declare. J.L. reports grants from Ansh Labs, Webster, Tx, USA, from Ferring, Hoofddorp, NL, from Dutch Heart Association, Utrecht, NL, from Zon MW, Amsterdam, NL, from Roche Diagnostics, Rothkreuz, Switzerland and personal fees from Ferring, Hoofddorp, NL, from Titus Healthcare, Hoofddorp, NL, from Gedeon Richter, Groot-Bijgaarden, Belgium and is an unpaid board member and president of the AE-PCOS Society outside the submitted work.

References

1. Teede, H.J.; Misso, M.L.; Costello, M.F.; Dokras, A.; Laven, J.; Moran, L.; Piltonen, T.; Norman, R.J.; on behalf of theInternational PCOS Network. Recommendations from the international evidence-based guideline for the assessment and management of polycystic ovary syndrome. *Fertil. Steril.* **2018**, *110*, 364–379. [CrossRef] [PubMed]
2. Lim, S.; Davies, M.; Norman, R.; Moran, L. Overweight, obesity and central obesity in women with polycystic ovary syndrome: A systematic review and meta-analysis. *Hum. Reprod. Update* **2012**, *18*, 618–637. [CrossRef]
3. Lim, S.S.; Norman, R.J.; Davies, M.J.; Moran, L.J. The effect of obesity on polycystic ovary syndrome: A systematic review and meta-analysis. *Obes. Rev.* **2013**, *14*, 95–109. [CrossRef] [PubMed]
4. Glueck, C.J.; Goldenberg, N. Characteristics of obesity in polycystic ovary syndrome: Etiology, treatment, and genetics. *Metabolism* **2019**, *92*, 108–120. [CrossRef] [PubMed]
5. Glueck, C.J.; Goldenberg, N. Fitness vs. Fatness on all-Cause Mortality: A Meta-Analysis. *Prog. Cardiovasc. Dis.* **2014**, *56*, 382–390.
6. Koivula, R.W.; Tornberg, A.B.; Franks, P.W. Exercise and diabetes-related cardiovascular disease: Systematic review of published evidence from observational studies and clinical trials. *Curr. Diab. Rep.* **2013**, *13*, 372–380. [CrossRef]
7. Nicolucci, A.; Balducci, S.; Cardelli, P.; Cavallo, S.; Fallucca, S.; Bazuro, A.; Simonelli, P.; Iacobini, C.; Zanuso, S.; Pugliese, G.; et al. Relationship of exercise volume to improvements of quality of life with supervised exercise training in patients with type 2 diabetes in a randomised controlled trial: The Italian Diabetes and Exercise Study (IDES). *Diabetologia* **2012**, *55*, 579–588. [CrossRef]
8. Caspersen, C.J.; Powell, K.E.; Christenson, G.M. Physical activity, exercise, and physical fitness: Definitions and distinctions for health-related research. *Public Health Rep.* **1985**, *100*, 126–131.
9. Lum, D.; Barbosa, T.M. Brief Review: Effects of Isometric Strength Training on Strength and Dynamic Performance. *Int. J. Sports Med.* **2019**, *40*, 363–375. [CrossRef]

10. Tremblay, M.S.; Aubert, S.; Barnes, J.D.; Saunders, T.J.; Carson, V.; Latimer-Cheung, A.E.; Chastin, S.F.M.; Altenburg, T.M.; Chinapaw, M.J.M. Sedentary Behavior Research Network (SBRN)–Terminology Consensus Project process and outcome. *Int. J. Behav. Nutr. Phys. Act.* **2017**, *14*, 75. [CrossRef]
11. Biddle, S.J.; Bennie, J.A.; Bauman, A.E.; Chau, J.Y.; Dunstan, D.; Owen, N.; Stamatakis, E.; van Uffelen, J.G.Z. Too much sitting and all-cause mortality: Is there a causal link? *BMC Public Health* **2016**, *16*, 635. [CrossRef]
12. Ekelund, U.; Steene-Johannessen, J. Does physical activity attenuate, or even eliminate, the detrimental association of sitting time with mortality? A harmonised meta-analysis of data from more than 1 million men and women. *Lancet* **2016**, *388*, 1302–1310. [CrossRef] [PubMed]
13. Tay, C.T.; Moran, L.J.; Harrison, C.L.; Brown, E.J. Physical activity and sedentary behaviour in women with and without polycystic ovary syndrome: An Australian population-based cross-sectional study. *Clin. Endocrinol.* **2020**, *93*, 154–162. [CrossRef] [PubMed]
14. Moran, L.J.; Ranasinha, S.; Zoungas, S.; McNaughton, S.; Brown, W.J.; Teede, H. The contribution of diet, physical activity and sedentary behaviour to body mass index in women with and without polycystic ovary syndrome. *Hum. Reprod* **2013**, *28*, 2276–2283. [CrossRef] [PubMed]
15. Dona, S.; Bacchi, E.; Moghetti, P. Is Cardiorespiratory Fitness Impaired in PCOS Women? A Review of the Literature. *J. Endocrinol. Investig.* **2017**, *40*, 463–469. [CrossRef]
16. Orio, F., Jr.; Giallauria, F.; Palomba, S.; Cascella, T.; Manguso, F.; Vuolo, L.; Russo, T.; Tolino, A.; Lombardi, G.; Colao, A.; et al. Cardiopulmonary Impairment in Young Women with Polycystic Ovary Syndrome. *J. Clin. Endocrinol. Metab.* **2006**, *91*, 2967–2971. [CrossRef]
17. Wang, Z.; Groen, H.; Cantineau, A.E.P.; van Elten, T.M.; Karsten, M.D.A.; van Oers, A.M.; Mol, B.W.J.; Roseboom, T.J.; Hoek, A. Dietary Intake, Eating Behavior, Physical Activity, and Quality of Life in Infertile Women with PCOS and Obesity Compared with Non-PCOS Obese Controls. *Nutrients* **2021**, *13*, 3526. [CrossRef]
18. Lim, S.; Smith, C.A.; Costello, M.F.; MacMillan, F.; Moran, L.; Ee, C. Barriers and facilitators to weight management in overweight and obese women living in Australia with PCOS: A qualitative study. *BMC Endocr. Disord* **2019**, *19*, 106. [CrossRef]
19. Lee, S.; Patel, P.; Myers, N.D.; Pfeiffer, K.A.; Smith, A.L. A Systematic Review of eHealth Interventions to Promote Physical Activity in Adults with Obesity or Overweight. *Behav. Med.* **2022**, 1–18. [CrossRef]
20. Fjeldsoe, B.S.; Marshall, A.L.; Miller, J.D. Behavior change interventions delivered by mobile telephone short-message service. *Am. J. Prev. Med.* **2009**, *36*, 165–173. [CrossRef]
21. Dijkstra, A.; de Vries, H. The development of computer-generated tailored interventions. *Patient. Educ. Couns.* **1999**, *36*, 193–203. [CrossRef] [PubMed]
22. Ryan, P.; Lauver, D.R. The efficacy of tailored interventions. *J. Nurs. Sch.* **2002**, *34*, 331–337. [CrossRef]
23. Jiskoot, G.; Benneheij, S.; Beerthuizen, A.; de Niet, J.; de Klerk, C.; Timman, R.; Busschbach, J.; Laven, J. A three-component cognitive behavioural lifestyle program for preconceptional weight-loss in women with polycystic ovary syndrome (PCOS): A protocol for a randomized controlled trial. *Reprod Health* **2017**, *14*, 34. [CrossRef] [PubMed]
24. Jiskoot, G.; Timman, R.; Beerthuizen, A.; De Loos, A.D.; Busschbach, J.; Laven, J. Weight Reduction Through a Cognitive Behavioral Therapy Lifestyle Intervention in PCOS: The Primary Outcome of a Randomized Controlled Trial. *Obesity* **2020**, *28*, 2134–2141. [CrossRef] [PubMed]
25. Rotterdam, E.A.; ASRM. Revised 2003 consensus on diagnostic criteria and long-term health risks related to polycystic ovary syndrome. *Fertil Steril.* **2004**, *81*, 19–25.
26. Brink, E.; van Rossum, C.; Postma-Smeets, A.; Stafleu, A.; Wolvers, D.; van Dooren, C.; Toxopeus, I.; Buurma-Rethans, E.; Geurts, M.; Ocké, M. Development of healthy and sustainable food-based dietary guidelines for the Netherlands. *Public Health Nutr.* **2019**, *22*, 2419–2435. [CrossRef]
27. WHO. *Global Recommendations on Physical Activity for Health*; World Health Organization: Geneva, Switzerland, 2010.
28. Craig, C.L.; Marshall, A.L.; Sjöström, M.; Bauman, A.E. International physical activity questionnaire: 12-country reliability and validity. *Med. Sci. Sport. Exerc.* **2003**, *35*, 1381–1395. [CrossRef]
29. Committee, I.R. Guidelines for Data Processing and Analysis of the International Physical Activity Questionnaire (IPAQ)-Short and Long Forms. 2005. Available online: http://www.ipaq.ki.se/scoring.pdf (accessed on 1 February 2023).
30. Thomas, S.; Reading, J.; Shephard, R.J. Revision of the Physical Activity Readiness Questionnaire (PAR-Q). *Can J. Sport. Sci.* **1992**, *17*, 338–345.
31. Van der Steeg, G.E.; Takken, T. Reference values for maximum oxygen uptake relative to body mass in Dutch/Flemish subjects aged 6-65 years: The LowLands Fitness Registry. *Eur. J. Appl. Physiol.* **2021**, *121*, 1189–1196. [CrossRef]
32. Tanaka, H.; Monahan, K.D.; Seals, D.R. Age-predicted maximal heart rate revisited. *J. Am. Coll. Cardiol.* **2001**, *37*, 153–156. [CrossRef]
33. Borg, G.A. Psychophysical bases of perceived exertion. *Med. Sci. Sport. Exerc.* **1982**, *14*, 377–381. [CrossRef]
34. Little, R.; Rubin, D. *Statistical Analysis with Missing Data*; John Wiley and Sons: New York, NY, USA, 1987.
35. Webb, M.A.; Mani, H.; Robertson, S.J.; Waller, H.L.; Webb, D.R.; Edwardson, C.L.; Bodicoat, D.H.; Yates, T.; Khunti, K.; Davies, M. Moderate increases in daily step count are associated with reduced IL6 and CRP in women with PCOS. *Endocr. Connect.* **2018**, *7*, 1442–1447. [CrossRef] [PubMed]

36. Nybacka, Å.; Carlström, K.; Ståhle, A.; Nyren, S.; Hellström, P.M.; Hirschberg, A.L. Randomized comparison of the influence of dietary management and/or physical exercise on ovarian function and metabolic parameters in overweight women with polycystic ovary syndrome. *Fertil. Steril.* **2011**, *96*, 1508–1513. [CrossRef] [PubMed]
37. Benham, J.L.; Booth, J.E.; Corenblum, B.; Doucette, S.; Friedenreich, C.M. Exercise training and reproductive outcomes in women with polycystic ovary syndrome: A pilot randomized controlled trial. *Clin. Endocrinol.* **2021**, *95*, 332–343. [CrossRef]
38. Roessler, K.K.; Birkebaek, C.; Ravn, P.; Andersen, M.S.; Glintborg, D. Effects of exercise and group counselling on body composition and VO2max in overweight women with polycystic ovary syndrome. *Acta Obs. Gynecol. Scand.* **2013**, *92*, 272–277. [CrossRef]
39. Patten, R.K.; McIlvenna, L.C.; Levinger, I.; Garnham, A.P.; Shorakae, S.; Parker, A.G.; McAinch, A.J.; Rodgers, R.J.; Hiam, D.; Moreno-Asso, A.; et al. High-intensity training elicits greater improvements in cardio-metabolic and reproductive outcomes than moderate-intensity training in women with polycystic ovary syndrome: A randomized clinical trial. *Hum. Reprod.* **2022**, *37*, 1018–1029. [CrossRef] [PubMed]
40. Patten, R.K.; Boyle, R.A.; Moholdt, T.; Kiel, I.; Hopkins, W.G.; Harrison, C.L.; Stepto, N.K. Exercise Interventions in Polycystic Ovary Syndrome: A Systematic Review and Meta-Analysis. *Front. Physiol.* **2020**, *11*, 606. [CrossRef]
41. Awoke, M.A.; Earnest, A.; Joham, A.E.; Hodge, A.M.; Teede, H.J.; Brown, W.J.; Moran, L.J. Weight gain and lifestyle factors in women with and without polycystic ovary syndrome. *Hum. Reprod.* **2021**, *37*, 129–141. [CrossRef]
42. Ashraf, S.; Aslam, R.; Bashir, I.; Majeed, I.; Jamshaid, M. Environmental determinants and PCOS symptoms severity: A cross-sectional study. *Health Care Women Int.* **2022**, *43*, 98–113. [CrossRef]
43. Nasiri, M.; Monazzami, A.; Alavimilani, S.; Asemi, Z. The Effect of High Intensity Intermittent and Combined (Resistant and Endurance) Trainings on Some Anthropometric Indices and Aerobic Performance in Women with Polycystic Ovary Syndrome: A Randomized Controlled Clinical Trial Study. *Int. J. Fertil. Steril.* **2022**, *16*, 268–274.
44. De Souza, S.A.F.; Faintuch, J.; Sant'Anna, A.F. Effect of weight loss on aerobic capacity in patients with severe obesity before and after bariatric surgery. *Obes. Surg.* **2010**, *20*, 871–875. [CrossRef] [PubMed]
45. Paluch, A.E.; Bajpai, S.; Bassett, D.R.; Carnethon, M.R.; Ekelund, U.; Evenson, K.R.; Galuska, D.A.; Jefferis, B.J.; Kraus, W.E.; Lee, I.-M.; et al. Daily steps and all-cause mortality: A meta-analysis of 15 international cohorts. *Lancet Public Health* **2022**, *7*, e219–e228. [CrossRef] [PubMed]
46. Ee, C.; Pirotta, S.; Mousa, A.; Moran, L.; Lim, S. Providing lifestyle advice to women with PCOS: An overview of practical issues affecting success. *BMC Endocr. Disord.* **2021**, *21*, 234. [CrossRef] [PubMed]
47. Qiang, C.Z.; Yamamichi, M.; Hausman, V.; Altman, D.; Unit, I.S. *Mobile Applications for the Health Sector*; World Bank: Washington, DC, USA, 2011; Volume 2.
48. Wang, L.; Guo, Y.; Wang, M.; Zhao, Y. A mobile health application to support self-management in patients with chronic obstructive pulmonary disease: A randomised controlled trial. *Clin. Rehabil.* **2021**, *35*, 90–101. [CrossRef]
49. Wang, L.; Liu, Y.; Tan, H.; Huang, S. Transtheoretical model-based mobile health application for PCOS. *Reprod. Health* **2022**, *19*, 117. [CrossRef]
50. Boyle, J.A.; Xu, R.; Gilbert, E.; Kuczynska-Burggraf, M.; Tan, B.; Teede, H.; Vincent, A.; Gibson-Helm, M.; Boyle, J.A. Ask PCOS: Identifying Need to Inform Evidence-Based App Development for Polycystic Ovary Syndrome. *Semin. Reprod. Med.* **2018**, *36*, 59–65.
51. Xie, J.; Burstein, F.; Teede, H.J.; Boyle, J.A.; Garad, R. Personalized Mobile Tool AskPCOS Delivering Evidence-Based Quality Information about Polycystic Ovary Syndrome. *Semin. Reprod. Med.* **2018**, *36*, 66–72. [CrossRef]
52. Althubaiti, A. Information bias in health research: Definition, pitfalls, and adjustment methods. *J. Multidiscip. Healthc* **2016**, *9*, 211–217. [CrossRef]
53. Fletcher, G.F.; Ades, P.A.; Kligfield, P.; Arena, P. Exercise standards for testing and training: A scientific statement from the American Heart Association. *Circulation* **2013**, *128*, 873–934. [CrossRef]
54. Kokkinos, P.; Kaminsky, L.A.; Arena, R.; Zhang, J.; Myers, J. A new generalized cycle ergometry equation for predicting maximal oxygen uptake: The Fitness Registry and the Importance of Exercise National Database (FRIEND). *Eur. J. Prev. Cardiol.* **2018**, *25*, 1077–1082. [CrossRef]

Disclaimer/Publisher's Note: The statements, opinions and data contained in all publications are solely those of the individual author(s) and contributor(s) and not of MDPI and/or the editor(s). MDPI and/or the editor(s) disclaim responsibility for any injury to people or property resulting from any ideas, methods, instructions or products referred to in the content.

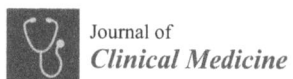 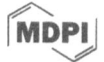

Article

How to Choose the Optimal Starting Dose of Clomiphene Citrate (50 or 100 mg per Day) for a First Cycle of Ovulation Induction in Anovulatory PCOS Women?

Lucie Huyghe [1], Camille Robin [1], Agathe Dumont [1], Christine Decanter [1], Maeva Kyheng [2,3], Didier Dewailly [4,5], Sophie Catteau-Jonard [1,4,5,6] and Geoffroy Robin [1,4,5,6,*]

[1] Department of Reproductive Medicine and Fertility Preservation, Lille University Hospital, 59000 Lille, France; doclhuyghe@gmail.com (L.H.); camille.robin@chu-lille.fr (C.R.); agathe.dumont@hotmail.fr (A.D.); sophie.jonard@chu-lille.fr (S.C.-J.)
[2] Department of Biostatistics, Lille University Hospital, 59000 Lille, France
[3] ULR 2694—METRICS: Evaluation des Technologies de Santé et des Pratiques Médicales, University of Lille, 59000 Lille, France
[4] Faculty of Medicine, University of Lille, 59000 Lille, France
[5] UMRS-1172, Laboratory of Development and Plasticity of the Neuroendocrine Brain, Jean-Pierre Aubert Research Centre, 59000 Lille, France
[6] Department of Medical Gynecology and Sexology, Lille University Hospital, 59000 Lille, France
* Correspondence: geoffroy.robin@chu-lille.fr

Abstract: Research question: Clomiphene citrate (CC) is one of the first-line treatments for ovulation induction in women with anovulatory polycystic ovary syndrome (PCOS). However, nearly 1 out of 2 women is resistant to 50 mg/day of CC. The objective of this study is to investigate the clinical, biological, and/or ultrasound factors that may predict the resistance to 50 mg/day of CC in the first cycle of treatment in women with anovulatory PCOS. This would make it possible to identify PCOS patients to whom the dose of 100 mg/day would be offered as of the first cycle. Design: A retrospective and monocentric study was conducted on 283 women with anovulatory PCOS who required the use of ovulation induction with CC (903 cycles). Results: During the first cycle of treatment, 104 patients (36.8%) were resistant to 50 mg/day of CC. Univariate regression analysis showed that patients who resisted 50 mg/day of CC had significantly higher BMI, waist circumference, serum levels of AMH, total testosterone, Δ4-androstenedione, 17-OHP, and insulin ($p < 0.05$), compared to patients ovulating with this dose. Serum levels of SHBG were significantly lower in patients resistant to 50 mg/day ($p < 0.05$). After multivariate analysis, only AMH and SHBG remained statistically significant ($p = 0.01$ and $p = 0.001$, respectively). However, areas under the ROC curves were weak (0.59 and 0.68, respectively). Conclusion: AMH and SHBG are the only two parameters significantly associated with the risk of resistance to 50 mg/day of CC. However, no satisfactory thresholds have been established to predict resistance to 50 mg CC.

Keywords: polycystic ovary syndrome; clomiphene citrate; ovulation induction; antimullerian hormone; sex hormone binding globulin

Citation: Huyghe, L.; Robin, C.; Dumont, A.; Decanter, C.; Kyheng, M.; Dewailly, D.; Catteau-Jonard, S.; Robin, G. How to Choose the Optimal Starting Dose of Clomiphene Citrate (50 or 100 mg per Day) for a First Cycle of Ovulation Induction in Anovulatory PCOS Women? *J. Clin. Med.* **2023**, *12*, 4943. https://doi.org/10.3390/jcm12154943

Academic Editor: Enrico Carmina

Received: 12 May 2023
Revised: 13 July 2023
Accepted: 26 July 2023
Published: 27 July 2023

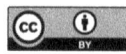

Copyright: © 2023 by the authors. Licensee MDPI, Basel, Switzerland. This article is an open access article distributed under the terms and conditions of the Creative Commons Attribution (CC BY) license (https://creativecommons.org/licenses/by/4.0/).

1. Introduction

Polycystic ovary syndrome (PCOS) is the most common endocrine disorder in women of childbearing age, with a prevalence ranging from 4% to 21%, depending on the diagnostic criteria used [1]. The presentation of this syndrome is very heterogeneous, with variable clinical expression, including usually menstrual cycle disorders, hyperandrogenism, and/or infertility [2]. Since 2004, the ESHRE/ASRM Rotterdam Consensus criteria are the most commonly used for the diagnosis of PCOS [3].

PCOS is the mean etiology of infertility due to anovulation [2,4,5]. Clomiphene citrate (CC) and letrozole are the first-line treatment for ovulation induction in PCOS [4–6]. Both

CC and letrozole are successful in inducing pregnancy. A recent meta-analysis confirms a moderate but significant superiority of letrozole over clomiphene citrate [7]. Thus, in countries where letrozole is off-label for ovulation induction, such as France, CC is used as a first-line treatment for ovulation induction in PCOS women [6].

CC is a selective modulator of estrogen receptors exerting anti-estrogenic activity at the hypothalamic level. CC enhances the pulsatile release of GnRH. This will result in an increase in the secretion of endogenous gonadotropins and especially follicle-stimulating hormone (FSH) by the anterior pituitary gland, allowing cyclic follicular growth [2,8–10]. The recommended starting dose of CC is 50 mg/day for 5 days. If ovulation is not achieved, the dose will then be increased by 50 mg/day for 5 days in the next cycle, up to a maximum dose of 150 mg/day for 5 days [11,12]. As reported by some authors, the ovulation rate with this treatment can be as high as 75–80% [10,11]. Despite the relatively high efficacy of CC, approximately 15–40% of patients will not respond to the maximum recommended dose of 150 mg/day for 5 days and will be considered resistant to this treatment [13–16].

Several studies have investigated factors that may potentially predict CC resistance, comparing treatment-sensitive patients with those resistant to CC 150 mg/day. Thus, obesity, insulin resistance, hyperandrogenism, and excess AMH are among the most common factors associated with CC resistance [4,17–19]. Genetic predisposition would also play a role in CC resistance [20]. However, all these studies failed to identify clinical, hormonal, metabolic, or ultrasound factors which could predict with certainty a complete resistance to CC. Thus, in countries where clomiphene citrate is the only first-line treatment available for ovulation induction in PCOS women, there is, therefore, no factor that would make it possible to immediately opt for second-line treatments (ovarian drilling or ovulation induction with gonadotropins) [4–6]. Therefore, it would be interesting to investigate clinical, biological, and/or ultrasound factors that may predict resistance to the initial CC dose of 50 mg/day. Indeed, nearly 1 in 2 women is resistant to 50 mg/day of CC [18,21]. Identifying this or these factor(s) would allow starting the treatment at a higher dose (100 mg/day) at once. This would save significant time for patients who are resistant to 50 mg/day of CC. Moreover, the fact of being able to achieve pregnancy more quickly also theoretically limits the risk of having to use second-line treatments: either injectable gonadotropins or laparoscopic ovarian drilling [4–6]. These two treatments are both more expensive and more prone to complications (e.g., higher risk of multiple pregnancies with injectable gonadotropins, requiring rigorous ultrasound and hormonal monitoring, or the operative and anesthetic risks of ovarian drilling) rather than first-line ovulation inducers such as clomiphene citrate [5,22]. To our knowledge, no study has investigated this issue.

The main objective of our study was, therefore, to investigate the clinical, biological, and/or ultrasound parameters which would predict resistance to CC at 50 mg/day in women with anovulatory PCOS. The secondary objective was to determine the effectiveness of anovulation management with this ovulation inducer in the whole cohort by trying to determine the optimal number of initiated cycles and ovulatory cycles to offer to these PCOS women.

2. Materials and Methods

2.1. Population

This is a retrospective, single-center study conducted between May 2003 and December 2020 in the Reproductive Medicine Department of Lille University Hospital in France. As this study was retrospective and without intervention, the opinion of the Ethics Committee on the study was not required. All patients had given prior consent for the use of their clinical, hormonal, and ultrasound records. On 16 December 2019, the Institutional Review Board of the Lille University Hospital gave unrestricted approval for the anonymous use of all patients' clinical, hormonal, and ultrasound records (reference DEC20150715-0002).

All anovulatory PCOS women treated with a starting dose of CC at 50 mg/day were included in the study. The diagnosis of PCOS was based on the Rotterdam criteria published in 2003 [3]. Two of the following three criteria had to be present for diagnosis:

(1) Oligo- or anovulation (OA): oligomenorrhea (<8 cycles per year), amenorrhea (absence of menses > 3 months) or regular anovulatory cycles (menstrual cycles between 26 and 34 days but with no progesterone increase above 3 ng/mL 7 to 8 days before menstruation [23]); all the women in our study suffer from OA. (2) Clinical hyperandrogenism (HA) (modified Ferriman and Gallwey score ≥ 7 in our Caucasian population [24] or biological hyperandrogenism (total testosteronemia ≥ 0.50 ng/mL, as previously described [25,26]). (3) Ultrasound polycystic ovaries (PCOM): ovarian volume ≥ 10 mL [27,28] and/or ovarian surface area ≥ 5.5 cm^2 [25], and/or FNPO (follicle number per ovary) ≥ 12 from 2003 to 2007 [3,27] (ultrasound scanner: General Electric Logic 400, Milwaukee, equipped with a 7 MHz endovaginal probe), then FNPO ≥ 19 from 2008 (ultrasound scanner: General Electric Voluson E8, equipped with a 5 to 9 MHz endovaginal probe) [26]. The presence of elevated AMH was considered equivalent to the presence of polycystic ovaries on ultrasound (serum AMH ≥ 35 pmol/L), as previously reported [26,29,30]. The PCOS phenotype was then identified for each patient, according to the NIH 2012 extension of the Rotterdam classification [1], as described above [30]: phenotype A (OA + HA + PCOM), phenotype B (OA + HA), phenotype D (OA + PCOM). Given our inclusion criteria, phenotype C (HA + PCOM = ovulatory PCOS) is not present in our population.

The exclusion criteria were women aged under 18 years or over 43 years, other etiologies of hyperandrogenism or dysovulation (hyperprolactinemia, nonclassical adrenal hyperplasia, organic or functional gonadotropic deficiencies, ovarian or adrenal tumors, Cushing's syndrome, thyroid dysfunctions, idiopathic dysovulation, and premature ovarian failure), endometriosis, alterations in tubal permeability, sperm abnormalities. We also excluded PCOS women with metformin treatment.

Clinical examination, hormonal and metabolic tests, and pelvic ultrasound examination were performed between the second and the fifth days of the menstrual cycle, either spontaneous or after a progestin challenge test (dydrogesterone, 10 mg/day for 7 to 10 days).

The clinical examination included a detailed interview, seeking, in particular, to specify the duration of menstrual cycles (regular cycles, oligomenorrhea, or amenorrhea), BMI calculation, waist circumference measurement, and assessment of hirsutism according to the modified Ferriman and Gallwey score [24]. The biological assessment carried out at the beginning of the follicular phase, between the second and the fifth days of the menstrual cycle, included measurements of estradiol, LH and FSH, AMH, total testosterone, Δ4-androstenedione, 17-hydroxy-progesteron, SDHEA, SHBG, TSH, prolactin, and insulin. As previously described [31–34], estradiol, LH, FSH, total testosterone, Δ4-androstenedione, 17-hydroxy-progesterone, SDHEA, SHBG, and prolactin were measured by immunoassays. Until January 2016, the AMH assay was performed using the second-generation AMH-EIA enzyme immunoassay kit from Beckman Coulter Immunotech (manual technique) as previously described [26,30]. From January 2016, AMH was measured using an automated method, Access Dxi, marketed by Beckman Coulter. We chose to perform the statistical analyses considering the values obtained with the AMH-EIA test. The conversion formula was applied for all AMH values obtained with the Access Dxi test, i.e., for all assays performed after January 2016: AMH-EIA = (AMH Dxi − 0.44)/0.775 (values expressed in pmol/L), as previously published [35]. The pelvic ultrasound was performed on the same day. In addition to the search for uterine or tubal pathologies, a count of antral follicles (follicles strictly less than 10 mm in diameter) was conducted during this examination. Antral follicular count (CFA) and follicle number per ovary (FNPO) was performed using "the Real-time 2D ultrasound" method [36], and ovarian surfaces using a manual ellipse, as described previously [25]. From 2002 to 2008, the ultrasound machine used was a General Electric Milwaukee Logic 400, with a 7 MHz endovaginal probe; then, from 2008, a General Electric Voluson 28, with a 5 to 9 MHz endovaginal probe. A complete infertility work-up was performed on both members of a couple before considering a CC ovulation induction treatment. Bilateral tubal patency was checked in the patient by hysterosalpingography or laparoscopy. The patient's partner had to perform at least one spermogram to ensure compatibility with spontaneous pregnancy.

2.2. Therapeutic

All patients were treated with simple CC ovulation induction therapy. In the first cycle, the initial dose was 50 mg/day, starting on the second day of a spontaneous cycle or triggered by sequential treatment with dydrogesterone, 10 mg/day for 7 to 10 days.

The ovarian response was systematically monitored by ovulation ultrasound monitoring, starting around D12 (±1 day), in the Reproductive Medicine Department of Lille University Hospital (France). No biological assay was performed during follicular growth monitoring.

The purpose of the ultrasound was to evaluate the response to CC by measuring the number of selected follicles ($\geq$10 mm) and to measure the endometrial thickness in order to identify a possible anti-estrogenic effect of CC on the endometrium [37].

The date of ovulation was estimated from the size of the dominant follicle measured on ultrasound. A progesterone assay was performed approximately 7–8 days after the estimated date of spontaneous ovulation. A significant increase in progesterone levels confirms spontaneous ovulation and, thus, a positive response to CC.

2.3. Cycle Outcome

In the absence of menstruation approximately 2 weeks after the estimated date of ovulation, a plasma hCG test was performed. If the blood pregnancy test was positive, a pelvic ultrasound was performed at about 6 weeks of amenorrhea to ensure that the pregnancy was ongoing and screen for multiple pregnancies. In the absence of pregnancy, however, the patient would start a new cycle of CC at the dose at which ovulation was achieved.

In case of the absence of follicular recruitment (confirmed by another ultrasound examination performed 5 to 7 days after the first), sequential treatment with 10 mg/day of dydrogesterone for 7 to 10 days was prescribed to induce menstruation. The dosage of CC was then increased to the next cycle in 50 mg increments, with a maximum dose of 150 mg/day. A maximum of 6 ovulatory cycles with CC was performed for achieving a clinical pregnancy.

2.4. Response to CC

The response to 50 mg CC was assessed by the presence or absence of ovulation via ultrasound monitoring and serum progesterone assay. The patient was considered sensitive to CC if the progesterone level in the second half of the cycle was $\geq$3 ng/mL. In the absence of follicular recruitment, the patient was then considered resistant to 50 mg CC.

Excessive responsiveness to CC was defined by the presence of three or more dominant follicles on ultrasound monitoring.

We have also evaluated the effectiveness of the current strategy of gradually increasing CC doses in the event of resistance to treatment by calculating the cumulative rates of progressive pregnancies per cycle initiated and per CC ovulatory cycle.

2.5. Statistical Analysis

Baseline characteristics were compared between the two groups using Chi-square tests (or Fisher's exact tests when expected cell frequency was <5) for categorical characteristics and the Student t-test (or Mann–Whitney U test for non-Gaussian distribution) for continuous characteristics.

To assess the independent predictors of the 50 mg resistance, baseline characteristics associated with a $p < 0.20$ in univariate analyses were implemented into a backward-stepwise multivariable logistic regression model using a removal criterion of $p > 0.05$. Results were expressed using Odds ratios (ORs) as effect sizes with 50 mg non-resistance as reference. Before developing the multivariable models, we examined the log-linearity assumption for continuous characteristics using restricted cubic spline functions [38], as well as the absence of colinearity between candidate predictors by calculating the variance inflation factors (VIFs). Because of the similarity and collinearity between SHBG and insulinemia, obesity and BMI, we decided to perform the multivariate model with SHBG and BMI. To avoid case deletion due to missing data on baseline characteristics and outcomes, missing data were imputed by multiple imputations using a regression-switching approach [39] (chained equations with m = 10) also before developing the multivariable model [39]. The imputation procedure was performed under the missing at random assumption using all baseline characteristics and study outcomes with a predictive mean matching method for continuous variables and logistic regression models (binary, ordinal or multinomial) for categorical variables. Estimates obtained in the different imputed data sets were combined using Rubin's rules [40].

Finally, we determined the optimal threshold value of factors associated with 50 mg resistance in the final models by maximizing the Youden index from the ROC curves. Statistical testing was conducted at the two-tailed α-level of 0.05. Data were analyzed using the SAS software version 9.4 (SAS Institute, Cary, NC, USA).

3. Results

A total of 283 patients with anovulatory PCOS were included in the study between May 2003 and December 2019, representing a total of 903 cycles of CC. The clinical, biological, and ultrasound characteristics of our population are detailed in Table 1.

Table 1. Clinical, biological, and ultrasound characteristics of the population (n = 283).

	Variables	Values *
	Age (years)	27.5 ± 3.7
	Regular anovulatory cycles	17 (5.9%)
Menstrual Cycles (%)	Oligomenorrhea	185 (65.5%)
	Amenorrhoea	81 (28.6%)
	BMI (kg/m^2)	25.8 ± 5.4
	Waist circumference (cm)	85.2 ± 15.2
	Modified Ferriman and Gallwey Score	5.0 (0 to 9.0)
	Estradiol (pg/mL)	37.0 (28.0 to 50.0)
	FSH (IU/L)	5.0 ± 1.3
	LH (IU/L)	5.9 (4.0 to 9.1)
	AMH (pmol/L)	71.8 (53.6 to 107.4)
	Total testosterone (ng/mL)	0.4 ± 0.2
	Δ4-androstenedione (ng/mL)	1.6 (1.2 to 2.2)
	17-OHP (ng/mL)	0.6 (0.5 to 0.9)
	SHBG (nmol/L)	38.4 (24.0 to 49.8)
	SDHEA (µmol/L)	4.6 (3.4 to 6.4)
	Fasting insulin (mUI/L)	6.0 (3.1 to 9.8)
	Mean ovarian surface (cm^2)	5.7 ± 1.6
	PCOM and/or elevated AMH	280 (99%)
	A = OA + HA + PCOM	225 (79.5%)
Phenotype PCOS (%)	B = OA + HA	3 (1.0%)
	D = OA + PCOM	55 (19.5%)

Table 1. *Cont.*

Variables	Values *
Mean number of CC cycles	3.2 ± 1.7
Mean number of CC ovulatory cycles	2.3 ± 1.5

* Qualitative variables are expressed as numbers (percentages). * Quantitative variables are expressed as mean ± standard deviation or median (inter-quartile range). Abbreviations: BMI = body mass index; FSH = Follicle Stimulating Hormone; LH = Luteinizing Hormone; AMH = Anti-Müllerian Hormone; 17-OHP = 17-hydroxy-progesterone; SHBG = Sex Hormone Binding Globulin; OA = Oligo or anovulation; HA = Hyperandrogenism; PCOM = Ultrasound polycystic ovaries; CC = Clomiphene Citrate.

Figure 1 illustrates the distribution of anovulatory PCOS women who do or do not ovulate after CC induction of ovulation in incremental daily doses of 50, 100, or 150 mg for 5 subsequent days. A total of 161 patients (56.9%) ovulated during the first cycle of CC treatment at 50 mg/day. Therefore, 122 patients (43.1%) were resistant to 50 mg/day of CC during the first cycle of treatment. Otherwise, 24 patients (8.5%) were hyperresponsive during the first cycle of CC at 50 mg/day. Finally, 49 patients (17.3%) were also resistant to the dose of 100 mg/day, and 13 patients (4.6%) were resistant to the dose of 150 mg/day.

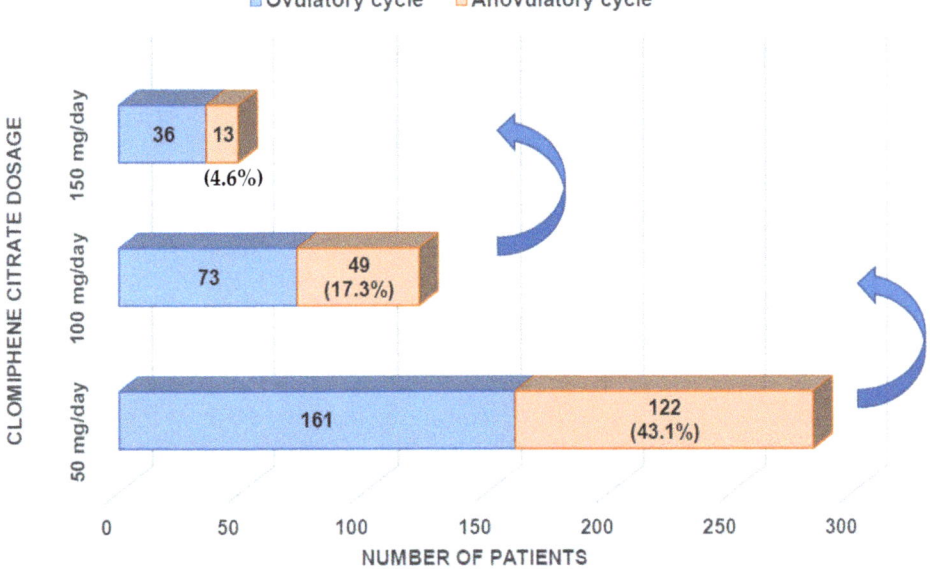

Figure 1. Distribution of anovulatory PCOS women who do or do not ovulate after CC induction of ovulation in incremental daily doses of 50, 100, or 150 mg for 5 subsequent days.

Figure 2 shows the cumulative clinical pregnancy rates per CC-initiated cycle and per CC ovulatory cycle at 50, 100, and 150 mg per day.

To investigate predictors of resistance to 50 mg CC in the first cycle of treatment, univariate regression analysis was performed to compare the clinical, biological, and ultrasound characteristics of patients sensitive to 50 mg CC versus those resistant to this dose. The results of the univariate regression analysis are presented in Table 2. Compared to patients ovulating at the 50 mg dose of CC in the first cycle, patients who were resistant to this same dose had significantly higher BMI, waist circumference, serum levels of AMH, total testosterone, ∆4-androstenedione, 17-OHP, and insulin. In contrast, serum levels of SHBG were significantly lower in patients resistant to 50 mg/day.

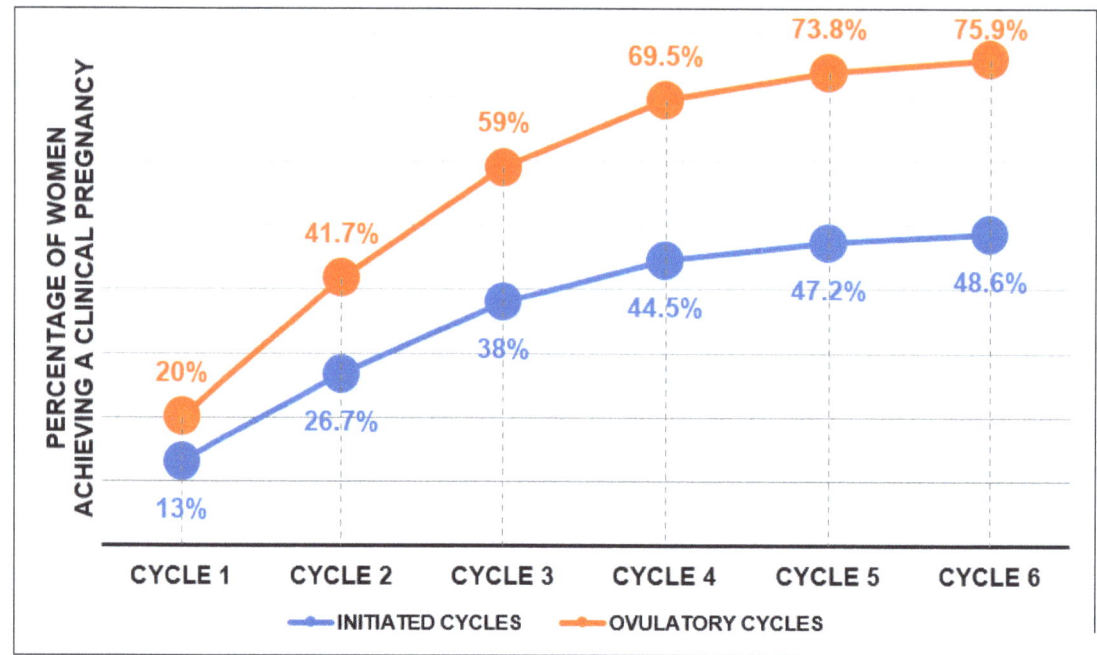

Figure 2. Cumulative rates of clinical pregnancy, per initiated and ovulatory CC cycle, at 50, 100, and 150 mg CC during 5 subsequent days.

Table 2. Factors associated with resistance to 50 mg CC in the first cycle of treatment in univariate analyzes.

		Sensitive to 50 mg (n = 179)	Resistant to 50 mg (n = 104)	p Value
	Age (years)	27.7 ± 3.8	27.0 ± 3.6	0.12
Menstrual cycles (%)	Regular anovulatory cycles	14 (7.8%)	3 (2.9%)	0.12
	Oligomenorrhea	119 (66.7%)	66 (63.5%)	
	Amenorrhoea	46 (25.5%)	35 (33.6%)	
	BMI (kg/m^2)	24.9 ± 5.2	27.1 ± 5.4	0.001
	Waist circumference (cm)	83.4 ± 15.8	88.3 ± 13.7	0.028
	Modified Ferriman and Gallwey Score	5.0 (0 to 9.0)	3.0 (0 to 9.0)	0.90
	Estradiol (pg/mL)	37.0 (28.0 to 49.5)	39.0 (28.0 to 50.0)	0.87
	FSH (IU/L)	5.01 ± 1.4	4.9 ± 1.1	0.48
	LH (IU/L)	5.7 (3.9 to 8.9)	6.2 (4.2 to 9.2)	0.33
	AMH (pmol/L)	69.4 (51.6 to 101.2)	89.5 (56.0 to 130.0)	0.014
	Total testosterone (ng/mL)	0.4 ± 0.2	0.4 ± 0.2	0.046
	Δ4-androstenedione (ng/mL)	1.5 (1.1 to 2.1)	1.7 (1.3 to 2.3)	0.023
	17-OHP (ng/mL)	0.6 (0.4 to 0.9)	0.7 (0.5 to 0.9)	0.046
	SHBG (nmol/L)	39.6 (28.7 to 53.7)	27.2 (18.0 to 40.5)	<0.001
	SDHEA (µmol/L)	4.4 (3.0 to 6.4)	4.8 (3.6 to 6.2)	0.43

Table 2. Cont.

		Sensitive to 50 mg (n = 179)	Resistant to 50 mg (n = 104)	p Value
Fasting insulin (mUI/L)		4.5 (2.9 to 7.1)	7.9 (3.9 to 11.6)	0.002
Mean ovarian surface (cm^2)		5.7 ± 1.7	5.9 ± 1.5	0.42
PCOS anovulatory phenotypes (%)	A + B	142 (79.3%)	86 (82.7%)	0.48
	D	37 (20.7%)	18 (17.3%)	

Qualitative variables are expressed as numbers (percentages). Quantitative variables are expressed as mean ± standard deviation or median (inter-quartile range). Abbreviations: BMI = body mass index; FSH = Follicle Stimulating Hormone; LH = Luteinizing Hormone; AMH = Anti-Müllerian Hormone; 17-OHP = 17-hydroxy-progesterone; SHBG = Sex Hormone Binding Globulin; OA = Oligo or anovulation; HA = Hyperandrogenism; PCOM = Ultrasound polycystic ovaries; CC = Clomiphene Citrate.

Table 3 shows the final model from the multivariate analysis. After multivariate analysis, higher levels of AMH and lower levels of SHBG were statistically associated with a higher risk of resistance at the dose of 50 mg/day of CC (OR = 1.08, 95% CI 1.03 to 1.14) and OR = 0.96, 95% CI 0.94 to 0.99, respectively).

Table 3. Independent factors of resistance to 50 mg CC in the first cycle of treatment after multivariate analysis.

Parameters	OR (95% CI)	p
AMH (pmol/L)	1.08 (1.03 to 1.14) *	0.002
SHBG (nmol/L)	0.96 (0.94 to 0.99)	0.002

Baseline characteristics associated with a $p < 0.20$ in univariate analyses (Table 2) were implemented into a backward-stepwise multivariable logistic regression model using a removal criterion of $p > 0.05$. Results were expressed using Odds ratios (ORs) as effect sizes with 50 mg non-resistance as reference. * OR expressed for the increase of 10 AMH units. Abbreviations: AMH = Anti-Müllerian Hormone; SHBG = Sex Hormone Binding Globulin.

We, therefore, sought to establish thresholds for AMH and SHBG that would potentially predict resistance to the 50 mg CC dose in the first cycle of treatment. ROC curves were produced for this purpose. These ROC curves are shown in Figure 3.

Finally, we estimated expected ovulation rates in the first cycle of ovulation induction by CC at the 50 mg/day dose according to the AMH thresholds, the SHBG thresholds, and the AMH and SHBG thresholds when these dosages are combined. The results are presented in Table 4.

Table 4. Predicted ovulation rates in the first cycle of ovulation induction by CC at 50 mg/day, based on the AMH threshold, the SHBG threshold, and the combined AMH and SHBG thresholds.

		No Ovulation	Ovulation
AMH tested alone	AMH > 86.1 pmol/L	46.12%	53.88%
	AMH < 86.1 pmol/L	29.86%	70.14%
SHBG tested alone	SHBG < 28.3 nmol/L	53,72%	46.28%
	SHBG > 28.3 nmol/L	27.93%	72.07%
AMH and SHBG combined	AMH > 86.1 pmol/L SHBG < 28.3 nmol/L	46.67%	53.33%
	AMH < 86.1 pmol/L SHBG > 28.3 nmol/L	19.42%	80.58%

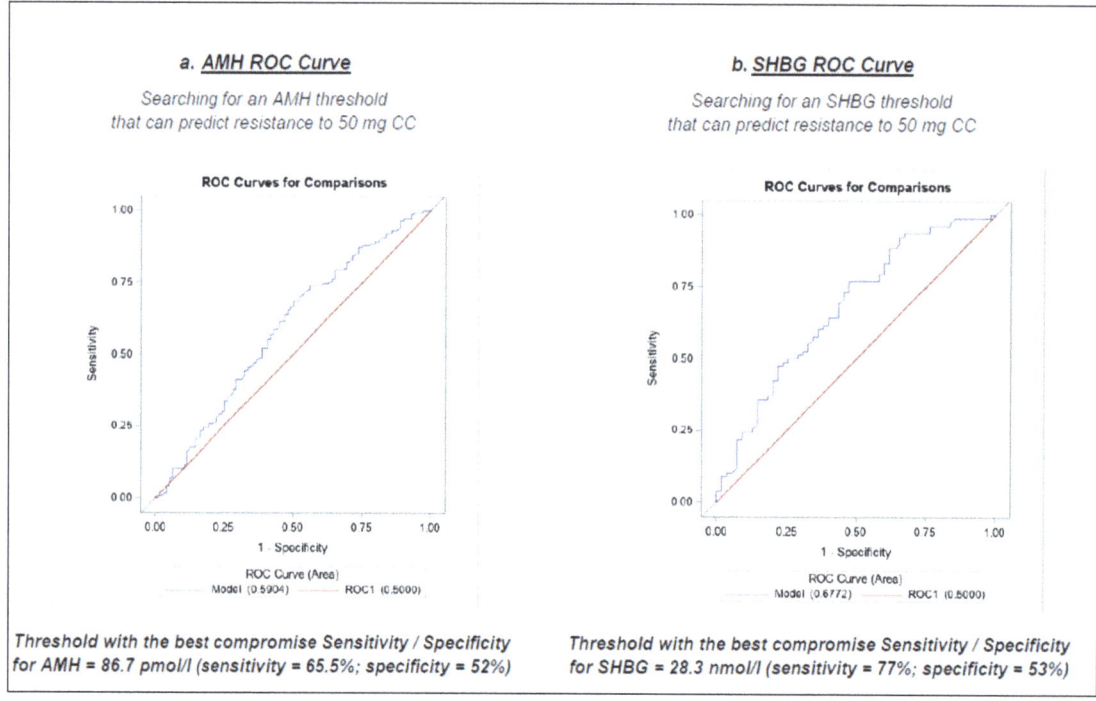

Figure 3. ROC analyses of AMH and SHBG and resistance to 50 mg CC.

4. Discussion

CC is an effective ovulation-inducing treatment for women with anovulatory PCOS, as highlighted by the good cumulative clinical pregnancy rates per ovulatory cycle in our study. However, in view of the stagnation of clinical pregnancy rates between rank 4 and rank 6, it seems wise not to continue this treatment beyond 4 consecutive ovulatory cycles. In addition, about a third of women will not respond to the 50 mg dose of CC. Thus, it could be of interest to identify women who present risk factors for resistance to the 50 mg dose of CC to accelerate the onset of clinical pregnancy. Indeed, it would then be relevant to immediately offer a dose of 100 mg/day of CC to these PCOS patients from the first cycle of ovulation induction.

Our study shows that AMH and SHBG appear to be predictive factors for resistance to 50 mg CC during the first cycle of ovulation induction in patients with anovulatory PCOS. Nevertheless, we failed to identify thresholds for both AMH and SHBG, which could be used to predict resistance to 50 mg CC, and thus, to initiate treatment at 100 mg/day.

To our knowledge, this is the first study to investigate predictive factors of resistance to 50 mg CC in the first cycle of ovulation induction in PCOS women. However, many authors have focused on predictors of resistance to 150 mg/day CC. Among these factors, AMH is a parameter frequently cited as a predictor of response to CC. Xi et al. [21] and Mahran et al. [41] consider AMH a good marker of CC response. According to Xi et al. [21], patients with a high AMH level, particularly above 55.5 pmol/L, have a significantly reduced chance of ovulation under CC. According to Mahran et al. [41], the AMH level may help determine the initial CC dose: the higher the AMH level, the greater the initial CC dose should be, with a proposed threshold of 24.3 pmol/L.

As AMH is produced in greater quantities in women with PCOS, its inhibitory action on FSH is therefore more pronounced [32,34,42–44]. This may explain the results of our study, which indicate that as serum AMH levels increase, the patient is more likely to be resistant to the initial 50 mg CC dose. The higher the AMH, the greater the doses of FSH required to achieve follicular growth and ovulation. This is in agreement with the results of Köninger et al. [45], suggesting that in CC-resistant women receiving recombinant FSH ovulation stimulation, the higher the patient's serum AMH level, the greater the doses of FSH required to achieve ovulation. Unfortunately, it was not possible to establish an AMH threshold predictive of resistance at the initial 50 mg CC dose. The selected AMH cut-off was 86.7 pmol/L, but sensitivity and specificity were not satisfactory for clinical application (65.5% and 52%, respectively). The AMH thresholds proposed in the literature to predict total resistance to CC (150 mg/day dose) are highly variable (from 24.3 pmol/L to 88.4 pmol/L) with no satisfactory relative sensitivities and specificities [21,41,46–48]. In addition, some authors found no significant difference in serum AMH levels between women ovulating on CC versus those resistant to treatment [49]. The latter explained the difference between these results and those of other teams by the difference in the AMH assay kits used in the different studies, which have different sensitivities. Indeed, there are several AMH test kits around the world, which makes the use of this test difficult to generalize [35,43].

A recent retrospective study has shown that in phenotype B of PCOS, ovarian volume did not have any predictive value of the dosage of CC required to induce ovulation [50]. This study is very interesting, but our population contains very few PCOS with phenotype B. In fact, as we have published previously, using AMH as a biological equivalent of PCOM, there are very few women with phenotype B of PCOS in our population [30]. Finally, to our knowledge, there are no studies demonstrating a clear statistical correlation between ovarian volume and serum AMH levels.

Furthermore, SHBG also appears to be a statistically significant parameter in the multivariate analysis of our study. The lower the SHBG, the greater the risk of resisting the dose of 50 mg/day of CC. Patients with confounding factors that may induce a decrease in SHBG, such as hypothyroidism, were excluded from our study. However, as with AMH, it was not possible to establish a satisfactory threshold for SHBG that would allow us to specify a starting dose of 100 mg CC. The selected cut-off of 28.3 nmol/L (sensitivity of 77% and specificity of 53%) is not useful in clinical practice. SHBG is a plasma transport glycoprotein produced by liver cells, whose role is to regulate the bioavailability of sex steroid hormones [51]. Abnormally low levels of SHBG are frequently observed in women with PCOS (especially in women with android obesity) and contribute to the symptoms of clinical hyperandrogenism observed in these patients by increasing the bioavailable (and therefore bioactive) fraction of circulating androgens (hirsutism, acne, androgenic alopecia) [52,53]. A low serum level of SHBG is considered a marker of insulin resistance (inhibition of hepatic synthesis of SHBG due to compensatory hyperinsulinism). A recent meta-analysis highlights the correlation between SHBG and metabolic dysregulation in PCOS women [54]. According to this meta-analysis, women with PCOS with low levels of SHBG were more likely to suffer from hyperandrogenism, insulin resistance, carbohydrate intolerance, type 2 diabetes, obesity, and cardiovascular disease. Therefore, the data in the literature, as well as the results of our study, demonstrate that a complete metabolic assessment and management of obesity are crucial before treatment in women with PCOS, both for the success of treatment and for the prevention of long-term complications. A recent prospective study indicates that women with more disturbed metabolic parameters were at greater risk of resistance to clomiphene citrate, even when the dose was increased to 150 mg/day for 5 consecutive days [55]. The meta-analysis by Deswal et al. [54] indicates that insulin-sensitizing agents, such as myo-inositol or metformin, can significantly improve the levels of SHBG in PCOS women. Moreover, several randomized clinical trials have shown a significant improvement in ovulation rates in women using the combination of metformin and CC compared to CC alone, although this probably applies more to PCOS women with insulin resistance [5].

The response to CC, used as a treatment for dysovulation in PCOS women, is therefore variable from woman to woman. Since there are no factors that can safely predict the response or not to CC at this time, some authors have suggested a genetic predisposition to explain resistance to treatment. Indeed, CC is metabolized primarily in the liver by cytochrome P450 2D6 (CYP2D6), and to a lesser extent, by cytochromes P450 3A4 and P450 3A5 [56–58]. CYP2D6 has a large genetic polymorphism responsible for several different metabolic profiles [59]. The impact of the genetic polymorphism of CYP2D6 on the clinical efficacy of clomiphene citrate is still controversial [56–61].

The main limitation of our study is its retrospective nature. The AMH assay was modified in 2016, but we applied a conversion formula for all assays performed after January 2016, thus homogenizing the results and avoiding any measurement bias [35]. Similarly, the ultrasound probe used for the pretherapeutic assessment and, therefore, for the evaluation of the AFC/FNPO was replaced in 2008. Therefore, we decided not to consider AFC/FNPO in the statistical analyses, preferring AMH levels, as previously demonstrated [26,30]. Indeed, the evaluation of AFC/FNPO is operator dependent and can evolve over time with the technical progress of ultrasound probes [28,36], unlike a biological assay such as the AMH assay, which is more reproducible [42,43].

To our knowledge, this study is the largest cohort of anovulatory PCOS patients treated with CC described in the literature and the only one which tries to investigate predictors of resistance to ovulation induction by CC initiated at 50 mg/day. The main strength of our study is, therefore, the large number of patients included. In addition, in this monocentric study, the diagnosis of PCOS and the procedure for monitoring ovulation during CC treatment were standardized. Our results suggest that AMH and SHBG are the only two parameters significantly associated with the risk of resistance to 50 mg/day of CC. However, no cut-off with satisfactory sensitivity and specificity could be established, both for AMH and SHBG, to predict resistance to 50 mg CC.

Author Contributions: L.H. contributed to study design, execution, acquisition, analysis and interpretation of data, manuscript drafting, and critical discussion. A.D., C.R., C.D., S.C.-J. and D.D. contributed to critical discussion. M.K. contributed to the statistical analysis and interpretation of data. G.R. contributed to the study design, execution, acquisition, analysis and interpretation of data, manuscript drafting, and critical discussion. All authors have read and agreed to the published version of the manuscript.

Funding: This research received no external funding.

Institutional Review Board Statement: As this study was retrospective and without intervention, the opinion of the Ethics Committee on the study was not required. All patients had given prior consent for the use of their clinical, hormonal, and ultrasound records. On 16 December 2019, the Institutional Review Board of the Lille University Hospital gave unrestricted approval for the anonymous use of all patients' clinical, hormonal, and ultrasound records (reference DEC20150715-0002).

Informed Consent Statement: Informed consent was obtained from all subjects involved in the study.

Data Availability Statement: The data that support the findings of this study are available from the corresponding author, G.R., upon reasonable request.

Acknowledgments: We thank our nurses, Lydie Lombardo and Sylvie Vanoverschelde, for their help in collecting the blood samples and caring for patients.

Conflicts of Interest: The authors have no conflict of interest.

References

1. Lizneva, D.; Suturina, L.; Walker, W.; Brakta, S.; Gavrilova-Jordan, L.; Azziz, R. Criteria, prevalence, and phenotypes of polycystic ovary syndrome. *Fertil. Steril.* **2016**, *106*, 6–15. [CrossRef]
2. Jayasena, C.N.; Franks, S. The management of patients with polycystic ovary syndrome. *Nat. Rev. Endocrinol.* **2014**, *10*, 624–636. [CrossRef]
3. The Rotterdam ESHRE/ASRM-Sponsored PCOS Consensus Workshop Group. Revised 2003 consensus on diagnostic criteria and long-term health risks related to polycystic ovary syndrome (PCOS). *Hum. Reprod.* **2004**, *19*, 41–47. [CrossRef]
4. The Thessaloniki ESHRE/ASRM-Sponsored PCOS Consensus Workshop Group. Consensus on infertility treatment related to polycystic ovary syndrome. *Hum. Reprod.* **2008**, *23*, 462–477. [CrossRef]

5. Balen, A.H.; Morley, L.C.; Misso, M.; Franks, S.; Legro, R.S.; Wijeyaratne, C.N.; Stener-Victorin, E.; Fauser, B.C.J.M.; Norman, R.J.; Teede, H. The management of anovulatory infertility in women with polycystic ovary syndrome: An analysis of the evidence to support the development of global WHO guidance. *Hum. Reprod. Update* **2016**, *22*, 687–708. [CrossRef]
6. Teede, H.J.; Misso, M.L.; Costello, M.F.; Dokras, A.; Laven, J.; Moran, L.; Piltonen, T.; Norman, R.J.; International PCOS Network. Recommendations from the international evidence-based guideline for the assessment and management of polycystic ovary syndrome. *Hum. Reprod.* **2018**, *33*, 1602–1618. [CrossRef]
7. Franik, S.; Le, Q.K.; Kremer, J.A.; Kiesel, L.; Farquhar, C. Aromatase inhibitors (letrozole) for ovulation induction in infertile women with polycystic ovary syndrome. *Cochrane Database Syst. Rev.* **2022**, *9*, CD010287. [CrossRef]
8. Hughes, E.; Collins, J.; Vandekerckhove, P. Clomiphene citrate for ovulation induction in women with oligo-amenorrhoea. *Cochrane Database Syst. Rev* **1996**, *22*, CD000056. [CrossRef]
9. Homburg, R. Clomiphene citrate—End of an era? A mini-review. *Hum. Reprod.* **2005**, *20*, 2043–2051. [CrossRef]
10. Homburg, R. Polycystic ovary syndrome. *Best. Pract. Res. Clin. Obs. Gynaecol.* **2008**, *22*, 261–274. [CrossRef]
11. Beck, J.I.; Boothroyd, C.; Proctor, M.; Farquhar, C.; Hughes, E. Oral anti-oestrogens and medical adjuncts for subfertility associated with anovulation. *Cochrane Database Syst. Rev.* **2005**, *25*, CD002249. [CrossRef]
12. Dewailly, D.; Hieronimus, S.; Mirakian, P.; Hugues, J.-N. Polycystic ovary syndrome (PCOS). *Ann. Endocrinol.* **2010**, *71*, 8–13. [CrossRef]
13. Balen, A.H. Ovulation induction in the management of anovulatory polycystic ovary syndrome. *Mol. Cell Endocrinol.* **2013**, *373*, 77–82. [CrossRef]
14. Brown, J.; Farquhar, C.; Beck, J.; Boothroyd, C.; Hughes, E. Clomiphene and anti-oestrogens for ovulation induction in PCOS. *Cochrane Database Syst. Rev.* **2009**, *7*, CD002249. [CrossRef]
15. Melo, A.S.; Ferriani, R.A.; Navarro, P.A. Treatment of infertility in women with polycystic ovary syndrome: Approach to clinical practice. *Clinics* **2015**, *70*, 765–769. [CrossRef]
16. Wang, L.; Qi, H.; Baker, P.N.; Zhen, Q.; Zeng, Q.; Shi, R.; Tong, C.; Ge, Q. Altered Circulating Inflammatory Cytokines Are Associated with Anovulatory Polycystic Ovary Syndrome (PCOS) Women Resistant to Clomiphene Citrate Treatment. *Med. Sci. Monit.* **2017**, *23*, 1083–1089. [CrossRef]
17. Ellakwa, H.E.; Sanad, Z.F.; Hamza, H.A.; Emara, M.A.; Elsayed, M.A. Predictors of patient responses to ovulation induction with clomiphene citrate in patients with polycystic ovary syndrome experiencing infertility. *Int. J. Gynecol. Obstet.* **2016**, *133*, 59–63. [CrossRef]
18. Imani, B.; Eijkemans, M.J.; te Velde, E.R.; Habbema, J.D.; Fauser, B.C. Predictors of patients remaining anovulatory during clomiphene citrate induction of ovulation in normogonadotropic oligoamenorrheic infertility. *J. Clin. Endocrinol. Metab.* **1998**, *83*, 2361–2365. [CrossRef]
19. Imani, B.; Eijkemans, M.J.; te Velde, E.R.; Habbema, J.D.; Fauser, B.C. Predictors of chances to conceive in ovulatory patients during clomiphene citrate induction of ovulation in normogonadotropic oligoamenorrheic infertility. *J. Clin. Endocrinol. Metab.* **1999**, *84*, 1617–1622. [CrossRef]
20. Overbeek, A.; Kuijper, E.A.M.; Hendriks, M.L.; Blankenstein, M.A.; Ketel, I.J.G.; Twisk, J.W.R.; Hompes, P.G.A.; Homburg, R.; Lambalk, C.B. Clomiphene citrate resistance in relation to follicle-stimulating hormone receptor Ser680Ser-polymorphism in polycystic ovary syndrome. *Hum. Reprod.* **2009**, *24*, 2007–2013. [CrossRef]
21. Xi, W.; Yang, Y.; Mao, H.; Zhao, X.; Liu, M.; Fu, S. Circulating anti-mullerian hormone as predictor of ovarian response to clomiphene citrate in women with polycystic ovary syndrome. *J. Ovarian Res.* **2016**, *9*, 3. [CrossRef]
22. Mercorio, A.; Della Corte, L.; De Angelis, M.C.; Buonfantino, C.; Ronsini, C.; Bifulco, G.; Giampaolino, P. Ovarian Drilling: Back to the Future. *Medicina* **2022**, *58*, 1002. [CrossRef]
23. Practice Committees of the American Society for Reproductive Medicine and the Society for Reproductive Endocrinology and Infertility. Diagnosis and treatment of luteal phase deficiency: A committee opinion. *Fertil. Steril.* **2021**, *115*, 1416–1423. [CrossRef]
24. Escobar-Morreale, H.F.; Carmina, E.; Dewailly, D.; Gambineri, A.; Kelestimur, F.; Moghetti, P.; Pugeat, M.; Qiao, J.; Wijeyaratne, C.N.; Witchel, S.F.; et al. Epidemiology, diagnosis and management of hirsutism: A consensus statement by the Androgen Excess and Polycystic Ovary Syndrome Society. *Hum. Reprod. Update* **2012**, *18*, 146–170. [CrossRef]
25. Jonard, S.; Robert, Y.; Dewailly, D. Revisiting the ovarian volume as a diagnostic criterion for polycystic ovaries. *Hum. Reprod.* **2005**, *20*, 2893–2898. [CrossRef]
26. Dewailly, D.; Gronier, H.; Poncelet, E.; Robin, G.; Leroy, M.; Pigny, P.; Duhamel, A.; Catteau-Jonard, S. Diagnosis of polycystic ovary syndrome (PCOS): Revisiting the threshold values of follicle count on ultrasound and of the serum AMH level for the definition of polycystic ovaries. *Hum. Reprod.* **2011**, *26*, 3123–3129. [CrossRef]
27. Balen, A.H.; Laven, J.S.E.; Tan, S.-L.; Dewailly, D. Ultrasound assessment of the polycystic ovary: International consensus definitions. *Hum. Reprod. Update* **2003**, *9*, 505–514. [CrossRef]
28. Dewailly, D.; Lujan, M.E.; Carmina, E.; Cedars, M.I.; Laven, J.; Norman, R.J.; Escobar-Morreale, H.F. Definition and significance of polycystic ovarian morphology: A task force report from the Androgen Excess and Polycystic Ovary Syndrome Society. *Hum. Reprod. Update* **2014**, *20*, 334–352. [CrossRef]
29. Robin, G.; Gallo, C.; Catteau-Jonard, S.; Lefebvre-Maunoury, C.; Pigny, P.; Duhamel, A.; Dewailly, D. Polycystic Ovary-Like Abnormalities (PCO-L) in women with functional hypothalamic amenorrhea. *J. Clin. Endocrinol. Metab.* **2012**, *97*, 4236–4243. [CrossRef]

30. Fraissinet, A.; Robin, G.; Pigny, P.; Lefebvre, T.; Catteau-Jonard, S.; Dewailly, D. Use of the serum anti-Müllerian hormone assay as a surrogate for polycystic ovarian morphology: Impact on diagnosis and phenotypic classification of polycystic ovary syndrome. *Hum. Reprod.* **2017**, *32*, 1716–1722. [CrossRef]
31. Jonard, S.; Robert, Y.; Cortet-Rudelli, C.; Pigny, P.; Decanter, C.; Dewailly, D. Ultrasound examination of polycystic ovaries: Is it worth counting the follicles? *Hum. Reprod.* **2003**, *18*, 598–603. [CrossRef]
32. Dewailly, D.; Pigny, P.; Soudan, B.; Catteau-Jonard, S.; Decanter, C.; Poncelet, E.; Duhamel, A. Reconciling the definitions of polycystic ovary syndrome: The ovarian follicle number and serum anti-Müllerian hormone concentrations aggregate with the markers of hyperandrogenism. *J. Clin. Endocrinol. Metab.* **2010**, *95*, 4399–4405. [CrossRef]
33. Pigny, P.; Jonard, S.; Robert, Y.; Dewailly, D. Serum anti-Mullerian hormone as a surrogate for antral follicle count for definition of the polycystic ovary syndrome. *J. Clin. Endocrinol. Metab.* **2006**, *91*, 941–945. [CrossRef]
34. Pigny, P.; Merlen, E.; Robert, Y.; Cortet-Rudelli, C.; Decanter, C.; Jonard, S.; Dewailly, D. Elevated serum level of anti-mullerian hormone in patients with polycystic ovary syndrome: Relationship to the ovarian follicle excess and to the follicular arrest. *J. Clin. Endocrinol. Metab.* **2003**, *88*, 5957–5962. [CrossRef]
35. Pigny, P.; Gorisse, E.; Ghulam, A.; Robin, G.; Catteau-Jonard, S.; Duhamel, A.; Dewailly, D. Comparative assessment of five serum antimüllerian hormone assays for the diagnosis of polycystic ovary syndrome. *Fertil. Steril.* **2016**, *105*, 1063–1069.e3. [CrossRef]
36. Coelho Neto, M.A.; Ludwin, A.; Borrell, A.; Benacerraf, B.; Dewailly, D.; da Silva Costa, F.; Condous, G.; Alcazar, J.L.; Jokubkiene, L.; Guerriero, S.; et al. Counting ovarian antral follicles by ultrasound: A practical guide. *Ultrasound Obstet. Gynecol.* **2018**, *51*, 10–20. [CrossRef]
37. Gadalla, M.A.; Huang, S.; Wang, R.; Norman, R.J.; Abdullah, S.A.; El Saman, A.M.; Ismail, A.M.; van Wely, M.; Mol, B.W.J. Effect of clomiphene citrate on endometrial thickness, ovulation, pregnancy and live birth in anovulatory women: Systematic review and meta-analysis. *Ultrasound Obstet. Gynecol.* **2018**, *51*, 64–76. [CrossRef]
38. Harrell, F.E.; Lee, K.L.; Mark, D.B. Multivariable prognostic models: Issues in developing models, evaluating assumptions and adequacy, and measuring and reducing errors. *Stat. Med.* **1996**, *15*, 361–387. [CrossRef]
39. Buuren, S.v.; Groothuis-Oudshoorn, K. Mice: Multivariate Imputation by Chained Equations in R. *J. Stat. Softw.* **2011**, *45*, 1–67. [CrossRef]
40. Segalas, C.; Leyrat, C.; Carpenter, J.R.; Williamson, E. Propensity score matching after multiple imputation when a confounder has missing data. *Stat. Med.* **2023**, *42*, 1082–1095. [CrossRef]
41. Mahran, A.; Abdelmeged, A.; El-Adawy, A.R.; Eissa, M.K.; Shaw, R.W.; Amer, S.A. The predictive value of circulating anti-Müllerian hormone in women with polycystic ovarian syndrome receiving clomiphene citrate: A prospective observational study. *J. Clin. Endocrinol. Metab.* **2013**, *98*, 4170–4175. [CrossRef]
42. Dewailly, D.; Andersen, C.Y.; Balen, A.; Broekmans, F.; Dilaver, N.; Fanchin, R.; Griesinger, G.; Kelsey, T.W.; La Marca, A.; Lambalk, C.; et al. The physiology and clinical utility of anti-Mullerian hormone in women. *Hum. Reprod. Update* **2014**, *20*, 370–385. [CrossRef] [PubMed]
43. Dumont, A.; Robin, G.; Catteau-Jonard, S.; Dewailly, D. Role of Anti-Müllerian Hormone in pathophysiology, diagnosis and treatment of Polycystic Ovary Syndrome: A review. *Reprod. Biol. Endocrinol.* **2015**, *13*, 137. [CrossRef]
44. Pellatt, L.; Rice, S.; Dilaver, N.; Heshri, A.; Galea, R.; Brincat, M.; Brown, K.; Simpson, E.R.; Mason, H.D. Anti-Müllerian hormone reduces follicle sensitivity to follicle-stimulating hormone in human granulosa cells. *Fertil. Steril.* **2011**, *96*, 1246–1251.e1. [CrossRef] [PubMed]
45. Köninger, A.; Sauter, L.; Edimiris, P.; Kasimir-Bauer, S.; Kimmig, R.; Strowitzki, T.; Schmidt, B. Predictive markers for the FSH sensitivity of women with polycystic ovarian syndrome. *Hum. Reprod.* **2014**, *29*, 518–524. [CrossRef]
46. Amer, S.A.; Li, T.C.; Ledger, W.L. The value of measuring anti-Mullerian hormone in women with anovulatory polycystic ovary syndrome undergoing laparoscopic ovarian diathermy. *Hum. Reprod.* **2009**, *24*, 2760–2766. [CrossRef]
47. Gülşen, M.S.; Ulu, İ.; Köpük, Y.Ş.; Kıran, G. The role of anti-Müllerian hormone in predicting clomiphene citrate resistance in women with polycystic ovarian syndrome. *Gynecol. Endocrinol.* **2019**, *35*, 86–89. [CrossRef]
48. Hestiantoro, A.; Negoro, Y.S.; Afrita, Y.; Wiweko, B.; Sumapradja, K.; Natadisastra, M. Anti-Müllerian hormone as a predictor of polycystic ovary syndrome treated with clomiphene citrate. *Clin. Exp. Reprod. Med.* **2016**, *43*, 207–214. [CrossRef]
49. Vaiarelli, A.; Drakopoulos, P.; Blockeel, C.; De Vos, M.; van de Vijver, A.; Camus, M.; Cosyns, S.; Tournaye, H.; Polyzos, N.P. Limited ability of circulating anti-Müllerian hormone to predict dominant follicular recruitment in PCOS women treated with clomiphene citrate: A comparison of two different assays. *Gynecol. Endocrinol.* **2016**, *32*, 227–230. [CrossRef]
50. Giampaolino, P.; Della Corte, L.; De Rosa, N.; Mercorio, A.; Bruzzese, D.; Bifulco, G. Ovarian volume and PCOS: A controversial issue. *Gynecol. Endocrinol.* **2018**, *34*, 229–232. [CrossRef]
51. Zhu, J.-L.; Chen, Z.; Feng, W.-J.; Long, S.-L.; Mo, Z.-C. Sex hormone-binding globulin and polycystic ovary syndrome. *Clin. Chim. Acta* **2019**, *499*, 142–148. [CrossRef]
52. Calzada, M.; López, N.; Noguera, J.A.; Mendiola, J.; Hernández, A.I.; Corbalán, S.; Sanchez, M.; Torres, A.M. AMH in combination with SHBG for the diagnosis of polycystic ovary syndrome. *J. Obstet. Gynaecol.* **2019**, *39*, 1130–1136. [CrossRef]
53. Simó, R.; Sáez-López, C.; Barbosa-Desongles, A.; Hernández, C.; Selva, D.M. Novel insights in SHBG regulation and clinical implications. *Trends Endocrinol. Metab.* **2015**, *26*, 376–383. [CrossRef]
54. Deswal, R.; Yadav, A.; Dang, A.S. Sex hormone binding globulin—An important biomarker for predicting PCOS risk: A systematic review and meta-analysis. *Syst. Biol. Reprod. Med.* **2018**, *64*, 12–24. [CrossRef]

55. Sachdeva, G.; Gainder, S.; Suri, V.; Sachdeva, N.; Chopra, S. Comparison of Clinical, Metabolic, Hormonal, and Ultrasound Parameters among the Clomiphene Citrate-Resistant and Clomiphene Citrate-Sensitive Polycystic Ovary Syndrome Women. *J. Hum. Reprod. Sci.* **2019**, *12*, 216–223. [CrossRef]
56. Ghobadi, C.; Amer, S.; Lashen, H.; Lennard, M.S.; Ledger, W.L.; Rostami-Hodjegan, A. Evaluation of the relationship between plasma concentrations of en- and zuclomiphene and induction of ovulation in anovulatory women being treated with clomiphene citrate. *Fertil. Steril.* **2009**, *91*, 1135–1140. [CrossRef]
57. Mürdter, T.E.; Kerb, R.; Turpeinen, M.; Schroth, W.; Ganchev, B.; Böhmer, G.M.; Igel, S.; Schaeffeler, E.; Zanger, U.; Brauch, H.; et al. Genetic polymorphism of cytochrome P450 2D6 determines oestrogen receptor activity of the major infertility drug clomiphene via its active metabolites. *Hum. Mol. Genet.* **2012**, *21*, 1145–1154. [CrossRef]
58. Ghobadi, C.; Gregory, A.; Crewe, H.K.; Rostami-Hodjegan, A.; Lennard, M.S. CYP2D6 is primarily responsible for the metabolism of clomiphene. *Drug Metab. Pharmacokinet.* **2008**, *23*, 101–105. [CrossRef]
59. Zhou, S.-F. Polymorphism of human cytochrome P450 2D6 and its clinical significance: Part II. *Clin. Pharmacokinet.* **2009**, *48*, 761–804. [CrossRef]
60. Robin, C.; Hennart, B.; Broly, F.; Gruchala, P.; Robin, G.; Catteau-Jonard, S. Could Cytochrome P450 2D6, 3A4 and 3A5 Polymorphisms Explain the Variability in Clinical Response to Clomiphene Citrate of Anovulatory PCOS Women? *Front. Endocrinol.* **2021**, *12*, 718917. [CrossRef]
61. Ji, M.; Kim, K.-R.; Lee, W.; Choe, W.; Chun, S.; Min, W.-K. Genetic Polymorphism of CYP2D6 and Clomiphene Concentrations in Infertile Patients with Ovulatory Dysfunction Treated with Clomiphene Citrate. *J. Korean Med. Sci.* **2016**, *31*, 310–314. [CrossRef]

Disclaimer/Publisher's Note: The statements, opinions and data contained in all publications are solely those of the individual author(s) and contributor(s) and not of MDPI and/or the editor(s). MDPI and/or the editor(s) disclaim responsibility for any injury to people or property resulting from any ideas, methods, instructions or products referred to in the content.

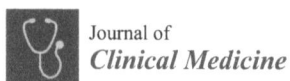

Article

Pregnancy Outcomes in Women with PCOS: Follow-Up Study of a Randomized Controlled Three-Component Lifestyle Intervention

Alexandra Dietz de Loos [1,*], Geranne Jiskoot [1,2], Yvonne Louwers [1], Annemerle Beerthuizen [2], Jan Busschbach [2] and Joop Laven [1]

[1] Division of Reproductive Endocrinology and Infertility, Department of Obstetrics and Gynaecology, Erasmus University Medical Center, 3015 GD Rotterdam, The Netherlands
[2] Department of Psychiatry, Section Medical Psychology and Psychotherapy, Erasmus University Medical Center, 3015 GD Rotterdam, The Netherlands
* Correspondence: a.dietzdeloos@erasmusmc.nl; Tel.: +31-622666365

Abstract: Women with polycystic ovary syndrome (PCOS) and excess weight often present with reproductive derangements. The first-line treatment for this population is a multi-component lifestyle intervention. This follow-up study of a randomized controlled trial based on data from the Dutch Perinatal registry was conducted to study the effect of a one-year three-component (cognitive behavioral therapy, healthy diet, and exercise) lifestyle intervention on pregnancy outcomes in women with PCOS and overweight or obesity. Women diagnosed with PCOS, a BMI ≥ 25 kg/m^2, and a wish to conceive were randomized to either three-component lifestyle intervention (LSI, n = 123), and care as usual (CAU, n = 60) where they were encouraged to lose weight autonomously. Conception resulting in live birth was 39.8% (49/123) within LSI and 38.3% (23/60) within CAU ($p = 0.845$). In total, 58.3% conceived spontaneously. Gestational diabetes (LSI: 8.2% vs. CAU: 21.7%, $p = 0.133$), hypertensive disorders (LSI: 8.2% vs. CAU 13.0%, $p = 0.673$), and preterm birth (LSI: 12.2% vs. CAU: 17.4%, $p = 0.716$) rates were all lower in LSI compared to CAU. This follow-up study showed no significant differences in conception resulting in live birth rates between LSI and CAU. Nonetheless, a large proportion eventually conceived spontaneously. Moreover, after LSI, the number of uneventful pregnancies was lower compared to care as usual.

Keywords: polycystic ovary syndrome; PCOS; obesity; conception; live birth; lifestyle intervention; multi-component

Citation: Dietz de Loos, A.; Jiskoot, G.; Louwers, Y.; Beerthuizen, A.; Busschbach, J.; Laven, J. Pregnancy Outcomes in Women with PCOS: Follow-Up Study of a Randomized Controlled Three-Component Lifestyle Intervention. *J. Clin. Med.* **2023**, *12*, 426. https://doi.org/10.3390/jcm12020426

Academic Editor: Enrico Carmina

Received: 9 December 2022
Revised: 30 December 2022
Accepted: 3 January 2023
Published: 5 January 2023

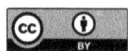

Copyright: © 2023 by the authors. Licensee MDPI, Basel, Switzerland. This article is an open access article distributed under the terms and conditions of the Creative Commons Attribution (CC BY) license (https://creativecommons.org/licenses/by/4.0/).

1. Introduction

Polycystic ovary syndrome (PCOS) is the most common endocrine disorder in women of reproductive age, and is defined by the presence of at least two of the following key characteristics according to the Rotterdam 2003 criteria: ovulatory dysfunction, hyperandrogenism, and polycystic ovarian morphology [1,2]. Moreover, PCOS is associated with overweight and obesity [3], and excess weight is known to have a positive correlation with the PCOS phenotypical severity status [4]. Overall, women with PCOS and overweight or obesity present with more pronounced clinical, metabolic, and reproductive derangements [5–7].

Reproductive problems in women with PCOS generally present as irregular or absent menstrual cycles (oligo- or amenorrhea respectively), which are signs of anovulatory subfertility. The ovulation rate is negatively affected by obesity, resulting in lower chances of spontaneous pregnancy [8]. Obesity also causes inferior outcomes with regard to infertility treatments when compared to women with a normal weight [9,10]. Moreover, when pregnant, complications such as gestational diabetes, hypertensive disorders, preterm birth, and stillbirth seem to be more prevalent in this population [11–15]. Hence, a wish to become pregnant is not so self-evident for women with PCOS, especially if they are overweight or obese.

The current first-line treatment for women with PCOS is a multicomponent lifestyle intervention (diet, exercise, behavioral therapies) in order to lose weight and to prevent excess weight gain [1]. Despite pregnancy not being the primary aim of many studies, some lifestyle intervention trials have reported on incidental pregnancy findings [16,17]. Nonetheless, a recent meta-analysis investigated reproductive outcomes after lifestyle interventions compared to minimal treatment in women with PCOS and concluded that there are no lifestyle studies available with live birth as a primary outcome [18]. Hence, the international PCOS guideline highlighted the critical need for more research with regard to pregnancy outcomes following lifestyle interventions [1].

In line with this PCOS guideline, we performed a randomized controlled long-term three-component lifestyle intervention, with or without additional short message service (SMS) support, in overweight or obese women with PCOS. Previous results on the primary outcome measure of weight loss demonstrated that our three-component lifestyle intervention program resulted in reasonable weight loss in women with PCOS, and adding SMS resulted in even more weight loss [19]. The aim of the current follow-up study was to evaluate conception resulting in live birth rates within 24 months after the start of the lifestyle intervention (LSI) compared to care as usual (CAU). Furthermore, time to conception after the start of the intervention, mode of conception, pregnancy complications, and neonatal outcomes were also evaluated. We hypothesized that pre-pregnancy weight loss and the adoption of a healthy lifestyle would cause more pregnancies, shorter time to conception, and less pregnancy complications.

2. Materials and Methods

2.1. Trial Design

This was a follow-up study from a randomized controlled trial (RCT) based on data from the Dutch Perinatal registry. The timeframe for data collection from the Dutch Perinatal registry per participant comprised a total of 24 months after the start of the study (0–12 months (during study period) and 12–24 months (post-study period)). The RCT was a one-year three-component lifestyle intervention study which was performed between August 2010 and March 2016. Three groups were compared: one-year lifestyle intervention with additional SMS support (SMS+), one-year lifestyle intervention without additional SMS support (SMS−), and one-year care as usual (CAU). We have previously published the study protocol [20]. For the current follow-up study, we combined the SMS+ and SMS− groups into one lifestyle intervention group (LSI). This RCT was approved by the Medical Research Ethics Committee of the Erasmus MC in Rotterdam (MEC 2008-337) and registered by clinical trial number: NTR2450 (www.trialsearch.who.int, accessed on 2 August 2010).

2.2. Participants

Women were included within the division of Reproductive Endocrinology and Infertility of the Department of Obstetrics and Gynaecology, at the Erasmus MC, the Netherlands, when they were actively trying to get pregnant, had a body mass index (BMI) > 25 kg/m^2, were between 18–38 years of age, and had a diagnosis of PCOS according to the Rotterdam 2003 consensus criteria [2]. Women were excluded when they had inadequate command of the Dutch language, severe mental illness, obesity due to another somatic cause, androgen excess caused by adrenal diseases or ovarian tumours, and other malformations of the internal genitalia.

The sample size calculation of the RCT was based on a notable difference in weight as the primary outcome measure. All participants provided written informed consent. Subsequently, participants were randomly assigned in a 1:1:1 ratio to one of the three groups of the study with the use of a computer-generated random numbers table. This procedure was executed by a research nurse who was not involved in the study. Assignment was made by sequentially numbered, identical, sealed envelopes, each containing a letter designating the allocation [20].

2.3. Three-Component Lifestyle Intervention (LSI) and Control Group (CAU)

The lifestyle intervention covered three main components during twenty 2.5 h group meetings over the period of one-year: (1) normo-caloric diet, as recommended by the "Dutch Food Guide" [21], (2) exercise according to the "Global Recommendations for physical activity by the World Health Organization" [22], (3) cognitive behavioral therapy, in order to create awareness and to restructure dysfunctional thoughts about, e.g., self-esteem and weight (loss). After three months the SMS+ group were sent weekly self-monitored information regarding their diet, physical activity, and emotions by SMS, and received patient-tailored SMS feedback by a semi-automated software program in order to provide social support and to encourage positive behavior. The LSI was first tested in a pilot group (n = 26) in order to get acquainted with the program and procedures. These data were not used for the study.

The control group received care as usual over the period of one year. The risk of excess weight for both mother and child, and the relation between overweight and infertility was discussed by their treating physician. Subsequently, weight loss was encouraged by publicly available services such as visiting a dietician or gym.

Participants in both groups (LSI and CAU) had a wish to become pregnant. They were encouraged to lose 5–10% of their initial body weight as their personal goal during the course of the study. Provided that they could sustain their weight loss for at least three months and complete the one-year study, participants received assisted reproductive care. In the meantime, spontaneous pregnancies could also occur during the one-year study and in the one-year follow-up period after the study. Participants did not receive further interventions if they became pregnant spontaneously during the course of the study.

2.4. Clinical and Endocrine Assessments

All participants received five standardized assessments from baseline till one year. These included general medical, obstetric and family history, and physical measurements (height, weight, BMI (kg/m^2), waist and hip circumference, and blood pressure). In addition, a transvaginal ultrasound (probe < 8 MHz) was performed and fasting blood samples were collected for an extensive endocrine assessment.

Pregnancy and neonatal outcomes were collected from the Dutch Central Bureau for Statistics (CBS) combined with the Dutch Perinatal registry (Perined). Maternal, neonatal and delivery characteristics are routinely registered by caregivers (midwives, gynecologists, and pediatricians) using electronic registration forms which are all collected by the Perined registry. This results in available population based data on approximately 96% of all deliveries and pregnancies in the Netherlands [23]. Information on miscarriages or deliveries < 16 weeks of gestational age is not available. Data from all participants were linked to the Perined registry by the Dutch CBS using pseudo-anonymization.

2.5. Outcome Measures

The primary outcome measure of the current follow-up study was conception within 24 months after the start of the intervention resulting in live birth. Live birth was defined as the delivery of a living child. Secondary outcome measures included time to conception (from start intervention until conception), mode of conception (spontaneous or by assisted reproductive technology (ART)), pregnancy complications such as (gestational) diabetes, hypertensive disorders (hypertension and/or (pre) eclampsia), and preterm birth (birth

<37 months of gestational age). Other secondary outcome measures included neonatal outcomes and complications such as neonatal intensive care unit (NICU) admission, small for gestational age (SGA) (birth weight < 10th percentile), large for gestational age (LGA) (birth weight > 90th percentile) and congenital abnormalities.

2.6. Statistical Methods

Data were analyzed according the intention-to-treat principle. Outcome measures were displayed as n (%) or median (interquartile range (IQR)). Differences between the groups (LSI (SMS+ and SMS− combined) vs CAU) were tested with the χ^2 test or Fishers exact test for categorical variables and with the Mann–Whitney U test for continuous outcomes.

A survival analysis was performed to calculate time to conception and differences between the groups were tested with the log rank test. Logistic regression analyses were used to evaluate the association between changes in weight within the groups and the chance to get pregnant.

Finally, different baseline characteristics were evaluated as predictors for conception within 24 months after the start of the intervention. These baseline characteristics were selected as potential predictors based on a literature search and included: study group, age, BMI, modified Ferriman–Gallwey score (mFG), waist circumference, time attempting to conceive before the start of the study, prior parity, smoking, testosterone, androstenedione, free androgen index (FAI), glucose, insulin, sex hormone-binding protein (SHBG), luteinizing hormone (LH), follicle stimulating hormone (FSH), estradiol, mean ovarian volume, mean ovarian follicle number, and menstrual cycle. Logistic regression analyses were used for the analyses of these potential predictors on conception. First, with univariate models we identified predictors with a significance of $p < 0.200$. Second, these identified potential predictors were entered in a multivariate model following a stepwise elimination of the least significant predictor until the final remaining variables reached a significance of $p < 0.05$. Outcomes were displayed as odds ratio (OR) with 95% confidence interval (CI). All models were corrected by including baseline weight as a covariate. Analyses were performed with IBM SPSS statistics version 25.0.

3. Results

A total of 561 women were eligible for the trial between 2 August 2010 and 11 March 2016. Figure 1 shows the participation selection flow-chart. To summarize, 26 women were included in the pilot study; 352 women could not participate because of various reasons; and finally 183 women were randomly assigned to one of the three arms of the study: (1) SMS+ group (n = 60), (2) SMS− group (n = 63); resulting in a total of n = 123 women in the LSI group, and (3) CAU group (n = 60). Baseline characteristics were presented in Table 1. Median age was 29 years (26–32)for LSI and 28 years (26–32) for CAU. BMI at baseline was 33.6 (30.8–36.6) for LSI and 30.6 (29.3–34.3) for CAU. Time attempting to conceive before the start of the study was 24 (15–38) and 23 (14–35) months for the LSI and CAU groups, respectively. The majority of the participants were nulliparous with 77.7% in LSI and 75.9% in CAU. Our previous results from this RCT demonstrated a statistically significant ($p < 0.001$) within-group mean weight loss of 7.87 kg in SMS+, 4.65 kg in SMS− and 2.32 kg in CAU after one year [19]. The following pregnancy results are based on calculations by the Erasmus MC using non-public microdata from Statistics Netherlands.

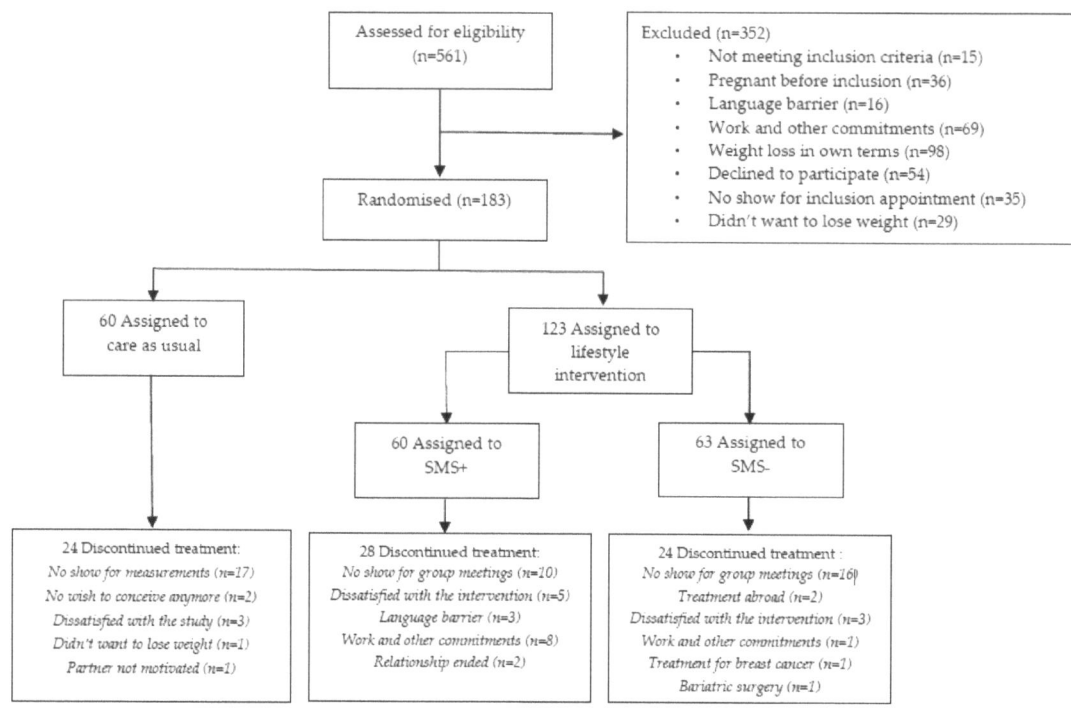

Figure 1. CONSORT flowchart.

Table 1. Baseline characteristics.

	Lifestyle Intervention (SMS+ and SMS−) n = 123	Care as Usual n = 60
	n (%)	n (%)
Nulliparous	94 (77.7)	44 (75.9)
Smoking	24 (19.7)	14 (23.7)
Alcohol consumption	27 (22.1)	19 (32.2)
Ethnicity		
Northern European	52 (42.6)	24 (40.0)
Mediterranean	18 (14.8)	12 (20.0)
Hindustani	15 (12.3)	6 (10.0)
African	27 (22.1)	17 (28.3)
Asian	6 (4.9)	0 (0.0)
Other	4 (3.3)	1 (1.7)
Education		
Low	10 (8.3)	8 (14.3)
Intermediate	67 (55.4)	35 (62.5)
High	44 (36.4)	13 (23.2)
PCOS characteristics		
OD	118 (96.7)	57 (95.0)
HA	97 (80.2)	47 (78.3)
PCOM	118 (98.3)	59 (98.3)
Phenotype classification		
A (OD + HA + PCOM)	89 (74.8)	43 (71.7)
B (OD + HA)	2 (1.7)	1 (1.7)
C (HA + PCOM)	4 (3.4)	3 (5.0)
D (OD + PCOM)	24 (20.2)	13 (21.7)

Table 1. Cont.

	Lifestyle Intervention (SMS+ and SMS−) n = 123	Care as Usual n = 60
	n (%)	n (%)
	Median (IQR)	Median (IQR)
Age (year)	29 (26–32)	28 (26–32)
Weight (kg)	92 (83–105)	84 (79–97)
BMI (kg/m^2)	33.6 (30.8–36.6)	30.6 (29.3–34.3)
Waist (cm)	101 (93–107)	96 (89–109)
Age of menarche (year)	12 (12–14)	12 (11–13)
Time attempting to conceive (months)	24 (15–38)	23 (14–35)

Note: Values are displayed as numbers (percentage) or as medians (interquartile range). Time attempting to conceive includes the time before the start of the study. Abbreviations: SMS+; lifestyle intervention with SMS support, SMS−; lifestyle intervention without SMS support, OD; ovulatory dysfunction, HA; hyperandrogenism, PCOM; polycystic ovarian morphology, IQR = interquartile range, BMI = body mass index.

3.1. Conception Resulting in Live Birth

Within 24 months after the start of the intervention, the conception resulting in live birth rate was 39.8% (49/123) within the LSI groups and 38.3% (23/60) within CAU. This was non-significant between the groups (p = 0.845), see Table 2. 26/49 (53.1%) of the offspring were male and 23/49 (46.9%) were female within the LSI groups. For the CAU group this was 13/23 (56.5%) and 10/23 (43.5%), respectively. Mean time to conception after the start of the study was illustrated in a Kaplan–Meier curve in Figure 2, with 18.7 and 19.4 months within the LSI and CAU groups, respectively (p = 0.646). Although weight loss had a positive effect on the chance to become pregnant (see Figure 3), this was non-significant (β = −0.038 SE 0.028, p = 0.169).

Table 2. Pregnancy outcomes within 24 months after the start of the intervention.

	Lifestyle Intervention (SMS+ and SMS−)	Care as Usual		Total
	n (%)	n (%)	p	n (%)
Conception resulting in live birth	49/123 (39.8)	23/60 (38.3)	0.845	72/183 (39.3)
Stillbirth (ante partum)	-	-	-	3/75 (4.0)
Mode of conception				
Spontaneous	27/49 (55.1)	15/23 (65.2)		42/72 (58.3)
After ART	16/49 (32.7)	7/23 (30.4)		23/72 (31.9)
Unknown	6/49 (12.2)	1/23 (4.3)	0.521	7/72 (9.7)
Method of delivery				
Vaginal birth	25/49 (51.0)	11/23 (47.8)		36/72 (50.0)
Instrument-assisted/caesarean section	22/49 (44.9)	12/23 (52.2)		34/72 (47.2)
Unknown	2/49 (4.1)	0/23 (0.0)	0.564	2/72 (2.8)
Pregnancy complications				
(gestational) diabetes	4/49 (8.2)	5/23 (21.7)	0.133	9/72 (12.5)
Hypertensive disorders	4/49 (8.2)	3/23 (13.0)	0.673	7/72 (9.7)
Preterm birth	6/49 (12.2)	4/23 (17.4)	0.716	10/72 (13.9)
Adverse postpartum outcomes				
Hemorrhage	-	-	-	5/72 (6.9)
Adverse neonatal outcomes				
Apgar score < 7 after 5 min	-	-	-	3/72 (4.2)
NICU admission	3/49 (6.1)	3/23 (13.0)	0.376	6/72 (8.3)
Small for gestational age	6/49 (12.2)	4/23 (17.4)	0.716	10/72 (13.9)
Large for gestational age	5/49 (10.6)	4/23 (17.4)	0.452	9/72 (12.5)
Congenital abnormalities	-	-	-	5/72 (6.9)
	Median (IQR)	Median (IQR)		
Birth weight (grams)	3350 (2915–3760)	3260 (2790–3870)	0.668	
Birth weight (percentile)	64 (24–83)	69 (22–86)	0.817	

Table 2. Cont.

	Lifestyle Intervention (SMS+ and SMS−)	Care as Usual	p	Total
	n (%)	n (%)		n (%)
	Median (IQR)	Median (IQR)		
Gestational age at delivery (days)	276 (264–283)	276 (267–283)	0.633	
Apgar 5 min	10 (9–10)	10 (9–10)	0.734	

Note: Results are based on calculations by the Erasmus MC using non-public microdata from Statistics Netherlands. Values are displayed as number/total (percentage) or as medians (interquartile range). Differences were tested with the use of the X^2 test or the Fishers exact test for categorical outcomes and with the use of the Mann–Whitney U test for continuous outcomes. There were no significant differences between the groups. Abbreviations: SMS+; lifestyle intervention with SMS support, SMS−; lifestyle intervention without SMS support, ART; assisted reproductive technology, NICU; neonatal intensive care unit, IQR = Interquartile range.

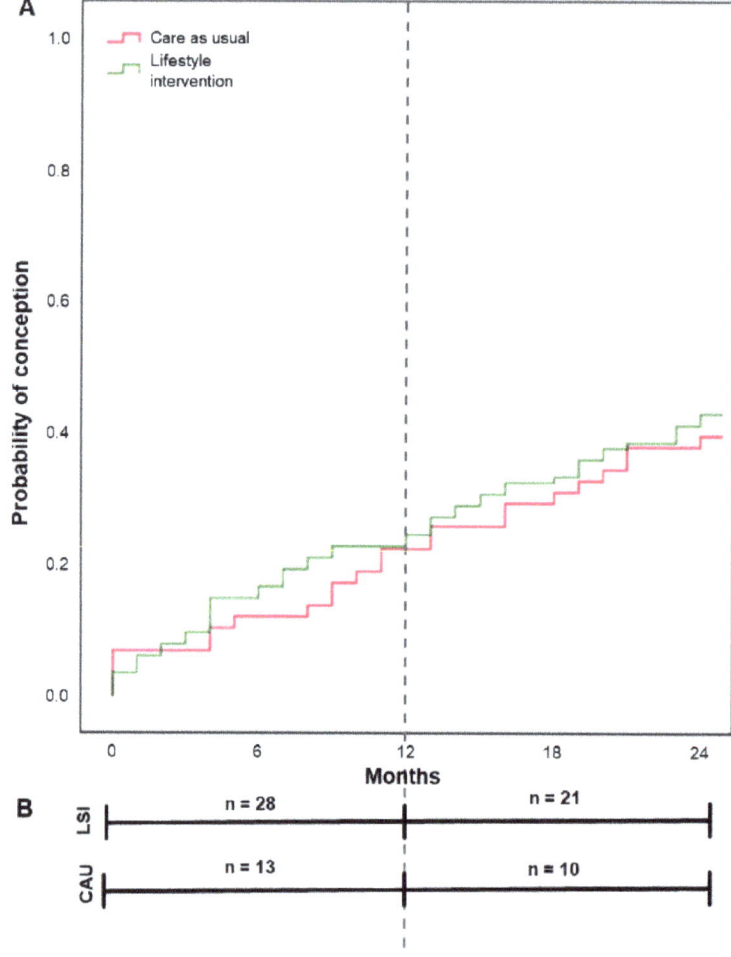

Figure 2. Time from the start of the study to conception resulting in live birth by group. Note: Results are based on calculations by the Erasmus MC using non-public microdata from Statistics Netherlands. (**A**) shows the Kaplan–Meier curve with mean time to conception resulting in live birth for lifestyle intervention (18.7 months), and care as usual (19.4 months). Differences were tested with the log rank test (p = 0.646). (**B**) shows the number of conceptions resulting in live birth within the given timeframe 0–12 months (during study period) and 12–24 months (post-study period) per study group.

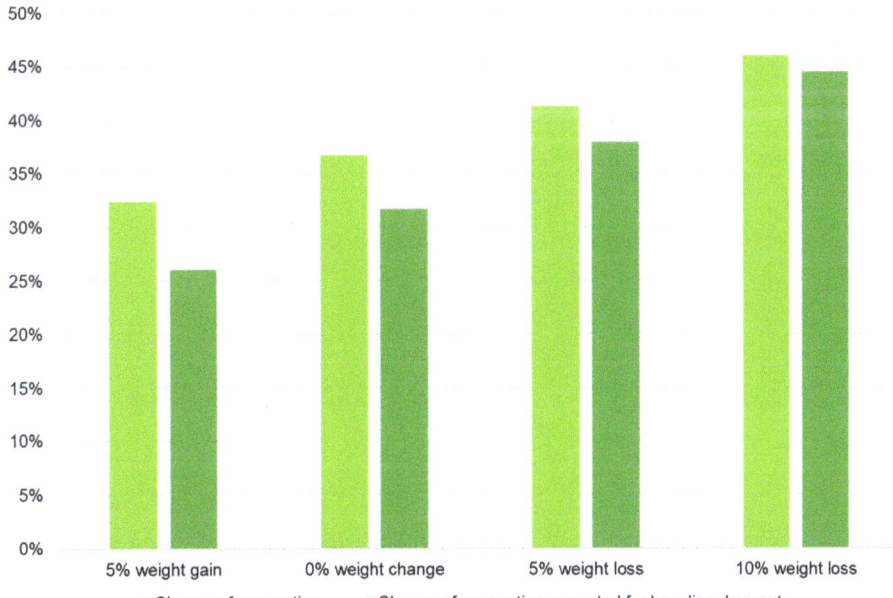

Figure 3. Logistic regression model for the effect of changes in weight on the chance of conception ≤ 24 months after the start of the intervention resulting in live birth. Note: Results are based on calculations by the Erasmus MC using non-public microdata from Statistics Netherlands. Logistic regression analyses; chance of conception: B = −0.038 SE 0.028, p = 0.169; chance of conception corrected for baseline drop-out: B = −0.055 SE 0.031, p = 0.081.

A large proportion of the participants conceived spontaneously (42/72, 58.3%), with 55.1% (27/49) in the LSI groups and 65.2% (15/23) in the CAU group (p = 0.521). Median birth weight was 3350 g (2915–3760) and 3260 g (2810–3848) for the LSI and CAU groups respectively (p = 0.668), with a median gestational age at delivery of 39 weeks (37–40)) for the LSI group and 39 weeks (38–40) for the CAU group (p = 0.830).

3.2. Pregnancy and Neonatal Complications

Both (gestational) diabetes (LSI 8.2% (4/49) and CAU 21.7% (5/23); p = 0.133), and hypertensive disorder rates (LSI 8.2% (4/49) and CAU 13.0% (3/23); p = 0.673) during pregnancy were non-significantly different between the groups, see Table 2. Preterm birth accounted for 12.2% (6/49) in the LSI groups, and for 17.4 (4/23) in the CAU group (p = 0.716). NICU admission rates were 6.1% (3/49) in the LSI groups, and 13.0% (3/23) within the CAU group (p = 0.376). Both groups combined contained 5 cases with a congenital abnormality. From our own data we encountered one neonatal death in total due to a severe congenital disorder.

3.3. Prediction of Conception

Twelve potentially predicting baseline variables, further specified in Table 3, were identified and joined in a multivariate model. The stepwise elimination process resulted in a model in which time attempting to conceive before the start of the study (OR 0.984 (95% CI 0.972–0.997), p = 0.017) and insulin (OR 0.991 (95% CI 0.986–0.997), p = 0.003) at baseline both had a negative predictive value for conception resulting in live birth within 24 months after the start of the intervention (see Table 3). The ROC curve for the final model is displayed in Figure 4 with an area under the curve of 0.691 (p < 0.001).

Table 3. Determinants of conception within 24 months after the start of the intervention.

Univariate Model	OR (95% CI)	p-Value
Age	0.939 (0.875–1.007)	0.078
Body mass index	0.877 (0.776–0.991)	0.035
Modified Ferriman–Gallwey score	0.959 (0.901–1.021)	0.191
Waist circumference	0.967 (0.930–1.006)	0.094
Time attempting to conceive	0.984 (0.971–0.997)	0.014
Androstenedione	0.906 (0.805–1.021)	0.105
Free androgen index	0.919 (0.852–0.992)	0.030
Glucose	0.564 (0.310–1.023)	0.060
Insulin	0.992 (0.986–0.997)	0.002
Sex hormone-binding globulin	1.020 (1.000–1.040)	0.049
Mean ovarian volume	0.925 (0.846–1.013)	0.091
Amenorrhea	0.535 (0.223–1.287)	0.163
Multivariate model	OR (95% CI)	p-value
Time attempting to conceive	0.984 (0.972–0.997)	0.017
Insulin	0.991 (0.986–0.997)	0.003

Note: Results are based on calculations by the Erasmus MC using non-public microdata from Statistics Netherlands. Logistic regression analyses, values are displayed as odds ratio (95% confidence interval), all model were corrected for baseline weight. Abbreviations: OR; odds ratio, CI; confidence interval.

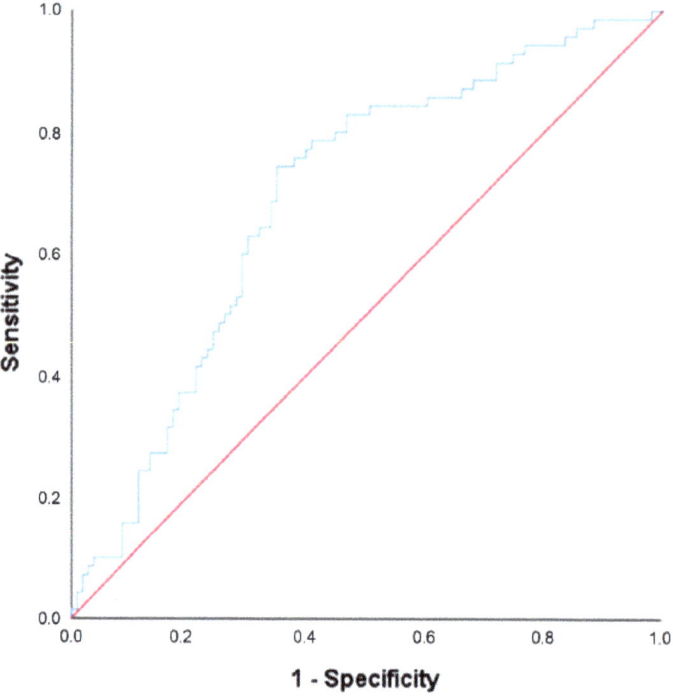

Figure 4. Receiver operating characteristic (ROC) curve for the model predicting conception within 24 months after the start of the intervention resulting in live birth. Note: Results are based on calculations by the Erasmus MC using non-public microdata from Statistics Netherlands. This final model included time attempting to conceive before the start of the study and insulin at baseline, area under the curve = 0.691 ($p < 0.001$).

3.4. Drop-Out Rate during Study Intervention Period

Finally, with the complete pregnancy data from the CBS and Dutch Perinatal registry we got more insight into participants who discontinued the intervention because of pregnancy or dropped out due to other causes. In previous publications we described a drop-out rate of 63.4% [19], which overestimated the number of true drop-outs as it included participants who dropped out due to pregnancy during the study period. With 28/123 pregnancies in the LSI group and 12/60 pregnancies in the CAU group there were a total of 40 (21.9%) pregnancies during the study intervention period, resulting in a true drop-out rate of 42.1%.

4. Discussion

This follow-up study from a randomized controlled one-year three-component lifestyle intervention reports on pregnancy outcomes based on data from the Dutch Perinatal registry. Conception rates and time to conception after the start of the study showed comparable non-significant results between the groups. It is worth mentioning that the majority of our population eventually conceived spontaneously. Pregnancy complications and outcomes were lower in the lifestyle intervention groups, and weight loss in general had a positive effect on the chance to conceive within 24 months after the start of the intervention. However, these findings were statistically non-significant. We also examined some predictors for pregnancy which resulted in a final model including baseline insulin level and time attempting to conceive before the start of the study.

Weight [19], emotional well-being [24], phenotypical characteristics [25], and metabolic health [26] all were shown to improve more in the LSI groups compared to CAU over the course of our study. It is believed that the pre-pregnancy optimization of these factors should improve reproductive and obstetric outcomes in women with PCOS as well as in their offspring [1]. Over the course of the study and follow-up period, women in all three groups got pregnant, either spontaneously or eventually aided by ART, as long as they reached their personal weight-loss goal at the end of the study. We observed coinciding increasing pregnancy rates and decreasing time to pregnancy after the start of the intervention in the lifestyle program. A similar trend was observed for pregnancy complications and adverse neonatal outcomes. It is interesting to see that the rates of pregnancy complications and adverse neonatal outcomes in the LSI group were, although still higher, more similar to the rates in the general Dutch population [27] when compared to the CAU group. However, the expected statistically significant differences were lacking. This could be explained by the fact that this study was powered on weight loss as the primary outcome [19], and not on pregnancy outcomes. Another explanation could be that the lifestyle intervention group was compared to care as usual, which also consisted of advice to lose weight. Although the amount of weight loss these women achieved was not as much as in the LSI group, this probably still had a positive influence on their chance to get pregnant.

Antenatal lifestyle interventions in the general population are associated with lower risks of adverse maternal and neonatal outcomes [28], which should be similar in women with PCOS. However, data on pregnancy outcomes reported from multi-component lifestyle interventions are lacking. A recent meta-analysis investigating the effect of lifestyle interventions in women with PCOS concluded that there were no studies which reported on live birth, miscarriage, or pregnancy [18]. However, Legro and colleagues did report on a preconception intervention (either 16 weeks of continuous oral contraceptive pills, lifestyle modification by low caloric diet, or both, followed by ovulation induction) in which live birth rates did not significantly differ between the groups [29]. The same group also demonstrated an improved live-birth rate as a benefit of delayed infertility treatment using clomiphene citrate (CC) when preceded by lifestyle modification with weight loss, compared to immediate treatment [30]. Furthermore, a few studies were performed on pregnancy outcomes in obese infertile women in general. These concluded that, although weight loss was achieved, lifestyle intervention preceding infertility treatment did not substantially affect live-birth rates [31–33]. However, we do have to keep in mind that success rates with fertility treatments are lower among obese infertile women when compared to normal-weight women [9,10], as well as the chance of natural conception [8]. Pregnancy and neonatal complications are also less common among non-obese women compared to obese women [34–36]. On top of this, women with PCOS have been found to be more prone to weight gain, which was most marked in those with unhealthy lifestyles [37]. Altogether, we would argue that recommending a lifestyle intervention in order to promote weight loss instead of immediately starting an infertility treatment in overweight or obese women with PCOS is the better choice. Moreover, a three-component lifestyle intervention aids in creating an overall healthier body composition in the metabolic, physical and mental domains which might as well result in a healthier pregnancy.

Based on our results, one could argue for the implementation of such a long-term and intensive lifestyle intervention for all women with PCOS, in order to improve fertility outcomes. Should we therefore look for other therapies to achieve even more weight loss, such as bariatric surgery? However, one should also keep in mind a treatment's impact, side-effects and cost-effectiveness. Bariatric surgery is an invasive procedure, and will cause a delay in fertility treatment because it is undesirable to conceive during a period of rapid weight loss. Furthermore, pregnancy complications due to nutrient malabsorption after bariatric surgery are also possible [1,38]. Other less invasive options, such as the use of insulin sensitizers like metformin or thiazolidinediones, are proven to be beneficial for weight loss and the treatment of infertility in women with PCOS [39]. However, these drugs can cause gastro-intestinal side effects or even weight gain, which may reduce patient compliance [40]. Inositol as an insulin sensitizer is currently recognized as a possible candidate for a non-invasive low-cost addition to lifestyle therapy with lack of significant adverse effects, even in pregnancy [41–43]. Benefits such as improving the ovulation rate as well as hormonal and insulin sensitivity indexes have been demonstrated [44]. However, further evidence will be necessary to confirm the efficacy of inositol to improve pregnancies and live birth in women with PCOS [45]. Finally, the use of anti-obesity drugs such as glucagon-like peptie-1 receptor agonists are currently an emerging area of interest and could also be considered while developing treatment strategies for overweight women with PCOS. Although contraindicated during pregnancy, these anti-obesity drugs simultaneously improve insulin sensitivity, reduce cardiovascular disease risk, and show promising potential in achieving and maintaining weight loss [46].

Baseline insulin levels and time attempting to get pregnant before the start of the study both had a negative predictive value on the chance to conceive. The same factors along with other predictors were reported in studies predicting the chances for live birth after ovulation induction using anti-estrogens [10,47,48], or using gonadotrophins [49–51]. In addition, a large proportion in our population conceived spontaneously, which again may be driven by different baseline predictors. Overall, given this spontaneous conception rate, and knowing most of them had a long time to pregnancy before they entered the study, which is a negative predictor, these study results are encouraging and may support the advice of lifestyle changes prior to infertility treatment in this population.

A strength of this follow-up study is the utilization of pregnancy data from the Dutch Perinatal registry. Because of this, we were sure to collect data on all conceptions resulting in live birth within the given timeframe, and we could even report on pregnancy outcomes from women who were lost to follow-up from the RCT. On top of this, we could make a distinction between the "real drop-out" and women who became pregnant during the study but were lost to follow-up, which resulted in a lower overall study drop-out rate than previously reported for this RCT [19].

However, a limitation of data from the CBS is the absent knowledge on miscarriages and pregnancies that ended before 16 weeks of gestation. Nonetheless, the final desired end-goal of couples will be an uneventful pregnancy and the birth of a living child, which is therefore in our eyes the most important study outcome. Furthermore, one should keep in mind that not all women in our study ultimately received fertility treatment, which could also be seen as a limitation. Participants in our study only received fertility treatment after achieving their personal weight loss goal, whereas other studies generally treated all participants [29,31–33]. This may cause an underestimation of pregnancies in our study when compared to other study designs. However, we believe that it was more desirable for participants to primarily achieve their weight loss goal and a healthy lifestyle before the start of an infertility treatment in order to decrease the chance on any possible iatrogenic induced pregnancy complications associated with overweight or obesity [52].

5. Conclusions

In total, 39.3% of the women conceived within 24 months after the start of the study, of which 58.3% were spontaneous conceptions. Women in het LSI groups lost more weight compared to CAU based on our previous data; however, this follow-up study showed no significant differences in conception resulting in live birth rates between LSI and CAU. These results should be interpreted with caution, because the study was not powered for pregnancy outcomes.

Author Contributions: Conceptualization, A.D.d.L., G.J., Y.L., A.B., J.B. and J.L.; data curation, A.D.d.L. and G.J.; formal analysis, A.D.d.L.; investigation, A.D.d.L. and G.J.; methodology, A.D.d.L., G.J., Y.L., A.B., J.B. and J.L.; project administration, A.D.d.L., G.J. and J.L.; supervision, J.L.; writing—original draft, A.D.d.L.; writing—review and editing, A.D.d.L., G.J., Y.L., A.B., J.B. and J.L. All authors have read and agreed to the published version of the manuscript.

Funding: This research received no external funding.

Institutional Review Board Statement: The study was conducted according to the guidelines of the Declaration of Helsinki, and approved by the Medical Research Ethics Committee of the Erasmus MC in Rotterdam (MEC-2008-337, date of approval: 4 December 2008).

Informed Consent Statement: Informed consent was obtained from all subjects involved in the study.

Data Availability Statement: Parts of the data presented in this study are available on request from the corresponding author. The data are not publicly available due to participant privacy reasons. Restrictions apply to the availability of the CBS/Perined data. Data was obtained from CBS/Perined and are only available from the authors with the permission of CBS/Perined.

Acknowledgments: We thank the entire PCOS team of the Erasmus MC.

Conflicts of Interest: A.D.d.L., G.J., Y.L., A.B. and J.B. have nothing to declare. J.L. reports grants from Ansh Labs, Webster, Tx, USA, from Ferring, Hoofddorp, NL, from Dutch Heart Association, Utrecht, NL, from Zon MW, Amsterdam, NL, from Roche Diagnostics, Rothkreuz, Switzerland and personal fees from Ferring, Hoofddorp, NL, from Titus Healthcare, Hoofddorp, NL, from Gedeon Richter, Groot-Bijgaarden, Belgium, and is an unpaid board member and president of the AE-PCOS Society, outside the submitted work.

References

1. Teede, H.J.; Misso, M.L.; Costello, M.F.; Dokras, A.; Laven, J.; Moran, L.; Piltonen, T.; Norman, R.J.; International, P.N. Recommendations from the international evidence-based guideline for the assessment and management of polycystic ovary syndrome. *Fertil. Steril.* **2018**, *110*, 364–379. [CrossRef]
2. The Rotterdam ESHRE/ASRM-Sponsored PCOS Consensus Workshop Group. Revised 2003 consensus on diagnostic criteria and long-term health risks related to polycystic ovary syndrome. *Fertil. Steril.* **2004**, *81*, 19–25. [CrossRef]
3. Lim, S.S.; Davies, M.J.; Norman, R.J.; Moran, L.J. Overweight, obesity and central obesity in women with polycystic ovary syndrome: A systematic review and meta-analysis. *Hum. Reprod. Update* **2012**, *18*, 618–637. [CrossRef] [PubMed]

4. Lizneva, D.; Suturina, L.; Walker, W.; Brakta, S.; Gavrilova-Jordan, L.; Azziz, R. Criteria, prevalence, and phenotypes of polycystic ovary syndrome. *Fertil. Steril.* **2016**, *106*, 6–15. [CrossRef] [PubMed]
5. Lim, S.S.; Norman, R.J.; Davies, M.J.; Moran, L.J. The effect of obesity on polycystic ovary syndrome: A systematic review and meta-analysis. *Obes. Rev.* **2013**, *14*, 95–109. [CrossRef] [PubMed]
6. Glueck, C.J.; Goldenberg, N. Characteristics of obesity in polycystic ovary syndrome: Etiology, treatment, and genetics. *Metabolism* **2019**, *92*, 108–120. [CrossRef]
7. Azziz, R.; Carmina, E.; Chen, Z.; Dunaif, A.; Laven, J.S.; Legro, R.S.; Lizneva, D.; Natterson-Horowtiz, B.; Teede, H.J.; Yildiz, B.O. Polycystic ovary syndrome. *Nat. Rev. Dis. Primers* **2016**, *2*, 16057. [CrossRef]
8. Silvestris, E.; de Pergola, G.; Rosania, R.; Loverro, G. Obesity as disruptor of the female fertility. *Reprod. Biol. Endocrinol.* **2018**, *16*, 22. [CrossRef]
9. Rittenberg, V.; Seshadri, S.; Sunkara, S.K.; Sobaleva, S.; Oteng-Ntim, E.; El-Toukhy, T. Effect of body mass index on IVF treatment outcome: An updated systematic review and meta-analysis. *Reprod. Biomed. Online* **2011**, *23*, 421–439. [CrossRef]
10. Imani, B.; Eijkemans, M.J.; te Velde, E.R.; Habbema, J.D.; Fauser, B.C. A nomogram to predict the probability of live birth after clomiphene citrate induction of ovulation in normogonadotropic oligoamenorrheic infertility. *Fertil. Steril.* **2002**, *77*, 91–97. [CrossRef]
11. Boomsma, C.M.; Eijkemans, M.J.; Hughes, E.G.; Visser, G.H.; Fauser, B.C.; Macklon, N.S. A meta-analysis of pregnancy outcomes in women with polycystic ovary syndrome. *Hum. Reprod. Update* **2006**, *12*, 673–683. [CrossRef] [PubMed]
12. Bahri Khomami, M.; Joham, A.E.; Boyle, J.A.; Piltonen, T.; Silagy, M.; Arora, C.; Misso, M.L.; Teede, H.J.; Moran, L.J. Increased maternal pregnancy complications in polycystic ovary syndrome appear to be independent of obesity-A systematic review, meta-analysis, and meta-regression. *Obes. Rev.* **2019**, *20*, 659–674. [CrossRef] [PubMed]
13. Qin, J.Z.; Pang, L.H.; Li, M.J.; Fan, X.J.; Huang, R.D.; Chen, H.Y. Obstetric complications in women with polycystic ovary syndrome: A systematic review and meta-analysis. *Reprod. Biol. Endocrinol.* **2013**, *11*, 56. [CrossRef]
14. Palomba, S.; de Wilde, M.A.; Falbo, A.; Koster, M.P.; La Sala, G.B.; Fauser, B.C. Pregnancy complications in women with polycystic ovary syndrome. *Hum. Reprod. Update* **2015**, *21*, 575–592. [CrossRef] [PubMed]
15. de Wilde, M.A.; Lamain-de Ruiter, M.; Veltman-Verhulst, S.M.; Kwee, A.; Laven, J.S.; Lambalk, C.B.; Eijkemans, M.J.C.; Franx, A.; Fauser, B.; Koster, M.P.H. Increased rates of complications in singleton pregnancies of women previously diagnosed with polycystic ovary syndrome predominantly in the hyperandrogenic phenotype. *Fertil. Steril.* **2017**, *108*, 333–340. [CrossRef] [PubMed]
16. Hoeger, K.M.; Kochman, L.; Wixom, N.; Craig, K.; Miller, R.K.; Guzick, D.S. A randomized, 48-week, placebo-controlled trial of intensive lifestyle modification and/or metformin therapy in overweight women with polycystic ovary syndrome: A pilot study. *Fertil. Steril.* **2004**, *82*, 421–429. [CrossRef] [PubMed]
17. Jedel, E.; Labrie, F.; Oden, A.; Holm, G.; Nilsson, L.; Janson, P.O.; Lind, A.K.; Ohlsson, C.; Stener-Victorin, E. Impact of electro-acupuncture and physical exercise on hyperandrogenism and oligo/amenorrhea in women with polycystic ovary syndrome: A randomized controlled trial. *Am. J. Physiol. Endocrinol. Metab.* **2011**, *300*, E37–E45. [CrossRef]
18. Lim, S.S.; Hutchison, S.K.; Van Ryswyk, E.; Norman, R.J.; Teede, H.J.; Moran, L.J. Lifestyle changes in women with polycystic ovary syndrome. *Cochrane Database Syst. Rev.* **2019**, *3*, CD007506. [CrossRef]
19. Jiskoot, G.; Timman, R.; Beerthuizen, A.; Dietz de Loos, A.; Busschbach, J.; Laven, J. Weight Reduction Through a Cognitive Behavioral Therapy Lifestyle Intervention in PCOS: The Primary Outcome of a Randomized Controlled Trial. *Obesity* **2020**, *28*, 2134–2141. [CrossRef]
20. Jiskoot, G.; Benneheij, S.H.; Beerthuizen, A.; de Niet, J.E.; de Klerk, C.; Timman, R.; Busschbach, J.J.; Laven, J.S. A three-component cognitive behavioural lifestyle program for preconceptional weight-loss in women with polycystic ovary syndrome (PCOS): A protocol for a randomized controlled trial. *Reprod. Health* **2017**, *14*, 34. [CrossRef]
21. Brink, E.; van Rossum, C.; Postma-Smeets, A.; Stafleu, A.; Wolvers, D.; van Dooren, C.; Toxopeus, I.; Buurma-Rethans, E.; Geurts, M.; Ocke, M. Development of healthy and sustainable food-based dietary guidelines for the Netherlands. *Public Health Nutr.* **2019**, *22*, 2419–2435. [CrossRef] [PubMed]
22. *Global Recommendations on Physical Activity for Health*; World Health Organization: Geneva, Switzerland, 2010.
23. Meray, N.; Reitsma, J.B.; Ravelli, A.C.; Bonsel, G.J. Probabilistic record linkage is a valid and transparent tool to combine databases without a patient identification number. *J. Clin. Epidemiol.* **2007**, *60*, 883–891. [CrossRef] [PubMed]
24. Jiskoot, G.; Dietz de Loos, A.; Beerthuizen, A.; Timman, R.; Busschbach, J.; Laven, J. Long-term effects of a three-component lifestyle intervention on emotional well-being in women with Polycystic Ovary Syndrome (PCOS): A secondary analysis of a randomized controlled trial. *PLoS ONE* **2020**, *15*, e0233876. [CrossRef] [PubMed]
25. Dietz de Loos, A.L.P.; Jiskoot, G.; Timman, R.; Beerthuizen, A.; Busschbach, J.J.V.; Laven, J.S.E. Improvements in PCOS characteristics and phenotype severity during a randomized controlled lifestyle intervention. *Reprod. Biomed. Online* **2021**, *43*, 298–309. [CrossRef]
26. Dietz de Loos, A.; Jiskoot, G.; Beerthuizen, A.; Busschbach, J.; Laven, J. Metabolic health during a randomized controlled lifestyle intervention in women with PCOS. *Eur. J. Endocrinol.* **2021**, *186*, 53–64. [CrossRef]

27. Perined. *Perinatale Zorg in Nederland Anno 2018: Landelijke Perinatale Cijfers en Duiding*; Perined: Utrecht, The Netherlands, 2019.
28. Teede, H.J.; Bailey, C.; Moran, L.J.; Bahri Khomami, M.; Enticott, J.; Ranasinha, S.; Rogozinska, E.; Skouteris, H.; Boyle, J.A.; Thangaratinam, S.; et al. Association of Antenatal Diet and Physical Activity-Based Interventions With Gestational Weight Gain and Pregnancy Outcomes: A Systematic Review and Meta-analysis. *JAMA Intern. Med.* **2022**, *182*, 106–114. [CrossRef]
29. Legro, R.S.; Dodson, W.C.; Kris-Etherton, P.M.; Kunselman, A.R.; Stetter, C.M.; Williams, N.I.; Gnatuk, C.L.; Estes, S.J.; Fleming, J.; Allison, K.C.; et al. Randomized Controlled Trial of Preconception Interventions in Infertile Women With Polycystic Ovary Syndrome. *J. Clin. Endocrinol. Metab.* **2015**, *100*, 4048–4058. [CrossRef]
30. Legro, R.S.; Dodson, W.C.; Kunselman, A.R.; Stetter, C.M.; Kris-Etherton, P.M.; Williams, N.I.; Gnatuk, C.L.; Estes, S.J.; Allison, K.C.; Sarwer, D.B.; et al. Benefit of Delayed Fertility Therapy With Preconception Weight Loss Over Immediate Therapy in Obese Women With PCOS. *J. Clin. Endocrinol. Metab.* **2016**, *101*, 2658–2666. [CrossRef]
31. Legro, R.S.; Hansen, K.R.; Diamond, M.P.; Steiner, A.Z.; Coutifaris, C.; Cedars, M.I.; Hoeger, K.M.; Usadi, R.; Johnstone, E.B.; Haisenleder, D.J.; et al. Effects of preconception lifestyle intervention in infertile women with obesity: The FIT-PLESE randomized controlled trial. *PLoS Med.* **2022**, *19*, e1003883. [CrossRef]
32. Einarsson, S.; Bergh, C.; Friberg, B.; Pinborg, A.; Klajnbard, A.; Karlstrom, P.O.; Kluge, L.; Larsson, I.; Loft, A.; Mikkelsen-Englund, A.L.; et al. Weight reduction intervention for obese infertile women prior to IVF: A randomized controlled trial. *Hum. Reprod.* **2017**, *32*, 1621–1630. [CrossRef]
33. Mutsaerts, M.A.; van Oers, A.M.; Groen, H.; Burggraaff, J.M.; Kuchenbecker, W.K.; Perquin, D.A.; Koks, C.A.; van Golde, R.; Kaaijk, E.M.; Schierbeek, J.M.; et al. Randomized Trial of a Lifestyle Program in Obese Infertile Women. *N. Engl. J. Med.* **2016**, *374*, 1942–1953. [CrossRef] [PubMed]
34. Ovesen, P.; Rasmussen, S.; Kesmodel, U. Effect of prepregnancy maternal overweight and obesity on pregnancy outcome. *Obstet. Gynecol.* **2011**, *118*, 305–312. [CrossRef]
35. Cnattingius, S.; Villamor, E.; Johansson, S.; Edstedt Bonamy, A.K.; Persson, M.; Wikstrom, A.K.; Granath, F. Maternal obesity and risk of preterm delivery. *JAMA* **2013**, *309*, 2362–2370. [CrossRef] [PubMed]
36. Aune, D.; Saugstad, O.D.; Henriksen, T.; Tonstad, S. Maternal body mass index and the risk of fetal death, stillbirth, and infant death: A systematic review and meta-analysis. *JAMA* **2014**, *311*, 1536–1546. [CrossRef] [PubMed]
37. Awoke, M.A.; Earnest, A.; Joham, A.E.; Hodge, A.M.; Teede, H.J.; Brown, W.J.; Moran, L.J. Weight gain and lifestyle factors in women with and without polycystic ovary syndrome. *Hum. Reprod.* **2021**, *37*, 129–141. [CrossRef]
38. Micic, D.D.; Toplak, H.; Micic, D.D.; Polovina, S.P. Reproductive outcomes after bariatric surgery in women. *Wien. Klin. Wochenschr.* **2022**, *134*, 56–62. [CrossRef]
39. Macut, D.; Bjekic-Macut, J.; Rahelic, D.; Doknic, M. Insulin and the polycystic ovary syndrome. *Diabetes Res. Clin. Pract.* **2017**, *130*, 163–170. [CrossRef]
40. Pasquali, R.; Gambineri, A. Insulin sensitizers in polycystic ovary syndrome. *Front. Horm. Res.* **2013**, *40*, 83–102. [CrossRef]
41. Unfer, V.; Nestler, J.E.; Kamenov, Z.A.; Prapas, N.; Facchinetti, F. Effects of Inositol(s) in Women with PCOS: A Systematic Review of Randomized Controlled Trials. *Int. J. Endocrinol.* **2016**, *2016*, 1849162. [CrossRef]
42. Mendoza, N.; Perez, L.; Simoncini, T.; Genazzani, A. Inositol supplementation in women with polycystic ovary syndrome undergoing intracytoplasmic sperm injection: A systematic review and meta-analysis of randomized controlled trials. *Reprod. Biomed. Online* **2017**, *35*, 529–535. [CrossRef]
43. Zheng, X.; Lin, D.; Zhang, Y.; Lin, Y.; Song, J.; Li, S.; Sun, Y. Inositol supplement improves clinical pregnancy rate in infertile women undergoing ovulation induction for ICSI or IVF-ET. *Medicine* **2017**, *96*, e8842. [CrossRef] [PubMed]
44. Pundir, J.; Psaroudakis, D.; Savnur, P.; Bhide, P.; Sabatini, L.; Teede, H.; Coomarasamy, A.; Thangaratinam, S. Inositol treatment of anovulation in women with polycystic ovary syndrome: A meta-analysis of randomised trials. *BJOG* **2018**, *125*, 299–308. [CrossRef] [PubMed]
45. Lagana, A.S.; Garzon, S.; Casarin, J.; Franchi, M.; Ghezzi, F. Inositol in Polycystic Ovary Syndrome: Restoring Fertility through a Pathophysiology-Based Approach. *Trends Endocrinol. Metab.* **2018**, *29*, 768–780. [CrossRef]
46. Siamashvili, M.; Davis, S.N. Update on the effects of GLP-1 receptor agonists for the treatment of polycystic ovary syndrome. *Expert. Rev. Clin. Pharmacol.* **2021**, *14*, 1081–1089. [CrossRef]
47. Rausch, M.E.; Legro, R.S.; Barnhart, H.X.; Schlaff, W.D.; Carr, B.R.; Diamond, M.P.; Carson, S.A.; Steinkampf, M.P.; McGovern, P.G.; Cataldo, N.A.; et al. Predictors of pregnancy in women with polycystic ovary syndrome. *J. Clin. Endocrinol. Metab.* **2009**, *94*, 3458–3466. [CrossRef] [PubMed]
48. Kuang, H.; Jin, S.; Hansen, K.R.; Diamond, M.P.; Coutifaris, C.; Casson, P.; Christman, G.; Alvero, R.; Huang, H.; Bates, G.W.; et al. Identification and replication of prediction models for ovulation, pregnancy and live birth in infertile women with polycystic ovary syndrome. *Hum. Reprod.* **2015**, *30*, 2222–2233. [CrossRef] [PubMed]
49. Mulders, A.G.; Eijkemans, M.J.; Imani, B.; Fauser, B.C. Prediction of chances for success or complications in gonadotrophin ovulation induction in normogonadotrophic anovulatory infertility. *Reprod. Biomed. Online* **2003**, *7*, 170–178. [CrossRef]
50. Mulders, A.G.; Laven, J.S.; Eijkemans, M.J.; Hughes, E.G.; Fauser, B.C. Patient predictors for outcome of gonadotrophin ovulation induction in women with normogonadotrophic anovulatory infertility: A meta-analysis. *Hum. Reprod. Update* **2003**, *9*, 429–449. [CrossRef]

51. Nyboe Andersen, A.; Balen, A.H.; Platteau, P.; Pettersson, G.; Arce, J.C. Prestimulation parameters predicting live birth in anovulatory WHO Group II patients undergoing ovulation induction with gonadotrophins. *Hum. Reprod.* **2010**, *25*, 1988–1995. [CrossRef]
52. Steegers-Theunissen, R.; Hoek, A.; Groen, H.; Bos, A.; van den Dool, G.; Schoonenberg, M.; Smeenk, J.; Creutzberg, E.; Vecht, L.; Starmans, L.; et al. Pre-Conception Interventions for Subfertile Couples Undergoing Assisted Reproductive Technology Treatment: Modeling Analysis. *JMIR Mhealth Uhealth* **2020**, *8*, e19570. [CrossRef]

Disclaimer/Publisher's Note: The statements, opinions and data contained in all publications are solely those of the individual author(s) and contributor(s) and not of MDPI and/or the editor(s). MDPI and/or the editor(s) disclaim responsibility for any injury to people or property resulting from any ideas, methods, instructions or products referred to in the content.

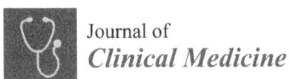

Article

Oral and Vaginal Hormonal Contraceptives Induce Similar Unfavorable Metabolic Effects in Women with PCOS: A Randomized Controlled Trial

Maria-Elina Mosorin [1,2,3], Terhi Piltonen [1,2,3], Anni S. Rantala [1,2,3], Marika Kangasniemi [1,2,3], Elisa Korhonen [1,2,3], Risto Bloigu [2,3], Juha S. Tapanainen [4,*] and Laure Morin-Papunen [1,2,3]

[1] Department of Obstetrics and Gynecology, Oulu University Hospital, Wellbeing Services County of North Ostrobothnia, 90220 Oulu, Finland
[2] Research Unit of Clinical Medicine, University of Oulu, 90220 Oulu, Finland
[3] Medical Research Center, University of Oulu, Oulu University Hospital, Wellbeing Services County of North Ostrobothnia, 90220 Oulu, Finland
[4] Department of Obstetrics and Gynecology, Helsinki University Hospital, University of Helsinki, 00290 Helsinki, Finland
* Correspondence: juha.tapanainen@helsinki.fi

Abstract: This clinical trial aims to compare hormonal and metabolic changes after a 9-week continuous use of oral or vaginal combined hormonal contraceptives (CHCs) in women with polycystic ovary syndrome (PCOS). We recruited 24 women with PCOS and randomized them to use either combined oral (COC, $n = 13$) or vaginal (CVC, $n = 11$) contraception. At baseline and 9 weeks, blood samples were collected and a 2 h glucose tolerance test (OGTT) was performed to evaluate hormonal and metabolic outcomes. After treatment, serum sex hormone binding globulin (SHBG) levels increased ($p < 0.001$ for both groups) and the free androgen index (FAI) decreased in both study groups (COC $p < 0.001$; CVC $p = 0.007$). OGTT glucose levels at 60 min ($p = 0.011$) and AUCglucose ($p = 0.018$) increased in the CVC group. Fasting insulin levels ($p = 0.037$) increased in the COC group, and insulin levels at 120 min increased in both groups (COC $p = 0.004$; CVC $p = 0.042$). There was a significant increase in triglyceride ($p < 0.001$) and hs-CRP ($p = 0.032$) levels in the CVC group. Both oral and vaginal CHCs decreased androgenicity and tended to promote insulin resistance in PCOS women. Larger and longer studies are needed to compare the metabolic effects of different administration routes of CHCs on women with PCOS.

Keywords: PCOS; oral combined hormonal contraception; vaginal combined hormonal contraception; metabolic effects; OGTT

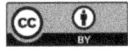

1. Introduction

Polycystic ovary syndrome (PCOS) is the most common endocrine disorder, affecting 5–18% of women of reproductive age [1,2]. According to the Rotterdam criteria [3] and the international evidence-based PCOS guideline [4], PCOS is defined by at least two of the following three features: (1) polycystic ovaries on gynecological ultrasonography, (2) oligo- or anovulation, and/or (3) clinical and/or biochemical hyperandrogenism (hirsutism or high serum testosterone or androgen levels). Women with PCOS display an increased risk for glucose metabolism disorders [5,6], obesity, hypertension, dyslipidemia, insulin resistance (IR), and metabolic syndrome [5–8].

Combined hormonal contraceptives (CHCs) are the first-line treatment for the most common PCOS-related clinical manifestations, namely menstrual irregularity and hirsutism [4,9]. However, CHCs are known to induce unfavorable metabolic effects, especially on glucose metabolism, in the general population [10–13]. Recommendations for CHC use by women with PCOS are generally based on studies of women without PCOS, with a limited number of studies on the use of CHCs in PCOS. Given the metabolic burden related to PCOS, it is plausible that CHCs may worsen already existing metabolic disorders related to the syndrome [14]. Some studies of women without PCOS have indicated that the use of combined vaginal contraception (CVC) causes fewer metabolic effects than combined oral contraception (COC) [12,15], although the findings are inconsistent [13]. Given the widespread use of CVC among women and possibly less adverse systemic effects of vaginal administration due to lower hepatic stress compared with oral administration, there is a necessity for studies to evaluate the metabolic effects of CVC use in women with PCOS.

Although the international evidence-based PCOS guideline recommends COCs in first-line pharmacological management for menstrual irregularity and hyperandrogenism, it does not provide specific recommendations for dosage, mode of administration, or specific preparation [4]. Earlier, the Amsterdam ESHRE/ASRM consensus on women's health aspects of PCOS concluded that there is a need to perform head-to-head trials comparing different CHC strategies, as well as longitudinal follow-up studies on CHC use in women with PCOS [3].

The aim of this randomized controlled trial was to compare the hormonal and metabolic effects of COC and CVC in women with PCOS after nine weeks.

2. Materials and Methods

This randomized, prospective, open-label, single-centered study was conducted at Oulu University Hospital, Finland, between 2011 and 2016. The study was approved by the Ethics Committee of Oulu University Hospital. All participants signed a written consent document. The study was registered at ClinicalTrials.gov (NCT01588873).

2.1. Study Population (Figure 1)

The participants were selected from the hospital register of Oulu University Hospital according to the ICD10 diagnosis code for PCOS (E 28.2). The women were eligible to participate if they were aged 18–40 years, healthy, and without medical contraindications for the use of CHCs (high blood pressure, migraine with focal aura, severe or multiple risk factors to thromboembolism, acute or chronic hepatocellular disease or hepatic adenomas or carcinomas, unexplained abnormal vaginal bleeding, diagnosed or suspected cancer, or an estrogen-dependent tumor), not using any medication, not smoking, not pregnant or breastfeeding, and had not used any hormonal or cortisone medicines for at least 2 months prior to study entry.

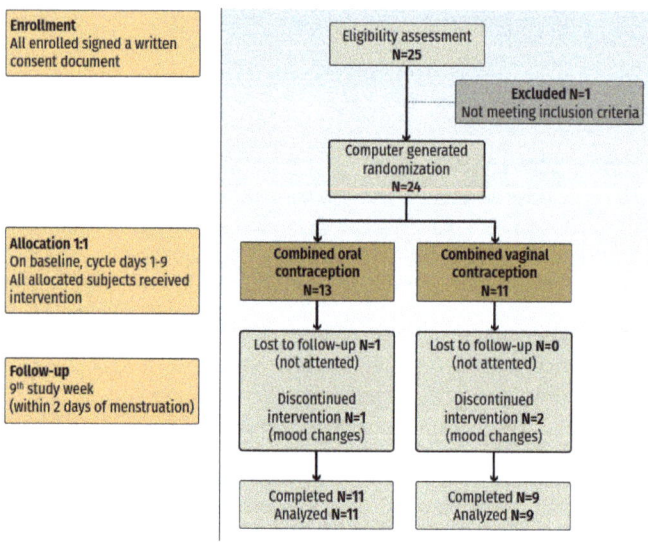

Figure 1. Flowchart of the study.

The participants were randomized to use either a combined hormonal oral contraceptive pill (COC group: ethinylestradiol, EE, 20 µg and desogestrel, 150 µg; Mercilon®; Organon Ltd., Dublin, Ireland) or a combined hormonal contraceptive vaginal ring (CVC group: EE, 15 µg/day and etonogestrel, an active metabolite of desogestrel, 120 µg/day; NuvaRing®; N.V.Organon, Oss, Netherlands) continuous for 9 weeks. The randomization list (allocation 1:1) was computer-generated. The participants went through two clinical examinations, the first at baseline and the second at 9 weeks of treatment, which included a gynecological examination, a transvaginal ultrasound (endometrium thickness, ovarian volumes, and the number of follicles), blood sampling for hormonal and metabolic parameters, and an oral glucose tolerance test (OGTT). At baseline, the clinical examination was performed between cycle days 1–3 and, at the ninth study week, within 3 days from the beginning of menstruation after discontinuation of the contraceptive preparation.

In all, 24 women with PCOS were recruited, 13 in the COC group and 11 in the CVC group (Figure 1). Diagnosis of PCOS was made according to the Rotterdam criteria. The baseline characteristics of the participants are described in Table 1.

Table 1. Baseline characteristics of the study population.

	COC	CVC	p-Value *
Age (years)	32.4 ± 6.6	30.8 ± 4.9	0.051
BMI (kg/m^2)	25.4 ± 3.3	23.2 ± 2.4	0.068
PCOM	13/13	11/11	0.287
oligomenorrhea	10/13	9/11	0.493
hirsutism/high testo	6/13	5/11	0.974

* p-value between the study groups at baseline. COC, combined oral contraceptive; CVC, combined vaginal contraceptive; BMI, body mass index; PCOM, polycystic ovarian morphology.

2.2. Oral Glucose Tolerance Test

The 75 g 2 h oral OGTT was performed after 12 h of fasting at baseline and 9 weeks. Blood samples were taken at 0, 30, 60, and 120 min. Glucose and insulin areas under the curve (glucose AUC and insulin AUC), the homeostatic model assessment of insulin resistance (HOMA-IR), the homeostatic model assessment of β-cell function (HOMA-2β), and whole-body insulin sensitivity (i.e., Matsuda index) [16] were calculated based on OGTT results to evaluate glucose tolerance, IR, and insulin sensitivity.

Although the hyperinsulinemic-euglycemic glucose clamp is the gold standard for evaluating insulin sensitivity, it is costly, time-consuming, invasive, and requires staff. The calculated indexes, such as HOMA-IR and Matsuda, have been shown to estimate insulin resistance and sensitivity more easily [16–18].

HOMA-IR (=insulin (mU/L) × glucose (mmol/L)/22.5) is a calculated index used to quantify IR from basal glucose and insulin levels and was first described in 1985 by Matthews et al. [18]. A strong linear correlation of HOMA-IR with the clamp has been found [17,18]. In women with PCOS, HOMA-IR has been used in various studies of different populations to assess IR [19–22] and has proven to be a robust clinical and epidemiological tool for assessing IR. HOMA-2β (=20 × fasting insulin (µIU/mL)/fasting glucose (mmol/mL) − 3.5) has been used as a marker of basal insulin secretion by pancreatic β-cells [21].

The Matsuda index (=[10,000/$\sqrt{\text{fasting glucose} \times \text{fasting insulin}}$] (mean glucose (OGTT) × mean insulin OGTT)]) was described by Matsuda and DeFronzo in 1999. It estimates whole-body physiological insulin sensitivity [16]. In women with PCOS, the Matsuda index correlates well with HOMA-IR and the quantitative insulin-sensitivity check index (QUICKI), which indicates its reliability in the detection of IR [23,24].

2.3. Assays

Serum samples for the assay of total testosterone (T) were conducted by using Agilent triple quadrupole 6410 liquid chromatography–mass spectrometry (LC-MS) equipment with an electrospray ionization source operating in positive-ion mode (Agilent Technologies, Wilmington, DE, USA). Multiple reaction monitoring was used to quantify T by using trideuterated T (d3-T) with the following transitions: m/z 289.2 to 97 and 289.2 to 109 for T and 292.2 to 97 and 292.2 to 109 for d3-T. The intra-assay coefficients of variation (CVs) of the method were 5.3%, 1.6%, and 1.2% for T at 0.6, 6.6, and 27.7 nmol/L, respectively.

Sex hormone binding globulin (SHBG) was analyzed by chemiluminometric immunoassays (Immulite 2000, Siemens Healthcare Diagnostics, Los Angeles, CA, USA) with a sensitivity of 0.02 nmol/L. Serum glucose, total cholesterol, low-density lipoprotein cholesterol (LDL-C), high-density lipoprotein cholesterol (HDL-C), and triglycerides were assayed using an automatic chemical analyzer (Advia, 1800; Siemens Healthcare Diagnostics, Tarrytown, NY, USA), insulin by using an automated a chemiluminescence system (Advia Centaur; Siemens Healthcare Diagnostics, Tarrytown, NY, USA), and high-sensitivity C-reactive protein (hs-CRP) by using an immunonephelometry (BN ProSpec; Siemens Healthcare Diagnostics, Marburg, Germany). All samples (baseline and 9 weeks) from the same subject were analyzed in the same assay.

2.4. Statistical Analyses

Power calculation was based on our previous study comparing the metabolic effects of the same preparations (Mercilon® and Nuvaring®) in young healthy women [13]. That study showed a significant increase of 0.44 mmol in serum triglyceride levels at 9 weeks of treatment with both preparations. The power analysis indicated that 17 women would have been needed in both study groups to reveal a similar increase in the serum level of triglycerides. To allow for dropouts, the planned sample size was 40 women (20 women in each group). Unfortunately, because of the strong criticism at the time of the recruitment raised in the media toward the thromboembolic risks linked to the use of hormonal contraception, the recruitment was extremely slow, and we managed eventually to recruit 24 women, 13 in the COC group and 11 in the CVC group.

All variables are present as means with standard deviation (SD) in Table 2. Paired samples t-tests were performed for normally distributed variables and Wilcoxon's tests were used for variables with a skewed distribution to explore changes in hormonal and metabolic levels within the same study group at the baseline and during the treatment. To analyze the differences between the study groups and the change from baseline to the 9th study week, we used a linear mixed model (repeated measures) with a random intercept. All results were adjusted with the BMI and age of the participants.

Table 2. Differences in the parameters of androgen secretion, glucose metabolism, lipid profile, and inflammation between the study groups. Analyses were performed with a linear mixed model with a random intercept.

Variable	Fixed Effect	Estimate	95%CI	p-Value	p Adjusted *
BMI (kg/m^2)	time	0.33	−0.08; 0.75	0.128	0.109
	CHC	−1.70	−4.20; 0.79	0.131	0.170
	time*CHC	−0.34	−0.95; 0.26	0.245	0.244
WC (cm)	time	−0.36	−3.32; 2.61	0.748	0.825
	CHC	−0.81	−8.22; 6.60	0.626	0.825
	time*CHC	0.42	−3.99; 4.83	0.812	0.843
sBP (mmHg)	time	−0.32	−5.77; 5.14	0.905	0.394
	CHC	−7.07	−16.41; 2.28	0.134	0.195
	time*CHC	−2.42	−10.76; 5.92	0.550	0.880
dBP (mmHg)	time	−0.63	−4.99; 3.73	0.425	0.762
	CHC	−2.78	−11.02; 5.45	0.109	0.495
	time*CHC	−1.53	−7.94; 4.88	0.613	0.618

Table 2. *Cont.*

Variable	Fixed Effect	Estimate	95%CI	p-Value	p Adjusted *
SHBG	time	−111.8	−144.98; −78.7	<0.001	<0.001
	CHC	37.8	−6.6; 81.9	0.019	0.093
	time*CHC	−39.2	−88.5; 10.1	0.080	0.113
Kol (mmol/L)	time	−111.8	−144.98; −78.7	<0.001	<0.001
	CHC	37.8	−6.6; 81.9	0.019	0.093
	time*CHC	−39.2	−88.5; 10.1	0.080	0.113
LDL-C (mmol/L)	time	−0.188	−0.61; 0.23	0.569	0.360
	CHC	0.113	−0.52; 0.75	0.766	0.718
	time*CHC	0.149	−0.48; 0.78	0.598	0.622
HDL-C (mmol/L)	time	−0.025	−0.34; 0.29	0.076	0.869
	CHC	0.291	−0.34; 0.92	0.574	0.351
	time*CHC	0.052	−0.42; 0.53	0.595	0.821
triglycerides (mmol/L)	time	−0.179	−0.4; 0.04	0.032	0.103
	CHC	0.236	−0.12; 0.59	0.919	0.182
	time*CHC	−0.333	−0.66; −0.01	0.542	0.046
CRP (mmol/L)	time	−0.538	−1.96; 0.88	0.403	0.432
	CHC	2.139	0.35; 3.93	0.109	0.021
	time*CHC	−1.350	−3.44; 0.74	0.376	0.190
fasting glucose (mmol/L)	time	−0.099	−0.36–0.17	0.700	0.440
	CHC	−0.181	−0.50–0.14	0.213	0.266
	time*CHC	0.131	−0.26–0.52	0.456	0.488
fasting insulin (mU/L)	time	−2.215	−4.8; 0.39	0.140	0.091
	CHC	3.127	−4.8; 0.39	0.718	0.108
	time*CHC	0.749	−3.13; 4.63	0.899	0.690
AUCglucose	time	−1.666	−3.52; 0.19	0.107	0.817
	CHC	0.283	−2.19; 2.75	0.065	0.076
	time*CHC	0.413	−2.42; 3.25	0.921	0.764
AUCinsulin	time	−27.11	−70.7; 16.5	0.260	0.206
	CHC	71.37	−1.8; 144.5	0.363	0.056
	time*CHC	−20.00	−86.7; 46.7	0.249	0.534
HOMA-IR	time	−0.430	−1.20; 0.34	0.404	0.266
	CHC	1.178	0.18; 2.18	0.295	0.022
	time*CHC	−0.292	−1.5;0.91	0.316	0.617
HOMA-2β	time	−26.61	−55.3; 2.05	0.269	0.067
	CHC	49.15	5.1; 93.2	0.065	0.030
	time*CHC	2.428	−40.2; 45.1	0.827	0.906
Matsuda index	time	1.835	0.29; 3.38	0.065	0.023
	CHC	0.302	−2.95; 3.55	0.673	0.850
	time*CHC	−0.968	−3.29; 1.36	0.717	0.759

* Adjusted with BMI and age. Time comparison between baseline and the ninth week of study. CHC, comparison between study groups. Time*CHC, comparison between study groups between baseline and week 9. COC, combined oral contraceptive; CVC, combined vaginal contraceptive; BMI, body mass index; WC, waist circumference; sBP, systolic blood pressure; dBP, diastolic blood pressure; SHBG, sex hormone binding globulin; FAI, free androgen index; HOMA-IR, homeostasis model assessment of insulin resistance; HOMA-2β, homeostasis model assessment of β-cell function; HDL-C, high-density lipoprotein cholesterol; LDL-C, low-density lipoprotein cholesterol; hs-CRP, high-sensitivity C-reactive protein.

Statistical analyses were performed using the Statistical Package for the Social Sciences (SPSS) software (version 28.0 for Windows, SPSS Inc., Chicago, IL, USA). The statistical significance level was set at $p \leq 0.05$.

3. Results

3.1. Anthropometric Parameters

At baseline, women in the COC group were older (32.4 vs. 30.8 years, $p = 0.051$), and their BMI tended to be higher (25.4 vs. 23.5, $p = 0.068$) compared to the CVC group (Table 1). At baseline and 9 weeks of treatment, there were no significant differences between the two study groups regarding BMI ($p = 0.245$), waist circumference (WC, $p = 0.812$), diastolic blood pressure (dBP, $p = 0.550$), or systolic blood pressure (sBP, $p = 0.613$) (Table 2).

3.2. Serum Levels of Androgens and SHBG

There were no significant differences in serum levels of testosterone at 9 weeks between the groups. However, SHBG levels increased significantly in both groups (COC $p < 0.001$, CVC $p < 0.001$) between baseline and week 9, and FAI was decreased in both groups (COC $p < 0.001$, CVC $p = 0.007$) (Table 3). The changes in SHBG and FAI between baseline and week 9 were similar within the groups (Table 2).

Table 3. Parameters (mean ± standard deviation, SD) related to androgen secretion, glucose metabolism, lipid profile, and inflammation in the study groups.

	COC					CVC				
	Week 0	Week 9	Change	Pcoc	Padj	Week 0	Week 9	Change	Pcvc	Padj
n	13	11				11	9			
BMI (kg/m^2)	25.4 ± 3.3	25.1 ± 3.0	−0.3 (−0.6; 0.1)	0.173	0.157	23.2 ± 2.4	23.5 ± 2.7	0.02 (−0.3; 0.4)	0.917	0.929
WC (cm)	82.3 ± 10.9	82.1 ± 8.6	−0.4 (−3.3; 2.5)	0.842	0.812	80.9 ± 7.5	80.5 ± 8.1	0.00 (−1.1; 1.1)	0.990	0.912
sBP (mmHg)	116.3 ± 9.4	116.4 ± 13.3	0.5 (−6.6; 7.5)	0.928	0.876	106.8 ± 10.1	111.1 ± 7.7	1.9 (−2.7; 6.4)	0.270	0.322
dBP (mmHg)	69.4 ± 8.2	70.5 ± 8.6	1.6 (−2.9; 6.1)	0.472	0.656	62.0 ± 9.2	65.9 ± 7.8	2.5 (−1.9; 6.9)	0.167	0.203
Testo (nmol/L)	1.31 ± 0.5	1.13 ± 0.6	−0.1 (−0.5; 0.2)	0.331	0.450	2.31 ± 2.1	1.20 ± 0.3	−1.3 (−3.2; 0.6)	0.140	0.195
SHBG (nmol/L)	48.54 ± 17.5	156.36 ± 1.6	109.8 (84.1; 135.6)	<0.001	<0.001	55.73 ± 22.3	208.84 ± 84.0	151.6 (101.1; 202.1)	<0.001	<0.001
FAI	2.88 ± 1.3	0.75 ± 0.4	−2.1 (−3.3; −1.0)	<0.001	<0.001	3.80 ± 2.9	0.61 ± 0.2	−3.5 (−6.0; −1.0)	0.005	0.007
Fasting glucose (mmol/L)	5.3 ± 0.3	5.3 ± 0.3	0.0 (−0.3; 0.3)	0.938	0.863	5.2 ± 0.5	5.1 ± 0.4	−0.2 (−0.4; 0.1)	0.166	0.324
Fasting insulin (mU/L)	10.1 ± 5.1	11.7 ± 4.1	1.58 (0.02; 3.1)	0.037	0.020	11.1 ± 6.2	12.8 ± 7.7	1.72 (−2.1; 5.6)	0.255	0.168
AUCglucose	12.2 ± 7.1	13.1 ± 10.6	1.5 (−1.4; 4.3)	0.129	0.281	10.7 ± 8.8	13.7 ± 11.5	1.5 (0.3; 2.7)	0.018	0.034
AUCinsulin	92.0 ± 286.6	129.0 ± 199.2	14.4 (−18.9; 47.6)	0.268	0.240	72.3 ± 402.0	212.7 ± 339.7	44.0 (−18.9; 106.8)	0.089	0.294
HOMA-IR	2.3 ± 1.3	2.7 ± 0.9	0.25 (−0.2; 0.7)	0.189	0.235	2.3 ± 1.5	3.4 ± 1.9	0.87 (−0.5; 2.3)	0.134	0.212
HOMA-2β	106.1 ± 41.7	137.0 ± 53.8	26.1 (6.2; 46.1)	0.011	0.010	130.0 ± 60.8	163.4 ± 81.5	30.7 (−9.4; 70.7)	0.098	0.532
Matsuda index	6.09 ± 3.4	4.91 ± 1.6	−1.2 (−2.4; 0.1)	0.066	0.089	6.18 ± 3.1	5.39 ± 3.6	−0.8 (−2.8; 1.1)	0.241	0.288
Cholesterol (mmol/L)	4.15 ± 0.6	4.33 ± 0.7	0.04 (−0.5; 0.6)	0.572	0.722	4.29 ± 0.5	4.36 ± 0.7	0.14 (−1.1; 1.4)	0.749	0.787
HDL-C (mmol/L)	1.44 ± 0.4	1.67 ± 0.5	−0.25 (−0.9; 0.4)	0.088	0.113	1.65 ± 0.3	1.65 ± 0.3	0.03 (−0.2; 0.3)	0.869	0.985
LDL-C (mmol/L)	2.56 ± 0.7	2.33 ± 0.8	0.19 (−0.04; 0.4)	0.959	0.988	2.60 ± 0.6	2.64 ± 0.7	−0.02 (−0.2; 0.3)	0.943	0.098
Triglycerides (mmol/L)	0.93 ± 0.4	1.29 ± 0.8	0.36 (−0.1; 0.8)	0.098	0.367	0.76 ± 0.3	1.28 ± 0.5	0.49 (0.3; 0.7)	<0.001	<0.001
Hs-CRP (mmol/L)	1.58 ± 1.8	2.00 ± 2.1	0.78 (−0.46; 2.0)	0.302	0.567	1.65 ± 1.5	3.50 ± 2.3	1.75 (−0.02; 3.6)	0.032	0.040

COC, combined oral contraceptive; CVC, combined vaginal contraceptive; BMI, body mass index; WC, waist circumference; sBP, systolic blood pressure; dBP, diastolic blood pressure; SHBG, sex hormone binding globulin; FAI, free androgen index; HOMA-IR, homeostasis model assessment of insulin resistance; HOMA-2β, homeostasis model assessment of β-cell function; HDL-C, high-density lipoprotein cholesterol; LDL-C, low-density lipoprotein cholesterol; hs-CRP, high-sensitivity C-reactive protein.

3.3. Oral Glucose Tolerance Test (OGTT)

In the OGTT, glucose levels at 60 min were higher after 9 weeks of treatment compared to baseline ($p = 0.008$, adjusted $p = 0.011$) in the CVC group. Further, glucose AUC was increased significantly in the CVC group ($p = 0.018$, adjusted $p = 0.034$) (Table 3, Figure 2).

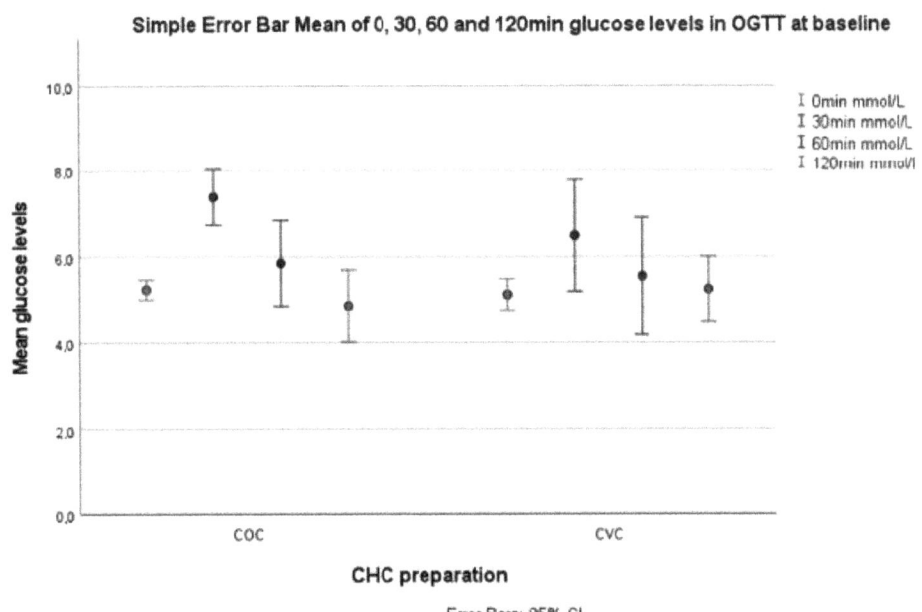

(a)

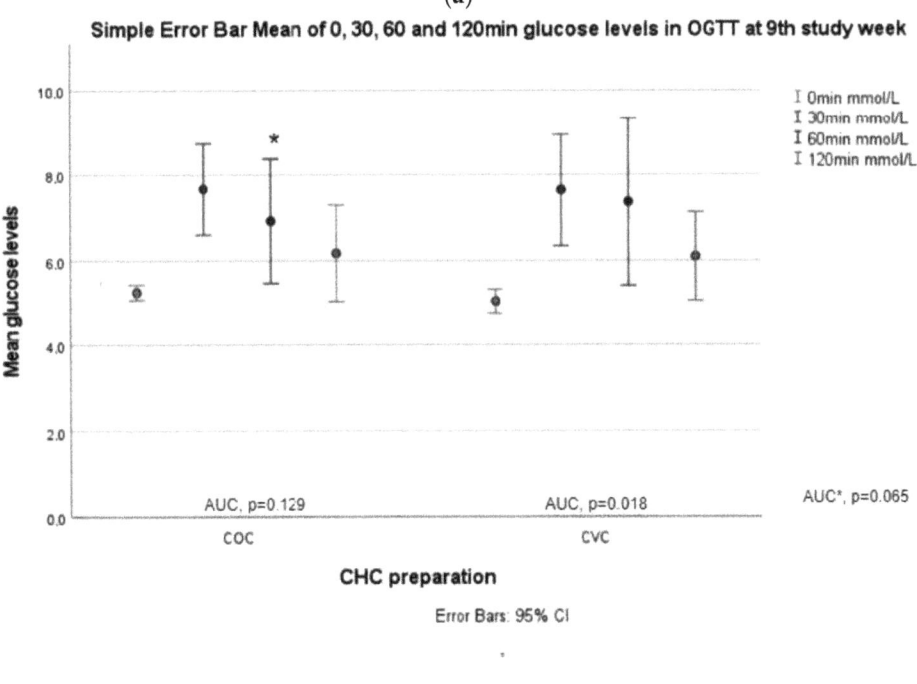

(b)

Figure 2. *Cont.*

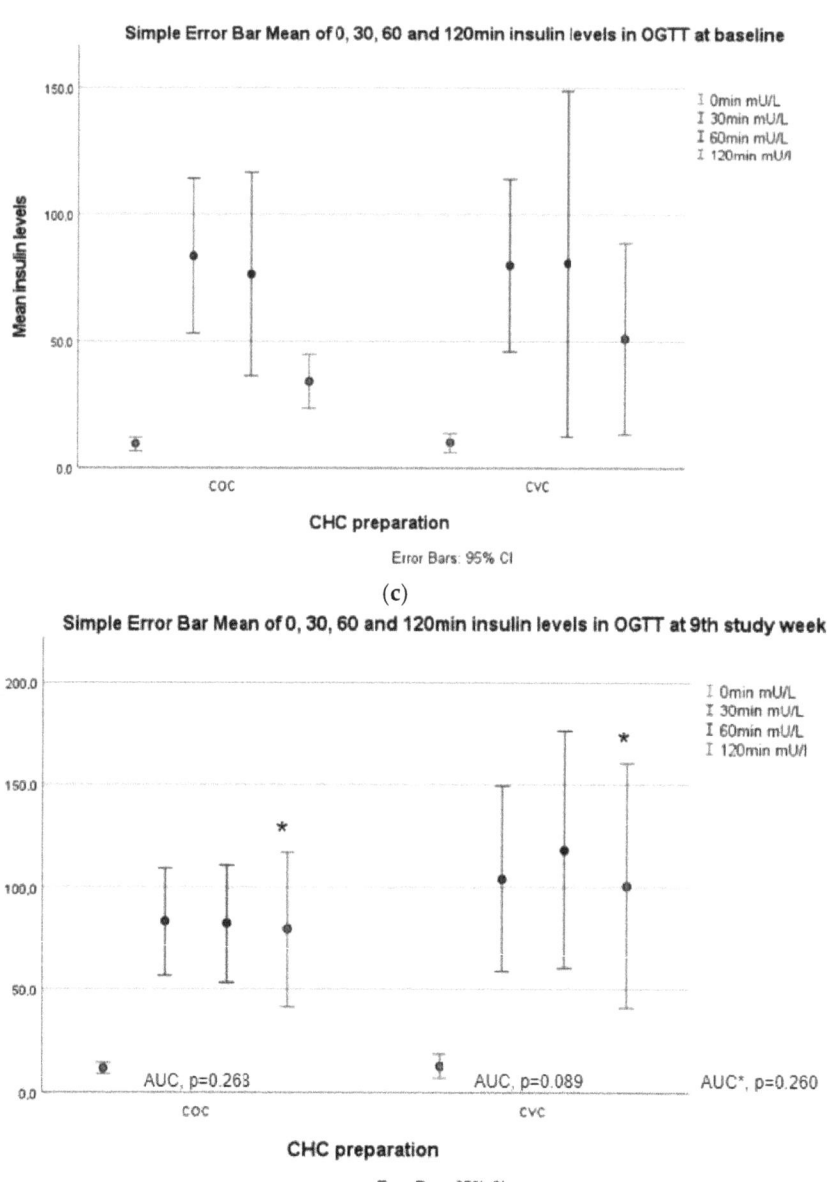

Figure 2. Glucose and insulin responses during OGTT. (**a**) Glucose values at 0, 30, 60, and 120 min in both study groups at baseline; (**b**) glucose values at 0, 30, 60, and 120 min in both study groups week 9. AUCglucose values between baseline and the ninth week in the COC and CVC groups. AUC * is AUCglucose between the study groups. An asterisk (*) marks a significant increase in 60 min glucose value in the CVC group compared to baseline; (**c**) insulin values at 0, 30, 60, and 120 min in both study groups at baseline.; (**d**) insulin values at 0, 30, 60, and 120 min in both study groups at baseline. AUCinsulin values between baseline and the ninth week in the COC and CVC groups. AUC * is AUCinsulin between the study groups at week 9. An asterisk (*) marks a significant increase in 120 min insulin values in both groups compared to baseline.

Fasting insulin levels ($p = 0.037$, adjusted $p = 0.023$) increased after 9 weeks of treatment in the COC group, and insulin levels at 120 min increased in both groups (COC $p = 0.005$, adjusted $p = 0.004$; CVC $p = 0.028$, adjusted $p = 0.042$) (Table 3, Figure 2).

HOMA-2β levels increased significantly in the COC group ($p = 0.011$), but the change became nonsignificant after adjustments (adjusted $p = 0.10$) (Table 3). HOMA-2β differed significantly between the two groups ($p = 0.037$, adjusted $p = 0.030$), but the increase in HOMA-2β levels was similar in both groups (Table 2).

3.4. Serum Lipids and hs-CRP

Serum levels of triglycerides ($p < 0.001$, adjusted $p < 0.001$) increased significantly at 9 weeks of treatment in the CVC group (Table 3). There were differences in triglyceride levels ($p = 0.030$, adjusted $p = 0.103$) between baseline and 9 weeks; the levels increased, and the change differed between the groups ($p = 0.542$, adjusted $p = 0.046$) (Table 2).

Hs-CRP levels ($p = 0.032$, adjusted $p = 0.040$) increased significantly after 9 weeks in the CVC group (Table 3). The levels differed between the groups after adjustments (adjusted $p = 0.021$), but the change in hs-CRP was similar in both groups ($p = 0.376$, adjusted 0.382) (Table 2).

4. Discussion

In this study, both COC and CVC decreased androgenicity but displayed only mild effects on glucose metabolism, IR, lipid profile, and chronic inflammation. Though the study failed to recruit the targeted number of women, the data contrasted with our hypothesis, as CVC did not seem to have a more beneficial hormonal or metabolic profile than COC in PCOS.

CHC preparations are the most used medical treatment for PCOS, as they reduce menstrual abnormalities and relieve manifestations of clinical hyperandrogenism (acne and hirsutism). In the present study, a 9-week use of 20 μg EE + DSG or 15 μg/d EE/EGS caused an approximately 200–270% increase in SHBG levels and a subsequent 74–84% decrease in FAI levels, in line with the results of previous studies [13,15,25]. Some studies have reported a greater increase in SHBG during oral CHC use [13,26], whereas others have found that SHBG increased more during CVC treatment [15,25]. The present results suggest that the routes are comparably efficient in improving hyperandrogenemia in PCOS.

In some studies, CVC was considered to cause fewer adverse changes in glucose metabolism and insulin sensitivity in general female populations [15]. In the present study, after 9 weeks of treatment, AUCglucose increased in the CVC group. A small compensatory increase in insulin secretion was observed in both groups. In the COC group, fasting insulin and 120 min insulin levels increased and, in the CVC group, there was an increase in 120 min insulin levels. These results are partly in line with those of our previous study, which demonstrated a reduction in insulin sensitivity and an increase in AUCglucose levels among 54 healthy young women who were given oral, vaginal, or transdermal CHCs continuously for 9 weeks [13]. However, not all studies agree on the detrimental effect of CHCs on glucose metabolism. In one study, CVC users did not experience any changes in carbohydrate metabolism compared to COC users over five cycles [15]. Furthermore, CVC for 24 months was found to be safe in women with type 1 diabetes when estimated by glycosylated hemoglobin levels [27]. Moreover, in the only randomized study performed with women with PCOS ($n = 37$), CVC improved insulin sensitivity and glucose tolerance, whereas COC (containing EE + drospirenone) worsened IR and insulin secretion at 6 months of treatment [28]. Comparisons with previous studies are challenging because studies differ regarding CHC preparations and the methods used to evaluate glucose metabolism and IR. The gold standard for assessing IR is the hyperinsulinemic-euglycemic glucose clamp technique. However, several measurements based on serum glucose and insulin response to glucose intake, such as HOMA-IR, HOMA-2β, and the Matsuda index, have been shown to be useful. These indexes have been shown to reliably reflect IR in several previous studies in women with PCOS [19–22]. On the other hand, it is unclear whether patients presenting mild IR (i.e., an altered response to a clamp but a normal HOMA-IR and a normal response to an oral glucose test) display any additional clinical problems when compared to patients with a normal response to the clamp. Indeed, there are also concerns that the evaluation of IR in women with PCOS is method-dependent, and there may be discrepancies between markers [29]. In addition, lean women with PCOS may be more easily misclassified as insulin sensitive [30]. Nonetheless, our results raise concerns that CVC may not be safer than COC in women with PCOS regarding its effects on glucose metabolism.

In the present study, changes in lipid profile showed an increase in triglyceride levels in the CVC group, and the increase was slightly greater in the CVC group. These results align with those of previous studies among women with PCOS, showing that COC use is associated with increased levels of triglycerides but also HDL and total cholesterol levels [14,31]. Similar results were generated in a study performed on healthy women treated with oral, transdermal, or vaginal CHCs for 9 weeks, showing an increase in triglycerides and HDL in all study groups [13]. Comparably, oral EE administration has been shown to result in increased total cholesterol, mainly due to increased HDL cholesterol and triglycerides [32–34]. A similar effect during the use of CVC has also been described [35]. High triglyceride levels seem to be an independent predictor of the future risk of myocardial infarction [36] and have been associated with elevated cardiovascular risks [37], specifically in women [37]. A meta-analysis of CHC effects on the lipid profile in PCOS women concluded that desogestrel containing CHCs increased triglyceride levels after 6 months of treatment [33]. In the present study, triglyceride levels e increased significantly in the CVC group. A 9-week study is too short for solid conclusions regarding lipid profile changes with COC or CVC use. However, our results do not support the recommendation that vaginal CHC be preferred to oral preparations to decrease the cardiovascular risks linked to PCOS. As an abnormal lipid profile is typically present in women with PCOS [38], larger, long-lasting follow-up studies and real-world register data analyses are needed to clarify whether the use of CHCs (either oral or vaginal) will increase the risk of cardiovascular morbidity and mortality in women with PCOS. It is possible that the alleviation of hyperandrogenemia with CHCs overcomes mild impairments in metabolic parameters.

Serum levels of hs-CRP increased in the CVC group after 9 weeks of treatment. Despite differences in CRP levels, the change in hs-CRP levels was similar between the two groups. This result is in line with studies performed with oral and vaginal preparations [39,40] and with our recently published data showing EE to be a strong promoter of chronic low-grade inflammation [13,41]. This is an important finding, as women with PCOS have been shown to display chronic inflammation [42,43], which, in turn, is associated with an increased risk of cardiovascular diseases and events, as well as overall mortality [44]. Of note, the findings of a recent study comparing estradiol valerate (EV) with EE among healthy women suggest that EV could display a more neutral effect on inflammation and lipids [41]. Further randomized studies are needed to clarify whether preparations containing EV instead of EE could be safer regarding cardiovascular risks in women with PCOS.

Strengths and Limitations

The main strengths of the present study are that PCOS diagnosis was made by a gynecologist and the participants were homogeneous concerning ethnicity, as all were Caucasians. All in all, the study provides important data for future meta-analyses. The weaknesses of the study are the failure to recruit enough participants to meet the power calculation criteria for a sufficient sample size and to engage participants to finish the study, which underscores the challenge of running a randomized clinical trial. Additionally, a slightly higher BMI (nonsignificant) and age at baseline in the COC group may have influenced the results. Further, the power calculation was based on changes in triglycerides, not on glucose metabolism parameters or inflammation markers, which must be taken into consideration when interpreting the results. Additionally, as discussed earlier, the hyperinsulinemic-euglycemic glucose clamp technique is the gold standard for IR measurement, but it is costly, time-consuming, invasive, and requires staff. We used basal and OGTT-derived calculated indexes (HOMA-IR, HOMA-2β, and the Matsuda index) to evaluate IR in women with PCOS. Lastly, the short follow-up period does not permit conclusions to be drawn on the long-term consequences of the use of COC or CVC, warranting future studies.

5. Conclusions

Contrary to our hypothesis, CVC did not seem to be metabolically safer than COC based on this short clinical study. As there are a limited number of studies assessing different administration routes of CHCs for women with PCOS, the results show some new data and underline the need for larger and longer studies comparing the metabolic effects of CHC administration routes in PCOS.

Author Contributions: Conceptualization, T.P., J.S.T. and L.M.-P.; methodology, T.P., J.S.T. and L.M.-P.; software, T.P. and L.M.-P.; validation, T.P., J.S.T. and L.M.-P.; formal analysis, M.-E.M., R.B. and E.K.; investigation, A.S.R., M.-E.M., T.P. and L.M.-P.; resources, T.P., J.S.T. and L.M.-P.; data curation, M.-E.M. and R.B.; writing—original draft preparation, M.-E.M.; writing—review and editing, M.-E.M., T.P., M.K., J.S.T. and L.M.-P.; visualization, M.-E.M., J.S.T. and L.M.-P.; supervision, J.S.T. and L.M.-P.; project administration, J.S.T. and L.M.-P.; funding acquisition, T.P., J.S.T. and L.M.-P. All authors have read and agreed to the published version of the manuscript.

Funding: This research was funded by grants from the Sigrid Juselius Foundation, the Academy of Finland (grant number 295760), and Oulu University Medical Research Center, and open access funding provided by University of Helsinki.

Institutional Review Board Statement: The study was conducted in accordance with the Declaration of Helsinki and approved by the Regional Ethics Committee of Northern Ostrobothnia Hospital District (number 106/2011, approval date 23 January 2012).

Informed Consent Statement: Written consent was obtained from all subjects involved in the study.

Data Availability Statement: Data cannot be shared openly but are available on request from authors upon reasonable request.

Acknowledgments: Open access funding provided by University of Helsinki.

Conflicts of Interest: The authors declare no conflict of interest.

References

1. Franks, S. Polycystic ovary syndrome. *N. Engl. J. Med.* **1995**, *333*, 853–861. [CrossRef] [PubMed]
2. March, W.A.; Moore, V.M.; Willson, K.J.; Phillips, D.I.W.; Norman, R.J.; Davies, M.J. The prevalence of polycystic ovary syndrome in a community sample assessed under contrasting diagnostic criteria. *Hum. Reprod.* **2010**, *25*, 544–551. [CrossRef] [PubMed]
3. Rotterdam ESHRE/ASRM-Sponsored PCOS Consensus Workshop Group. Revised 2003 consensus on diagnostic criteria and long-term health risks related to polycystic ovary syndrome. *Fertil. Steril.* **2004**, *81*, 19–25. [CrossRef] [PubMed]
4. Teede, H.J.; Misso, M.L.; Costello, M.F.; Dokras, A.; Laven, J.; Moran, L.; Piltonen, T.; Norman, R.J.; Internatiol PCOS Network. Recommendations from the international evidence-based guideline for the assessment and management of polycystic ovary syndrome. *Fertil. Steril.* **2018**, *110*, 364–379. [CrossRef] [PubMed]
5. Kakoly, N.S.; Khomami, M.B.; Joham, A.E.; Cooray, S.D.; Misso, M.L.; Norman, R.J.; Harrison, C.L.; Ranasinha, S.; Teede, H.J.; Moran, L.J. Ethnicity, obesity and the prevalence of impaired glucose tolerance and type 2 diabetes in PCOS: A systematic review and meta-regression. *Hum. Reprod. Update* **2018**, *24*, 455–467. [CrossRef]
6. Teede, H.; Deeks, A.; Moran, L. Open Access REVIEW Polycystic ovary syndrome: A complex condition with psychological, reproductive and metabolic manifestations that impacts on health across the lifespan. *BMC Med.* **2010**, *8*, 41. [CrossRef]
7. Ollila, M.M.E.; West, S.; Keinänen-Kiukaanniemi, S.; Jokelainen, J.; Auvinen, J.; Puukka, K.; Ruokonen, A.; Järvelin, M.-R.; Tapanainen, J.S.; Franks, S.; et al. Overweight and obese but not normal weight women with PCOS are at increased risk of Type 2 diabetes mellitus-a prospective, population-based cohort study. *Hum. Reprod.* **2017**, *32*, 423–431. [CrossRef]
8. Fauser, B.C.J.M.; Tarlatzis, B.C.; Rebar, R.W.; Legro, R.S.; Balen, A.H.; Lobo, R.; Carmina, E.; Chang, J.; Yildiz, B.O.; Laven, J.S.E.; et al. Consensus on women's health aspects of polycystic ovary syndrome (PCOS): The Amsterdam ESHRE/ASRM-Sponsored 3rd PCOS Consensus Workshop Group. *Fertil. Steril.* **2012**, *97*, 28–38. [CrossRef]
9. Sanches De Melo, A.; Maria, R.; Rui, R.; Vieira, C.S. Hormonal contraception in women with polycystic ovary syndrome: Choices, challenges, and noncontraceptive benefits. *Open Access J. Contracept.* **2017**, *8*, 13–23. [CrossRef]
10. Chasan-Taber, L.; Stampfer, M.J. Epidemiology of oral contraceptives and cardiovascular disease. *Ann. Intern. Med.* **1998**, *128*, 467–477. [CrossRef]

11. Morin-Papunen, L.; Martikainen, H.; McCarthy, M.I.; Franks, S.; Soivio, U.; Hartikainen, A.-L.; Ruokonen, A.; Leinonen, M.; Laitinen, J.; Järvelin, M.R.; et al. Comparison of metabolic and inflammatory outcomes in women who used oral contraceptives and the levonorgestrel-releasing intrauterine device in a general population. *Am. J. Obs. Gynecol.* **2008**, *199*, 529.e1–529.e10. [CrossRef] [PubMed]
12. Cagnacci, A.; Ferrari, S.; Tirelli, A.; Zanin, R.; Volpe, A. Route of administration of contraceptives containing desogestrel/etonorgestrel and insulin sensitivity: A prospective randomized study. *Contraception* **2009**, *80*, 34–39. [CrossRef] [PubMed]
13. Piltonen, T.; Puurunen, J.; Hedberg, P.; Ruokonen, A.; Mutt, S.J.; Herzig, K.H.; Nissinen, A.; Morin-Papunen, L.J.; Tapanainen, J.S. Oral, transdermal and vaginal combined contraceptives induce an increase in markers of chronic inflammation and impair insulin sensitivity in young healthy normal-weight women: A randomized study. *Hum. Reprod.* **2012**, *27*, 3046–3056. [CrossRef]
14. Halperin, I.J.; Sujana Kumar, S.; Stroup, D.F.; Laredo, S.E. The association between the combined oral contraceptive pill and insulin resistance, dysglycemia and dyslipidemia in women with polycystic ovary syndrome: A systematic review and meta-analysis of observational studies. META-ANALYSIS Reproductive endocrinology. *Hum. Reprod.* **2011**, *26*, 191–201. [PubMed]
15. Elkind-Hirsch, K.E.; Darensbourg, C.; Ogden, B.; Ogden, L.F.; Hindelang, P. Contraceptive vaginal ring use for women has less adverse metabolic effects than an oral contraceptive. *Contraception* **2017**, *76*, 348–356. [CrossRef] [PubMed]
16. Matsuda, M.; DeFronzo, R.A. Insulin sensitivity indices obtained from oral glucose tolerance testing: Comparison with the euglycemic insulin clamp. *Diabetes Care* **1999**, *22*, 1462–1470. [CrossRef]
17. Bonora, E.; Targher, G.; Alberiche, M.; Bonadonna, R.C.; Saggiani, F.; Zenere, M.B.; Monauni, T.; Muggero, M. Homeostasis model assessment closely mirrors the glucose clamp technique in the assessment of insulin sensitivity: Studies in subjects with various degrees of glucose tolerance and insulin sensitivity. *Diabetes Care* **2000**, *23*, 57–63. [CrossRef]
18. Matthews, D.R.; Hosker, J.P.; Rudenski, A.S.; NAylor, B.A.; Treacher, D.F.; Turner, R.C. Homeostasis model assessment: Insulin resistance and beta-cell function from fasting plasma glucose and insulin concentrations in man. *Diabetologia* **1985**, *28*, 412–419. [CrossRef]
19. Amisi, C.; Mputu, L.; Mboloko, E.; Pozzili, P. Biological insulin resistance in Congolese woman with polycystic ovary syndrome (PCOS). *Gynecol. Obs.* **2013**, *41*, 707–710.
20. Amisi, C.A.; Ciccozzi, M.; Pozzili, P. Wrist circumference: A new marker for insulin resistance in African women with polycystic ovary syndrome. *World J. Diabetes* **2020**, *11*, 42–51. [CrossRef]
21. DeUgarte, C.M.; Bartolucci, A.A.; Azziz, R. Prevalence of insulin resistance in the polycystic ovary syndrome using the homeostasis model assessment. *Fertil. Steril.* **2005**, *83*, 1454–1460. [CrossRef] [PubMed]
22. Wei, H.J.; Young, R.; Kuo, I.L.; Liaw, C.M.; Chiang, H.S.; Yeh, C.Y. Prevalence of insulin resistance and determination of risk factors for glucose intolerance in Polycystic ovary syndrome: A cross-sectional study of Chinese infertility patients. *Fertil. Steril.* **2009**, *91*, 1864–1868. [CrossRef] [PubMed]
23. Rizzo, M.; Berneis, K.; Spinas, G.; Rini, G.B.; Carmina, E. Long-term consequences of polycystic ovary syndrome on cardiovascular risk. *Fertil. Steril.* **2009**, *91*, 1563–1567. [CrossRef] [PubMed]
24. Ciampelli, M.; Leoni, F.; Cucinelli, F.; Mancuso, S.; Panunzi, S.; De Gaetano, A.; Lanzone, A. Assessment of insulin sensitivity from measurements in the fasting state and during an oral glucose tolerance test in polycystic ovary syndrome and menopausal patients. *J. Clin. Endocrinol. Metab.* **2005**, *90*, 1398–1406. [CrossRef]
25. Tuppurainen, M.; Klimscheffskij, R.; Venhola, M.; Dieben, T.O.M. The combined contraceptive vaginal ring (NuvaRing) and lipid metabolism: A comparative study. *Contraception* **2004**, *69*, 389–394. [CrossRef]
26. van den Heuvel, M.W.; van Bragt, A.J.M.; Alnabawy, A.K.M.; Kaptein, M.C.J. Comparison of ethinylestradiol pharmacokinetics in three hormonal contraceptive formulations: The vaginal ring, the transdermal patch and an oral contraceptive. *Contraception* **2005**, *72*, 168–174. [CrossRef]
27. Duijkers, I.; Killick, S.; Bigrigg, A.; Diebem, T. A comparative study on effects of a contraceptive vaginal ring Nuvaring and an oral contraceptive on carbohydrate metabolism and adrenal and thyroid function. *Eur. J. Contracept. Reprod. Health Care* **2004**, *9*, 131–140. [CrossRef]
28. Grodnitskaya, E.E.; Grigoryan, O.R.; Klinyshkova, E.V.; Andreeva, E.N.; Melnichenko, G.A.; Dedov, I.I. Effect on carbohydrate metabolism and analysis of acceptability (menstrual cycle control) of extended regimens of the vaginally inserted hormone-releasing system "NuvaRing" as compared with the standard 21/7 regime in reproductive-age women with type 1 d. *Gynecol. Endocrinol.* **2010**, *26*, 663–668. [CrossRef]
29. Battaglia, C.; Mancini, F.; Cianciosi, A.; Busacchi, P.; Facchinetti, F.; Marchesini, G.R.; Marzocchi, R.; de Aloysio, D. Vascular risk in young women with polycystic ovary and polycystic ovary syndrome. *Obstet. Gynecol.* **2008**, *111*, 385–395. [CrossRef]
30. Battaglia, C.; Mancini, F.; Fabbri, R.; Persico, N.; Busacchi, P.; Facchinetti, F.; Venturoli, S. Polycystic ovary syndrome and cardiovascular risk in young patients treated with drospirenone-ethinylestradiol or contraceptive vaginal ring. A prospective, randomized, pilot study. *Fertil. Steril.* **2010**, *94*, 1417–1425. [CrossRef]
31. Lewandowski, K.C.; Skowrońska-Jóźwiak, E.; Łukasiak, K.; Gałuszko, K.; Dukowicz, A.; Cedro, M.; Lewiński, A. How much insulin resistance in polycystic ovary syndrome? Comparison of HOMA-IR and insulin resistance (Belfiore) index models. *Arch. Med. Sci.* **2019**, *15*, 613–618. [CrossRef] [PubMed]
32. Tosi, F.; Bonora, E.; Moghetti, P. Insulin resistance in a large cohort of women with polycystic ovary syndrome: A comparison between euglycaemic-hyperinsulinaemic clamp and surrogate indexes. *Hum. Reprod.* **2017**, *1*, 2515–2521. [CrossRef] [PubMed]

33. Amiri, M.; Ramezani Tehrani, F.; Nahidi, F.; Kabir, A.; Azizi, F.; Carmina, E. Effects of oral contraceptives on metabolic profile in women with polycystic ovary syndrome: A meta-analysis comparing products containing cyproterone acetate with third generation progestins. *Metabolism* **2017**, *73*, 22–35. [CrossRef] [PubMed]
34. Åkerlund, M.; Almström, E.; Högstedt, S.; Nabrink, M. Oral contraceptive tablets containing 20 and 30 micrograms of ethinyl estradiol with 150 micrograms desogestrel. Their influence on lipids, lipoproteins, sex hormone binding globulin and testosterone. *Acta Obstet. Gynecol. Scand.* **1994**, *73*, 136–143. [CrossRef] [PubMed]
35. Guazzelli, C.A.; Barreiros, F.A.; Torloni, M.R.; Barbieri, M. Effects of extended regimens of the contraceptive vaginal ring on carbohydrate metabolism. *Contraception* **2012**, *85*, 253–256. [CrossRef] [PubMed]
36. Wiegratz, I.; Stahlberg, S.; Manthey, T.; Sänger, N.; Mittmann, K.; Palombo-Kinne, E.; Mellinger, U.; Lange, E.; Kuhl, H. Effects of an oral contraceptive containing 30 mcg ethinyl estradiol and 2 mg dienogest on lipid metabolism during 1 year of conventional or extended-cycle use. *Contraception* **2010**, *81*, 57–61. [CrossRef]
37. Toth, P.P.; Fazio, S.; Wong, N.D.; Hull, M.; Nichols, G.A. Risk of cardiovascular events in patients with hypertriglyceridaemia: A review of real-world evidence. *Diabetes Obes. Metab.* **2020**, *22*, 279–289. [CrossRef]
38. Contreras-Manzano, A.; Villalpando, S.; García-Diaz, C.; Flores-Aldana, M. Cardiovascular risk factors and their association with vitamin D deficiency in Mexican women of reproductive age. *Nutrients* **2019**, *11*, 1211. [CrossRef]
39. Cauci, S.; Di Santolo, M.; Culhane, J.F.; Stel, G.; Gonano, F.; Guaschino, S. Effects of third-generation oral contraceptives on high-sensitivity C-reactive protein and homocysteine in young women. *Obs. Gynecol.* **2008**, *111*, 857–864. [CrossRef]
40. Divani, A.A.; Luo, X.; Datta, Y.H.; Flaherty, J.D.; Panoskaltsis-Mortari, A. Effect of oral and vaginal hormonal contraceptives on inflammatory blood biomarkers. *Mediat. Inflamm.* **2015**, *2015*, 379501. [CrossRef]
41. Kangasniemi, M.H.; Haverinen, A.; Luiro, K.; Hiltunen, K.; Komsi, E.K.; Arffman, R.K.; Heikinheimo, O.; Tapanainen, J.S.; Piltonen, T.T. Estradiol Valerate in COC Has More Favorable Inflammatory Profile Than Synthetic Ethinyl Estradiol: A Randomized Trial. *J. Clin. Endocrinol. Metab.* **2020**, *105*, e2483–e2490. [CrossRef] [PubMed]
42. Dehdashtihaghighat, S.; Mehdizadehkashi, A.; Arbabi, A.; Pishgahroudsari, M.; Chaichian, S. Assessment of C-reactive Protein and C3 as Inflammatory Markers of Insulin Resistance in Women with Polycystic Ovary Syndrome: A Case-Control Study. *J. Reprod. Infertil.* **2013**, *14*, 197–201. [PubMed]
43. Güdücü, N.; İşçi, H.; Yiğiter, A.B.; Dünder, I. C-reactive protein and lipoprotein-a as markers of coronary heart disease in polycystic ovary syndrome. *J. Turk.-German Gynecol. Assoc.* **2012**, *13*, 227–259. [CrossRef] [PubMed]
44. The Emerging Risk Factors Collaboration. C-reactive protein concentration and risk of coronary heart disease, stroke and mortality: An individual participant meta-analysis. *Lancet* **2010**, *375*, 132–140. [CrossRef] [PubMed]

Disclaimer/Publisher's Note: The statements, opinions and data contained in all publications are solely those of the individual author(s) and contributor(s) and not of MDPI and/or the editor(s). MDPI and/or the editor(s) disclaim responsibility for any injury to people or property resulting from any ideas, methods, instructions or products referred to in the content.

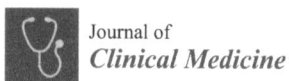 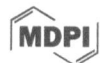

Article

Reactive Hypoglycemia: A Trigger for Nutrient-Induced Endocrine and Metabolic Responses in Polycystic Ovary Syndrome

Sidika E. Karakas [1,2]

[1] Division of Endocrinology, Diabetes and Metabolism, School of Medicine, University of California Davis, Davis, CA 95616, USA; sekarakas@ucdavis.edu
[2] University of California Medical Center Sacramento, Sacramento, CA 95817, USA

Abstract: Polycystic ovary syndrome (PCOS) is an insulin-resistant state compensated for by the body via hyperinsulinemia. More than 50% of women with PCOS are obese and/or have metabolic syndrome. Weight loss improves both metabolic and reproductive outcomes. Energy/caloric content as well as the nutrient composition of one's diet may also be important. This article will present a series of studies from our research comparing the effects of dietary protein vs. simple carbohydrates (CHOs). The results of the acute challenge studies demonstrate that simple CHO intake causes reactive hypoglycemia in one third of women with PCOS, especially among obese and insulin-resistant individuals. Symptoms of hypoglycemia are associated with secretion of cortisol and adrenal androgens. Simple CHOs suppress the hunger signal ghrelin for a shorter period. During weight loss, women who receive protein supplementation achieve more significant weight and fat mass losses. The amino acid compositions of the protein supplements do not affect the improvements in weight and insulin resistance. It is plausible that simple CHO intake leads to weight gain, or interferes with weight loss, by causing reactive hypoglycemia, triggering adrenal steroid secretion and thus leading to snacking. Since obese women with PCOS are more susceptible to reactive hypoglycemia, a vicious cycle is established. Restriction of simple CHOs may break this cycle.

Keywords: reactive hypoglycemia; postprandial hypoglycemia; polycystic ovary syndrome; protein supplements; whey protein; weight loss; adrenal steroids; ghrelin

Citation: Karakas, S.E. Reactive Hypoglycemia: A Trigger for Nutrient-Induced Endocrine and Metabolic Responses in Polycystic Ovary Syndrome. *J. Clin. Med.* **2023**, *12*, 7252. https://doi.org/10.3390/jcm12237252

Academic Editor: Enrico Carmina

Received: 3 November 2023
Accepted: 17 November 2023
Published: 23 November 2023

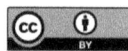

Copyright: © 2023 by the author. Licensee MDPI, Basel, Switzerland. This article is an open access article distributed under the terms and conditions of the Creative Commons Attribution (CC BY) license (https://creativecommons.org/licenses/by/4.0/).

1. Introduction

Characteristic features of polycystic ovary syndrome (PCOS) include oligomenorrhea/amenorrhea/anovulation, hyperandrogenemia and cystic ovaries. In addition, women with PCOS have insulin resistance and hyperinsulinemia even in the absence of obesity. In the USA, 69% of women with PCOS are obese and 64% have metabolic syndrome [1,2]. Weight loss improves both metabolic and reproductive outcomes in PCOS [3–6]. Our earlier research in women without PCOS demonstrated that replacement of dietary fat with carbohydrates (CHOs) can lead to weight loss in free-living conditions [7]. However, those women who do not lose weight on a low-fat/high-CHO diet experience worsening of dyslipidemia and a rise in inflammatory risk factors [8]. This article will summarize the results of our nutrition research in women with PCOS. Potential links between the nutrient composition of their diets and the changes in anthropometric and metabolic outcomes will be discussed. A unifying conceptual framework for a dietary approach to PCOS will be presented.

A notable finding of our studies was that simple CHO intake was associated with reactive hypoglycemia in a significant number of PCOS patients [9,10] and triggered adrenal steroid secretion. Hypoglycemia is defined as low blood glucose concentrations that can cause harm to an individual. Glucose levels below 70 mg/dL are considered mild, and those below 54 mg/dL are considered serious hypoglycemia. Mild hypoglycemia leads to adrenergic symptoms such as tremors, palpitations, sweating, hunger and paresthesia. Serious hypoglycemia causes additional neuroglycopenic symptoms such as headache, dizziness, confusion, amnesia, seizure and coma [11].

Hypoglycemia occurring within four hours after a meal is called reactive or postprandial hypoglycemia [12]. This condition is frequently undermined by the medical community for several reasons: Hypoglycemic symptoms can occur without biochemical evidence of low blood glucose. There is no accurate method of diagnosing postprandial hypoglycemia. The oral glucose tolerance test (OGTT) overestimates the problem since 10% of individuals tested with an extended (5 h) OGTT develop blood glucose below 50 mg/dL. A mixed-meal challenge can elicit neuroglycopenic symptoms in the absence of hypoglycemia. Because of these limitations, reactive hypoglycemia is considered significant when it develops after bariatric surgery, significant alcohol intake or in the rare case of hereditary fructose intolerance or insulinoma.

The goal of our research was to determine the optimal weight loss diet for women with PCOS. All the studies presented here were approved by the Institutional Review Boards, peer-reviewed and published. We addressed the following questions:

1. Does replacement of dietary fat with CHOs vs. protein influence the amount of weight loss and body composition?
2. What are the acute metabolic and endocrine effects of CHO and protein intake on PCOS?
3. Do the amino acid compositions of dietary proteins affect weight loss and/or insulin resistance?

1.1. Comparing Low-Fat/High-CHO vs. Low-Fat/High-Protein Diets during Weight Loss in Women with PCOS

Acute Effects of Simple CHOs vs. Protein

Thirty-three women who fulfilled the National Institutes of Health criteria for PCOS participated in this 2-month-long, free-living, randomized, single-blinded study [13]. To achieve a final energy reduction of 450 kcal/day, their daily energy intake was reduced by 700 kcal, and a 240 kcal supplement containing either whey protein (WP) or simple CHOs was added. The powdered supplements contained either sugar-free WP isolate (96% pure) or simple sugars (glucose plus maltose) and were packaged in individual, identical-looking pouches to allow blinding. Because whey is naturally calcium-enriched, and calcium can independently promote weight loss, the calcium contents of the supplements were equalized by adding tricalcium phosphate to the carbohydrate supplement. Whey protein supplement was sweetened by adding a non-caloric sugar substitute; both supplements were similarly flavored. Most participants consumed the supplements as a partial meal replacement for breakfast.

First, the effects of oral whey protein (WP) vs. simple sugar intakes were examined during 5 h challenge studies [10]. Even though WP did not change plasma glucose concentrations (Figure 1a), it increased plasma insulin 5-fold (Figure 1b), indicating that WP is a potent insulin secretagogue. Another significant difference was seen in plasma ghrelin levels. Ghrelin is a gastrointestinal hormone secreted in the stomach and duodenum. It is a "hunger signal". It is suppressed by food intake and rises to signal hunger when the stomach empties. While both simple sugar and WP similarly suppressed ghrelin, after simple sugar intake, ghrelin started to rise after two hours, whereas after WP intake, ghrelin remained suppressed throughout the five-hour test (Figure 1c). This observation suggested that protein intake may provide satiety for a longer period as compared to simple sugar.

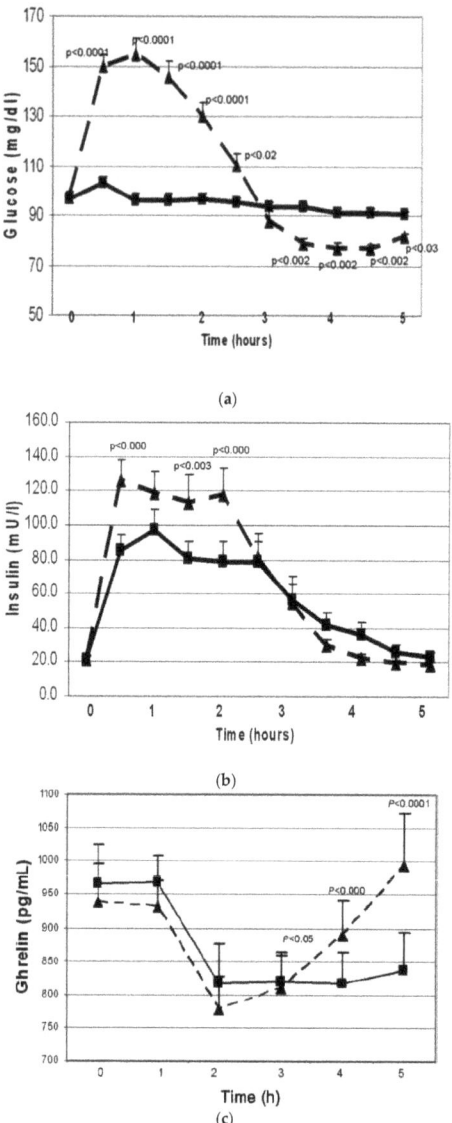

Figure 1. Changes in plasma glucose (**a**), insulin (**b**) and total plasma ghrelin (**c**) (mean ± SEM) during oral glucose tolerance (*n* = 28, dashed line) and protein challenge (*n* = 23, solid line) tests. Differences between responses to the two treatments are expressed through the treatment-by-time interaction effect. Overall, the interaction effect was highly significant (*p* < 0.001). Key timepoint *p* values are shown on the graph. All tests were based on the Wald test performed by using a linear mixed model applied to all available data (from reference [10]).

1.2. Postprandial Hypoglycemia after Simple Sugar vs. Protein Intake

During the previous studies, a significant number of PCOS patients developed the symptoms of hypoglycemia after simple sugar consumption. It is well known that hypoglycemia stimulates the secretion of several pituitary hormones, including ACTH, and triggers the secretion of adrenal hormones [14,15]. Therefore, the next study focused on hypoglycemic symptoms as they relate to adrenal function [9]. Since the standard test used to evaluate this is the 5 h oral glucose test (OGTT), responses to glucose vs. WP were compared. The adrenal response was defined based on cortisol changes during the OGTT. Subjects who had a minimum increase of 7.2 µg/dL (200 nM) in cortisol were defined as "responders" because such a response is considered positive during cortrysin stimulation testing. In total, 9 subjects had a 10.7 ± 1.0 µg/dL increase in cortisol (responders); 10 subjects had a 3.5 ± 0.6 µg/dL decrease (non-responders); and 11 subjects had an intermediate response of a 4.3 ± 1.0 µg/dL increase ($p < 0.0001$). The changes in DHEA concentrations followed a similar pattern: $\Delta = 14.4 \pm 1.7$ ng/mL in the responders, $\Delta = 0.4 \pm 0.9$ ng/mL in the non-responders and $\Delta = 3.6 \pm 1.2$ ng/mL in the intermediates ($p = 0.0003$) (Figure 2a).

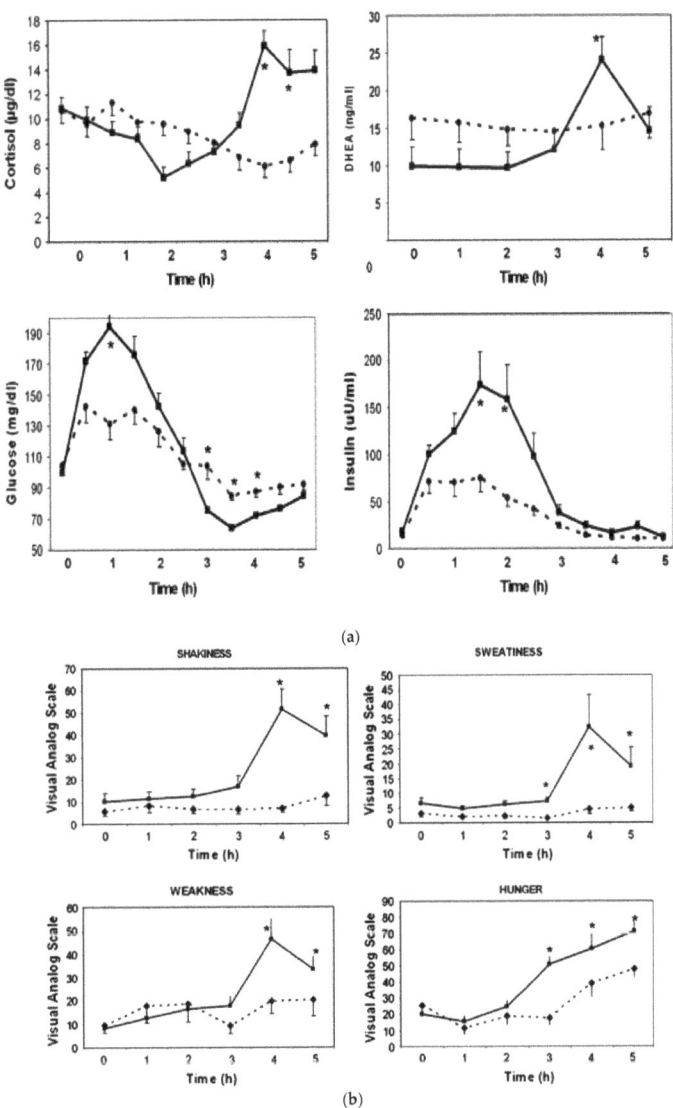

Figure 2. Changes in cortisol and DHEA, glucose and insulin (a) and clinical symptoms (b) in responders ($n = 9$, solid line) vs. non-responders ($n = 10$, dashed line) during oral glucose tolerance test (mean ± SEM, *; $p < 0.05$ when responders are compared to non-responders) (from reference [9]).

Responders had higher glucose levels at 1 h (194 ± 13 vs. 131 ± 12 mg/dL, $p < 0.05$) but lower nadir glucose levels later during the test (61.4 ± 2.2 vs. 70.2 ± 2.3 mg/dL, $p = 0.0002$). Responders also had a higher insulin response at 2 h as compared to non-responders (159 ± 31 vs. 54 ± 29 mU/mL, $p < 0.05$) (Figure 2a).

The key clinical symptoms related to the autonomic response, neuroglycopenia and malaise (sweating, shaking, hunger, weakness, confusion, drowsiness, behavior, speech difficulty, incoordination, nausea and headache) were monitored using the Hypoglycemia Symptoms Logs program developed in collaboration with William Horn and Nancy Keim, PhD [9]. The symptoms were recorded hourly on a 0–100 scale on hand-held tablets. The data were transferred from the tablets to an Excel spreadsheet for analysis and were plotted against time. When responders were compared to non-responders, the symptoms diverged at the 3rd hour. The responders had higher scores in shakiness, sweatiness, weakness and hunger (Figure 2b).

When the baseline characteristics of responders were compared to those of non-responders, the responders were more obese (BMI: 37.0 ± 1.6 vs. 31.7 ± 1.8 kg/m^2, $p < 0.05$) and had higher serum leptin levels (28.9 ± 1.7 vs. 24.1 ± 1.1 ng/mL, $p < 0.03$). The responders also had lower and sex hormone-binding globulin (SHBG) levels (33.9 ± 3.1 vs. 58.6 ± 6.7 nmol/L, $p = 0.022$).

These results indicate that one third of the women with PCOS developed physiologically significant reactive hypoglycemia stimulating adrenal steroid secretion. These patients were more obese and insulin-resistant as compared to those who did not develop hypoglycemia.

1.3. Effects of Dietary CHOs vs. Protein on Anthropometric Outcomes during Weight Loss Intervention

These studies compared the effects of WP vs. simple CHOs on changes in weight and body composition [13]. Twenty-four women who fulfilled the National Institutes of Health criteria for PCOS completed the 2-month, free-living, randomized, single-blinded study. Habitual energy intake was reduced by 700 kcal, and a 240 kcal supplement containing either WP or simple CHOs was added. The final energy restriction was −450 kcal/day. After randomization, 13 participants first received the simple CHO supplement, and 11 participants received the WP supplement. Seven-day food records were analyzed using NutritionistPro (v7.9, Redmond, WA, USA).

The baseline energy intakes were similar (1947 ± 166 kcal/d in the WP; 1770 ± 157 kcal/d in the simple CHO groups). Energy intake decreased similarly (by 476 and 400 kcal/day, respectively). Protein intake increased from 20% to 33% in the WP group and decreased from 22% to 17% in the simple CHO group. Body composition was determined using electrical bioimpedance.

Those receiving WP lost more weight (−3.3 +/−0.8 kg vs. −1.1 +/−0.6 kg, $p < 0.03$) and more fat mass (−3.1 +/−0.9 kg vs. −0.5 +/−0.6 kg, $p < 0.03$). Serum leptin was determined to be an independent measure of fat mass, and it decreased from 37.2 ± 3.9 μg/L to 31.3 ± 3.4 μg/L in the WP group but did not change in the simple CHO group (Figure 3). The effects of weight loss on the insulin resistance parameters, endocrine hormones and plasma lipids are shown on Table 1.

Table 1. Changes in metabolic, inflammatory and endocrine variables (mean ± SEM) before and two months after weight loss program in patients supplemented with either whey protein ($n = 11$) or simple carbohydrate ($n = 13$).

	Baseline	2 mo.	Change	P1	P2
Fasting glucose (mg/dL)					
Whey protein	111 ± 5	110 ± 5	−1.5 ± 3.3	(log)	
Simple carbohydrates	102 ± 6	97 ± 4	−4.5 ± 2.9	0.561	0.513

Table 1. Cont.

	Baseline	2 mo.	Change	P1	P2
Fasting insulin (mIU/mL)					
Whey protein	31.8 ± 4.2	28.6 ± 4.6	−3.2 ± 2.1		
Simple carbohydrates	23.9 ± 5.0	22.0 ± 5.4	−1.9 ± 2.1	0.664	0.664
Adiponectin (μg/L) (log)					
Whey protein	8.6 ± 1.2	6.7 ± 0.6	−1.9 ± 0.8 [a]	(log)	
Simple carbohydrates	8.6 ± 1.5	8.0 ± 1.2	−0.6 ± 0.8	0.159	0.126
HOMA					
Whey protein	9.0 ± 1.3	7.3 ± 1.6	−1.7 ± 1.0		
Simple carbohydrates	6.1 ± 1.8	5.5 ± 1.6	−0.6 ± 0.6	0.306	0.298
HgBA1 (%)					
Whey protein	5.7 ± 0.1	5.5 ± 0.2	−0.1 ± 0.1		
Simple carbohydrates	5.4 ± 0.1	5.2 ± 0.1	−0.1 ± 0.1	0.855	0.855
Triglyceride (mg/dL)					
Whey protein	149 ± 16	117 ± 19	−32 ± 21		
Simple carbohydrates	92 ± 11	94 ± 12	2 ± 8	0.15	0.0974
Cholesterol (mg/dL)					
Whey protein	201 ± 8	168 ± 10	−33 ± 8.4 [b]		
Simple carbohydrates	164 ± 6	162 ± 7	−2.3 ± 6.8	**0.0089**	**0.0053**
HDL cholesterol (mg/dL)					
Whey protein	38 ± 2	34 ± 2	−4.5 ± 1.3 [b]		
Simple carbohydrates	37 ± 1	36 ± 2	−0.4 ± 1.3	**0.0395**	**0.024**
Apo B (mg/dL)					
Whey protein	117 ± 4	97 ± 7	−20 ± 5 [b]		
Simple carbohydrates	90 ± 5	93 ± 6	3 ± 5	**0.0045**	**0.0045**
hs-CRP (ng/mL)					
Whey protein	4.7 ± 0.9	3.7 ± 0.8	−1.0 ± 0.6		
Simple carbohydrates	4.5 ± 1.2	3.6 ± 1.1	−0.9 ± 0.6	0.887	0.881
Total testosterone (ng/mL)					
Whey protein	0.95 ± 0.19	0.79 ± 0.11	−0.16 ± 0.16	(log)	
Simple carbohydrates	0.70 ± 0.07	0.73 ± 0.09	0.04 ± 0.04	0.817	0.791
SHBG (nmol/L)					
Whey protein	37.8 ± 8.5	32.7 ± 8.5	−5.1 ± 4.0	(log)	
Simple carbohydrates	48.3 ± 10.4	41.0 ± 7.2	−7.4 ± 6.6	0.774	0.755
Free androgen index					
Whey protein	15.8 ± 4.8	14.6 ± 3.0	−1.2 ± 3.9	(log)	
Simple carbohydrates	7.5 ± 1.5	9.2 ± 1.8	1.7 ± 1.2	0.943	0.941
DHEAS (ng/mL)					
Whey protein	203.8 ± 34.1	256.8 ± 57.1	53.1 ± 43.8		
Simple carbohydrates	261.8 ± 45.2	275.7 ± 50.6	14.0 ± 22.6	0.425	0.425

Raw data were analyzed. Selected variables were log-transformed to satisfy distributional assumptions. [a] $p < 0.05$, baseline vs. 2 months within group. [b] $p < 0.01$, baseline vs. 2 months within group. P1: significance of the changes between the whey protein and simple carbohydrate groups based on a 2-sample t-test. P2: significance of the changes between the whey protein and simple carbohydrate groups based on a mixed-model analysis of variance that adjusts for the baseline values.

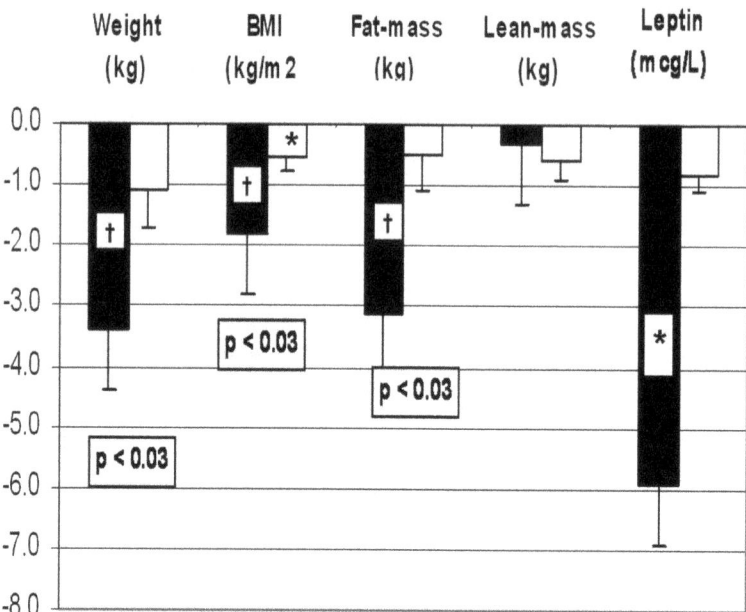

Figure 3. Effects of whey protein (WP: black columns) vs. simple carbohydrate (CHO: white columns) supplements on weight, body mass index (BMI), fat mass and plasma leptin concentrations during two months of weight loss intervention. *: $p < 0.05$ and †: $p < 0.01$ when compared to before-weight-loss baseline; numeric p values indicate the differences between the WP vs. simple CHO supplements. Changes in the variables over time were analyzed using mixed-model analysis of variance methods. Post hoc comparisons between timepoints were conducted using paired t-tests. A significance level of 0.05 was used to determine statistical significance of observed differences. Post hoc comparisons between the treatment groups with respect to contemporaneous changes in the same response measures were based on two-sample t-tests. From reference [13]).

Whey protein recipients had significantly larger decreases in serum cholesterol (-33.0 $+/-8.4$ mg/dL vs. $-2.3 +/-6.8$ mg/dL), high-density lipoprotein cholesterol ($-4.5 +/-1.3$ mg/dL vs. $-0.4 +/-1.3$ mg/dL) and apoprotein B ($-20 +/-5$ mg/dL vs. $3 +/-5$ mg/dL) as compared to the simple CHO group (Table 1).

These results indicate that women with PCOS may lose more weight and fat mass on a hypocaloric high-protein diet as compared to those on a high-simple-CHO diet.

1.4. Effects of Amino Acid Composition of Dietary Protein on Weight Loss and Metabolic Parameters in Women with PCOS

Whey protein comprises 60% essential amino acids (EAAs) and 23% branched-chain amino acids (BCAAs) [16]. The literature-reported measurements of plasma metabolome indicated that plasma BCAA concentrations correlate with insulin resistance [17,18]. Since PCOS and metabolic syndrome are insulin-resistant states, it is important to determine whether WP, a rich source of BCAAs, can exacerbate insulin resistance. To evaluate this possibility, WP was compared to gelatin (a form of collagen) during weight loss in women with metabolic syndrome. Gelatin differs from WP significantly in its AA content [19]. It is an incomplete protein missing the essential AA tryptophan, while it is enriched with proline and hydroxyproline. Whey protein contains three times more BCAAs as compared to gelatin.

In an 8-week double-blinded, placebo-controlled, randomized weight loss intervention, 29 women with metabolic syndrome received either gelatin-based or WP-based supplements (Glanbia, Inc., Twin Falls, ID, USA), 20 g/day. The metabolome of 27 participants

(WP: n = 16) and (gelatin: n = 11) was investigated at the beginning and at the end of the intervention using GC–time-of-flight mass spectrometry [20].

Before the intervention, plasma BCAA levels correlated with the homeostasis model assessment of insulin resistance (HOMA) (r = 0.52, 0.43 and 0.49 for Leu, Ile and Val, respectively; all p < 0.05). However, after the weight loss intervention, these correlations disappeared. There was no difference in plasma abundances (reported as quantifier ion peak height $\div$ 100) of BCAAs between the WP and gelatin supplementation groups (Ile: gelatin: 637 $\pm$ 18 vs. WP: 744 $\pm$ 65), (Leu: gelatin: 1210 $\pm$ 33; WP: 1380 $\pm$ 79) and (Val: gelatin: 2080 $\pm$ 59; WP: group: 2510 $\pm$ 230).

These findings suggest the composition of dietary protein did not affect the anthropometric or metabolic outcomes. Whey protein supplementation did not cause insulin resistance when compared to gelatin. Weight loss was the most important determinant of insulin resistance.

2. Discussion and a Unifying Hypothesis

Our studies indicated that (Table 2):

1. One third of the women with PCOS developed physiologically significant reactive hypoglycemia after simple sugar intake and secretion of cortisol and adrenal androgens.
2. Adrenal steroid secretion coincided with hypoglycemic symptoms.
3. Whey protein intake stimulated insulin secretion but did not cause hypoglycemia.
4. Whey protein supplementation suppressed the hunger signal ghrelin for a longer period as compared to simple CHO supplement.
5. A weight loss diet containing a WP supplement was associated with greater weight loss and fat mass loss and a decrease in leptin when compared to the diet containing a simple CHO supplement.
6. When the WP supplement was compared to the gelatin supplement, there was no difference in the amount of weight loss or the improvement in insulin sensitivity, despite the lower essential AA- and BCAA content of gelatin.

The literature supports that women with PCOS are susceptible to reactive hypoglycemia. Altuntas et al. tested 64 lean subjects with PCOS with an extended OGTT and reported the prevalence of reactive hypoglycemia to be 50% [21]. Mumm et al. compared 88 women with PCOS to 34 age- and BMI-matched controls using a 5 h OGTT [22]. Seventeen percent of the women with PCOS but none of the controls developed hypoglycemia. Obese women with PCOS who developed reactive hypoglycemia had a higher cumulative insulin response as compared to those who did not develop hypoglycemia.

It is well known that hypoglycemia stimulates the secretion of several pituitary hormones including ACTH [15]. Insulin-induced hypoglycemia is used to test central stimulation of adrenal function [14]. It is not known, however, whether reactive hypoglycemia can trigger adrenal hormone secretion as well. The literature suggests that women with PCOS may respond to hypoglycemia differently than control women. Sam et al. compared 10 women with PCOS to 9 age-, BMI- and ethnicity-matched controls using hypoglycemic clamp and found that women with PCOS had a three-fold higher glucagon response [23]. The other counter-regulatory hormones, such as growth hormone and cortisol, did not show differential responses. Gennarelli et al. used insulin-induced hypoglycemia to compare the counter-regulatory hormones in women with PCOS vs. control women [24]. Obese women with PCOS were less symptomatic and had a blunted noradrenaline response as compared to the obese controls. Lean women with PCOS had a greater increase in growth hormone as compared to lean controls.

Our studies focused on the clinical presentation of hypoglycemia. We showed that one third of women with PCOS developed hypoglycemic symptoms during the 5 h OGTT. The symptomatic patients had lower nadir glucose levels and secreted cortisol and adrenal androgens while experiencing symptoms. They were also more obese and insulin-resistant than the asymptomatic women with PCOS. The link between hypoglycemic symptoms and adrenal hormone secretion indicates that the clinical symptoms are important clues pointing to the triggering of the adrenals. The link between hypoglycemic symptoms and obesity suggests that hypoglycemia may alter eating/snacking behavior, as observed by Kishimoto in men with subclinical hypoglycemia [25].

Table 2. Summary of the intervention studies comparing dietary proteins and simple carbohydrates (WP: whey protein; CHOs: carbohydrate).

	WP vs. Simple-CHO		WP vs. Gelatin
Acute Challenge Studies (Reference [10])	WP	Simple-CHO	-----
	Glucose: No change	Increased	
	Insulin: Increased	Increased	
	Ghrelin: Suppressed 5 h	Suppressed 3 h	
Adrenal-Steroid Response to Acute Challenge (Reference [9])	Responders	Non-Responders	-----
	Cortisol: Increased	No change	
	DHEA: Increased	No change	
	Hypoglycemia: Yes	No	
Weight Loss studies Reference [13]	WP	Simple-CHO	WP Gelatin
	Weight: Decreased	Decreased less	Similar decreases in weight, BMI, and plasma glucose, insulin, and lipids in both groups
	BMI: Decreased	Decreased less	
	Fat mass: Decreased	No change	
	Leptin: Decreased	No change	
Plasma Metabolome Changes (Reference [18])	------------		Before, but not after, weight loss, branch chain amino acids (Leu, Ile, Val) correlated with homeostasis model assessment of insulin resistance (HOMA) ($p < 0.05$ for all). Proline and cystine related pathways discriminated WP vs. gelatin supplementations.

Since PCOS is an insulin-resistant state and a significant number of patients may have obesity and metabolic syndrome, several studies attempted to identify the optimal diet for weight loss and maintenance in PCOS. We found that a high-protein diet containing WP was superior to a high-CHO diet in achieving weight loss and fat mass loss. Studies of plasma metabolome by Ooi et al. showed that branched-chain AA supplementation may increase fat oxidation [26], offering a potential mechanism for our observation. A meta-analysis including 24 studies by Wycherley et al. compared energy-restricted high-protein/low-fat vs. standard-protein weight loss diets and found that high-protein diets caused more significant weight loss and fat mass loss and lowered plasma triglyceride levels more than the standard-protein diets [27]. There were no differences in changes in plasma insulin and other lipids. Even though all these studies included obese, insulin-resistant patients, only two focused on PCOS. One of these was our study, which, as summarized earlier, found favorable effects of a high-protein diet [13]. The other study, which was conducted by Stames et al., did not find any difference between the high-protein vs. high-CHO diets [28]. Moran et al. reviewed the results of five studies in 137 women with PCOS [29]. The differences in study populations and dietary interventions did not permit a meta-analysis. It appeared that a monounsaturated-fat-enriched diet caused greater weight loss. Low-glycemic-index and/or low-CHO diets improved menstrual regularity and quality of life and elicited greater reductions in insulin resistance, fibrinogen and total as well as high-density lipoprotein cholesterol [30,31]. A high-protein diet improved depression and self-esteem [32], whereas a high-CHO diet increased the free androgen index. Most importantly, regardless of dietary composition, weight loss improved the presentation of PCOS. Sorensen et al. compared high-protein vs. standard-protein diets in a 6-month study of 27 women with PCOS and reported greater weight and fat mass losses with the high-protein diet [33].

Our initial high-protein weight loss studies used WP supplementation. Whey protein contains high amounts of essential AAs and BCAAs. Studies of the plasma metabolome indicated that plasma BCAAs correlated with insulin resistance [17,18]. Therefore, we compared WP to gelatin, a protein which is relatively poor in BCAAs; there was no difference in weight or fat mass loss or the change in insulin sensitivity [20]. It appeared that the protein content of the diet but not the AA composition of the protein was an important factor for weight loss.

In clinical practice, symptoms suggesting reactive hypoglycemia occur mostly during mid-morning and/or mid-afternoon and may include "getting hungry; craving sugar/carbohydrate", "losing concentration/getting sleepy" and "developing headaches/sweating". Typically, these complaints are preceded by a breakfast or a lunch enriched with simple CHOs. Patients attempt to relieve the symptoms by eating CHO-rich snacks. We propose that this frequent snacking behavior contributes to obesity.

Here, we present a unifying concept linking simple CHO intake to reactive hypoglycemia and hunger, which in turn leads to frequent snacking and obesity (Figure 4).

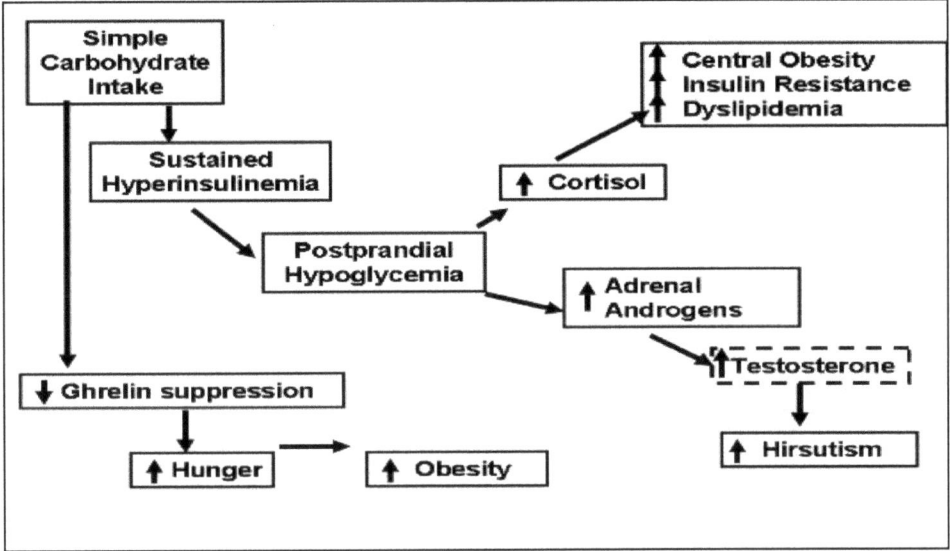

Figure 4. Simple carbohydrate intake can trigger secretion of cortisol and adrenal androgens by causing sustained hyperinsulinemia and postprandial hypoglycemia, which causes sugar craving and frequent snacking. Cortisol secretion leads to central obesity and insulin resistance, and adrenal androgens may worsen hirsutism by converting to testosterone. Simple carbohydrates suppress the hunger signal ghrelin for a shorter period when compared to protein intake, decreasing satiety.

The following mechanisms are proposed:

1. Polycystic ovary syndrome is an insulin-resistant state, compensated for by the body via hyperinsulinemia. Simple CHO intake results in large amounts of insulin secretion. Insulin levels in the circulation remain elevated after emptying of the stomach, and this causes reactive hypoglycemia. Protein intake also stimulates insulin secretion but does not cause hypoglycemia, possibly because protein intake stimulates glucagon, which facilitates glycogenolysis in the liver [34]. In addition, amino acids, especially alanine, serve as glucose precursors for gluconeogenesis [35].

2. Reactive hypoglycemia triggers an adrenergic response, as evidenced by the symptoms of tremors and sweating and stimulates steroid hormone secretion from the adrenals. Cortisol causes central fat deposition, insulin resistance and dyslipidemia. This concept is supported by our observation that the women with hypoglycemic symptoms were more obese and insulin-resistant. Adrenal androgens are converted to testosterone in the peripheral tissues and increase hirsutism. We found that the women with hypoglycemic symptoms had a 1.7-times higher testosterone level/DHEAS molar ratio as compared to those without hypoglycemic symptoms.
3. Even though protein and CHOs are equally effective in suppressing the hunger signal ghrelin, the effect of CHOs does not last as long. Moran et al. reported no difference between the suppressive effects of oral protein vs. CHO challenges during a 3 h test [36]. We saw that the suppressive effects of CHO vs. protein intakes differed after the 3rd hour. After protein intake, ghrelin remained suppressed for 5 h; after simple CHO intake, ghrelin started to rise by the 3rd hour and returned to baseline by the 5th hour.

In summary, the evidence from our research suggests that simple CHO intake causes reactive hypoglycemia in a significant number of women with PCOS. Reactive hypoglycemia leads to hypoglycemic symptoms and triggers adrenal steroid secretion. In addition, simple CHO intake suppresses the hunger signal for a short time. All these factors may encourage snacking between meals and lead to obesity. Since obesity increases the risk of reactive hypoglycemia, a vicious cycle emerges. Limiting simple CHO intake and increasing protein intake can break this vicious cycle by preventing reactive hypoglycemia and frequent snacking and consequently may improve the anthropometric, endocrine and metabolic outcomes in PCOS.

Funding: This manuscript was not supported with any external funding.

Data Availability Statement: Data were contained in the individual articles.

Conflicts of Interest: The author declares no conflict of interest.

References

1. Carmina, E.; Legro, R.S.; Stamets, K.; Lowell, J.; Lobo, R.A. Difference in body weight between American and Italian women with polycystic ovary syndrome: Influence of the diet. *Hum. Reprod.* **2003**, *18*, 2289–2293. [CrossRef] [PubMed]
2. Glueck, C.J.; Papanna, R.; Wang, P.; Goldenberg, N.; Sieve-Smith, L. Incidence and treatment of metabolic syndrome in newly referred women with confirmed polycystic ovarian syndrome. *Metabolism* **2003**, *52*, 908–915. [CrossRef] [PubMed]
3. Haase, C.L.; Varbo, A.; Laursen, P.N.; Schnecke, V.; Balen, A.H. Association between body mass index, weight loss and the chance of pregnancy in women with polycystic ovary syndrome and overweight or obesity: A retrospective cohort study in the UK. *Hum. Reprod.* **2023**, *38*, 471–481. [CrossRef] [PubMed]
4. Marzouk, T.M.; Sayed Ahmed, W.A. Effect of Dietary Weight Loss on Menstrual Regularity in Obese Young Adult Women with Polycystic Ovary Syndrome. *J. Pediatr. Adolesc. Gynecol.* **2015**, *28*, 457–461. [CrossRef]
5. Ravn, P.; Haugen, A.G.; Glintborg, D. Overweight in polycystic ovary syndrome. An update on evidence based advice on diet, exercise and metformin use for weight loss. *Minerva Endocrinol.* **2013**, *38*, 59–76.
6. Thomson, R.L.; Buckley, J.D.; Moran, L.J.; Noakes, M.; Clifton, P.M.; Norman, R.J.; Brinkworth, G.D. The effect of weight loss on anti-Mullerian hormone levels in overweight and obese women with polycystic ovary syndrome and reproductive impairment. *Hum. Reprod.* **2009**, *24*, 1976–1981. [CrossRef]
7. Mueller-Cunningham, W.M.; Quintana, R.; Kasim-Karakas, S.E. An ad libitum, very low-fat diet results in weight loss and changes in nutrient intakes in postmenopausal women. *J. Am. Diet Assoc.* **2003**, *103*, 1600–1606. [CrossRef]
8. Kasim-Karakas, S.E.; Tsodikov, A.; Singh, U.; Jialal, I. Responses of inflammatory markers to a low-fat, high-carbohydrate diet: Effects of energy intake. *Am. J. Clin. Nutr.* **2006**, *83*, 774–779. [CrossRef]
9. Gurusinghe, D.; Gill, S.; Almario, R.U.; Lee, J.; Horn, W.F.; Keim, N.L.; Kim, K.; Karakas, S.E. In polycystic ovary syndrome, adrenal steroids are regulated differently in the morning versus in response to nutrient intake. *Fertil. Steril.* **2010**, *93*, 1192–1199. [CrossRef]
10. Kasim-Karakas, S.E.; Cunningham, W.M.; Tsodikov, A. Relation of nutrients and hormones in polycystic ovary syndrome. *Am. J. Clin. Nutr.* **2007**, *85*, 688–694. [CrossRef]
11. Field, J.B. Hypoglycemia. Definition, clinical presentations, classification, and laboratory tests. *Endocrinol. Metab. Clin. N. Am.* **1989**, *18*, 27–43. [CrossRef]
12. Brun, J.F.; Fedou, C.; Mercier, J. Postprandial reactive hypoglycemia. *Diabetes Metab.* **2000**, *26*, 337–351. [PubMed]

13. Kasim-Karakas, S.E.; Almario, R.U.; Cunningham, W. Effects of protein versus simple sugar intake on weight loss in polycystic ovary syndrome (according to the National Institutes of Health criteria). *Fertil. Steril.* **2009**, *92*, 262–270. [CrossRef]
14. Drummond, J.B.; Soares, B.S.; Pedrosa, W.; Ribeiro-Oliveira, A., Jr. Revisiting peak serum cortisol response to insulin-induced hypoglycemia in children. *J. Endocrinol. Investig.* **2021**, *44*, 1291–1299. [CrossRef] [PubMed]
15. Streeten, D.H.; Anderson, G.H., Jr.; Dalakos, T.G.; Seeley, D.; Mallov, J.S.; Eusebio, R.; Sunderlin, F.S.; Badawy, S.Z.A.; King, R.B. Normal and abnormal function of the hypothalamic-pituitary-adrenocortical system in man. *Endocr. Rev.* **1984**, *5*, 371–394. [CrossRef]
16. Gorissen, S.H.M.; Crombag, J.J.R.; Senden, J.M.G.; Waterval, W.A.H.; Bierau, J.; Verdijk, L.B.; van Loon, L.J.C. Protein content and amino acid composition of commercially available plant-based protein isolates. *Amino Acids* **2018**, *50*, 1685–1695. [CrossRef]
17. Newgard, C.B. Interplay between lipids and branched-chain amino acids in development of insulin resistance. *Cell Metab.* **2012**, *15*, 606–614. [CrossRef]
18. Newgard, C.B.; An, J.; Bain, J.R.; Muehlbauer, M.J.; Stevens, R.D.; Lien, L.F.; Haqq, A.M.; Shah, S.H.; Arlotto, M.; Slentz, C.A.; et al. A branched-chain amino acid-related metabolic signature that differentiates obese and lean humans and contributes to insulin resistance. *Cell Metab.* **2009**, *9*, 311–326. [CrossRef]
19. Eastoe, J.E. The amino acid composition of mammalian collagen and gelatin. *Biochem. J.* **1955**, *61*, 589–600. [CrossRef]
20. Piccolo, B.D.; Comerford, K.B.; Karakas, S.E.; Knotts, T.A.; Fiehn, O.; Adams, S.H. Whey protein supplementation does not alter plasma branched-chained amino acid profiles but results in unique metabolomics patterns in obese women enrolled in an 8-week weight loss trial. *J. Nutr.* **2015**, *145*, 691–700. [CrossRef]
21. Altuntas, Y.; Bilir, M.; Ucak, S.; Gundogdu, S. Reactive hypoglycemia in lean young women with PCOS and correlations with insulin sensitivity and with beta cell function. *Eur. J. Obstet. Gynecol. Reprod. Biol.* **2005**, *119*, 198–205. [CrossRef]
22. Mumm, H.; Altinok, M.L.; Henriksen, J.E.; Ravn, P.; Glintborg, D.; Andersen, M. Prevalence and possible mechanisms of reactive hypoglycemia in polycystic ovary syndrome. *Hum. Reprod.* **2016**, *31*, 1105–1112. [CrossRef]
23. Sam, S.; Vellanki, P.; Yalamanchi, S.K.; Bergman, R.N.; Dunaif, A. Exaggerated glucagon responses to hypoglycemia in women with polycystic ovary syndrome. *Metabolism* **2017**, *71*, 125–131. [CrossRef]
24. Gennarelli, G.; Holte, J.; Stridsberg, M.; Niklasson, F.; Berne, C.; Backstrom, T. The counterregulatory response to hypoglycaemia in women with the polycystic ovary syndrome. *Clin. Endocrinol.* **1997**, *46*, 167–174. [CrossRef]
25. Kishimoto, I. Subclinical Reactive Hypoglycemia with Low Glucose Effectiveness-Why We Cannot Stop Snacking despite Gaining Weight. *Metabolites* **2023**, *13*, 754. [CrossRef] [PubMed]
26. Ooi, D.S.Q.; Ling, J.Q.R.; Ong, F.Y.; Tai, E.S.; Henry, C.J.; Leow, M.K.S.; Khoo, E.Y.H.; Tan, C.S.; Chong, M.F.F.; Khoo, C.M.; et al. Branched Chain Amino Acid Supplementation to a Hypocaloric Diet Does Not Affect Resting Metabolic Rate but Increases Postprandial Fat Oxidation Response in Overweight and Obese Adults after Weight Loss Intervention. *Nutrients* **2021**, *13*, 4245. [CrossRef] [PubMed]
27. Wycherley, T.P.; Moran, L.J.; Clifton, P.M.; Noakes, M.; Brinkworth, G.D. Effects of energy-restricted high-protein, low-fat compared with standard-protein, low-fat diets: A meta-analysis of randomized controlled trials. *Am. J. Clin. Nutr.* **2012**, *96*, 1281–1298. [CrossRef]
28. Stamets, K.; Taylor, D.S.; Kunselman, A.; Demers, L.M.; Pelkman, C.L.; Legro, R.S. A randomized trial of the effects of two types of short-term hypocaloric diets on weight loss in women with polycystic ovary syndrome. *Fertil. Steril.* **2004**, *81*, 630–637. [CrossRef] [PubMed]
29. Moran, L.J.; Ko, H.; Misso, M.; Marsh, K.; Noakes, M.; Talbot, M.; Frearson, M.; Thondan, M.; Stepto, N.; Teede, H.J. Dietary composition in the treatment of polycystic ovary syndrome: A systematic review to inform evidence-based guidelines. *J. Acad. Nutr. Dietetics* **2013**, *113*, 520–545. [CrossRef]
30. Douglas, C.C.; Gower, B.A.; Darnell, B.E.; Ovalle, F.; Oster, R.A.; Azziz, R. Role of diet in the treatment of polycystic ovary syndrome. *Fertil. Steril.* **2006**, *85*, 679–688. [CrossRef]
31. Marsh, K.A.; Steinbeck, K.S.; Atkinson, F.S.; Petocz, P.; Brand-Miller, J.C. Effect of a low glycemic index compared with a conventional healthy diet on polycystic ovary syndrome. *Am. J. Clin. Nutr.* **2010**, *92*, 83–92. [CrossRef] [PubMed]
32. Galletly, C.; Moran, L.; Noakes, M.; Clifton, P.; Tomlinson, L.; Norman, R. Psychological benefits of a high-protein, low-carbohydrate diet in obese women with polycystic ovary syndrome—A pilot study. *Appetite* **2007**, *49*, 590–593. [CrossRef] [PubMed]
33. Sorensen, L.B.; Soe, M.; Halkier, K.H.; Stigsby, B.; Astrup, A. Effects of increased dietary protein-to-carbohydrate ratios in women with polycystic ovary syndrome. *Am. J. Clin. Nutr.* **2012**, *95*, 39–48. [CrossRef] [PubMed]
34. Ichikawa, R.; Takano, K.; Fujimoto, K.; Kobayashi, M.; Kitamura, T.; Shichiri, M.; Miyatsuka, T. Robust increase in glucagon secretion after oral protein intake, but not after glucose or lipid intake in Japanese people without diabetes. *J. Diabetes Investig.* **2023**, *14*, 1172–1174. [CrossRef]

35. Ishikawa, E.; Aikawa, T.; Matsutaka, H. The roles of alanine as a major precursor among amino acids for hepatic gluconeogenesis and as a major end product of the degradation of amino acids in rat tissues. *J. Biochem.* **1972**, *71*, 1097–1099. [CrossRef]
36. Moran, L.J.; Noakes, M.; Clifton, P.M.; Wittert, G.A.; Le Roux, C.W.; Ghatei, M.A.; Stephen, R.B.; Robert, J.N. Postprandial ghrelin, cholecystokinin, peptide, Y.Y.; and appetite before and after weight loss in overweight women with and without polycystic ovary syndrome. *Am. J. Clin. Nutr.* **2007**, *86*, 1603–1610. [CrossRef]

Disclaimer/Publisher's Note: The statements, opinions and data contained in all publications are solely those of the individual author(s) and contributor(s) and not of MDPI and/or the editor(s). MDPI and/or the editor(s) disclaim responsibility for any injury to people or property resulting from any ideas, methods, instructions or products referred to in the content.

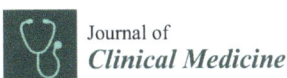
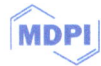

Review

The Role of Sodium-Glucose Cotransporter-2 Inhibitors in the Treatment of Polycystic Ovary Syndrome: A Review

Rachel Porth [1,†], Karina Oelerich [1,†] and Mala S. Sivanandy [1,2,*]

1 Department of Medicine, Beth Israel Deaconess Medical Center, Boston, MA 02215, USA; rporth@bidmc.harvard.edu (R.P.); koeleric@bidmc.harvard.edu (K.O.)
2 PCOS Center, Division of Endocrinology, Beth Israel Deaconess Medical Center, Harvard Medical School, Boston, MA 02115, USA
* Correspondence: msivanan@bidmc.harvard.edu
† These authors contributed equally to this work.

Abstract: Polycystic ovary syndrome (PCOS) is the most common endocrine disorder in reproductive-age women impacting their reproductive, mental, and metabolic health. Insulin resistance is a major driver of the pathophysiology of PCOS. There are several challenges with the management of this complex disorder including insufficient treatment options. Over the past 88 years, multiple hormonal and non-hormonal medications have been tried to treat the various components of this syndrome and there is no FDA (Food and Drug Administration)-approved medication specifically for PCOS yet. Sodium-glucose cotransporter-2 (SGLT-2) inhibitors have a unique mechanism of inhibiting the coupled reabsorption of sodium and glucose in renal proximal convoluted tubules. This review aims to examine the efficacy and side-effect profile of SGLT-2 inhibitors in patients with PCOS. In a limited number of studies, SGLT-2 inhibitors appear to be effective in improving menstrual frequency, reducing body weight and total fat mass, lowering total testosterone and DHEAS levels, and improving some glycemic indices in women with PCOS. SGLT2 inhibitors are generally well tolerated. With future research, it is possible that SGLT-2 inhibitors could become a key therapeutic option for PCOS.

Keywords: SGLT-2 inhibitors; polycystic ovary syndrome; treatment

Citation: Porth, R.; Oelerich, K.; Sivanandy, M.S. The Role of Sodium-Glucose Cotransporter-2 Inhibitors in the Treatment of Polycystic Ovary Syndrome: A Review. *J. Clin. Med.* **2024**, *13*, 1056. https://doi.org/10.3390/jcm13041056

Academic Editor: Enrico Carmina

Received: 15 December 2023
Revised: 1 February 2024
Accepted: 6 February 2024
Published: 13 February 2024

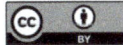

Copyright: © 2024 by the authors. Licensee MDPI, Basel, Switzerland. This article is an open access article distributed under the terms and conditions of the Creative Commons Attribution (CC BY) license (https://creativecommons.org/licenses/by/4.0/).

1. Introduction

1.1. Polycystic Ovary Syndrome

Polycystic ovary syndrome (PCOS) is the most common endocrinopathy in women in the reproductive age group, with a worldwide prevalence of 10–13% depending upon the diagnostic criteria used. This disorder is also a common cause of infertility. The pathogenesis of PCOS involves genetic [1], epigenetic [2], neuroendocrine [3], reproductive, and metabolic alterations [4] and is not completely understood. It is hypothesized that aberrant activity of the GnRH (Gonadotropic-releasing hormone) pulse generator results in preferential secretion of the Luteinizing hormone over the Follicle-stimulating hormone, leading to increased androgen production in the theca cells and diminished testosterone-to-estrogen conversion in the granulosa cells of ovaries [5]. Insulin receptor binding defects and a decrease in Glut4 receptors lead to hyperglycemia and hyperinsulinemia, which further stimulates ovarian androgen production [6]. About 38–88% of women with PCOS are either overweight or obese [7], which substantially exacerbates insulin resistance and contributes to multiple other metabolic abnormalities. Though there are multiple commonly recognized phenotypes of PCOS (Type A, B, C, and D), insulin resistance and hyperinsulinemia are thought to be core features [8]. Insulin resistance is also a major driver of the pathophysiology of PCOS, leading to inflammation, metabolic complications, and reproductive dysfunction.

Management of PCOS includes treatment of oligo/anovulation, hyperandrogenic symptoms, and metabolic risks including prediabetes, type 2 diabetes, dyslipidemia, obesity, NAFLD, and obstructive sleep apnea [9]. Since polycystic ovary syndrome is associated with a multitude of symptoms, women with this disorder are often treated with more than one medication, both approved and off-label [10]. There are multiple treatment options and include hormonal preparations [11], antiandrogens, topical agents, laser photo epilation, electrolysis, diet, exercise, behavioral strategies, and insulin sensitizers. PCOS women are often treated with more than one medication and there is ongoing curiosity in finding novel treatment options to provide relief from the various issues associated with the syndrome.

Insulin resistance is a core component of PCOS, hence insulin sensitizers such as Metformin have been commonly used to treat overweight and obese women with PCOS to improve anthropometric and metabolic outcomes. In a review of 24 randomized controlled trials, metformin was associated with a reduction in body weight, BMI, fasting blood glucose, total testosterone, androstenedione, 17-hydroxyprogesterone levels, and an increase in the likelihood of pregnancy rate in women with PCOS [12]. It is equally effective as an active lifestyle intervention. The common side effects of metformin are gastrointestinal, such as nausea or abdominal discomfort, as well as B12 deficiency [13] in patients with pernicious anemia or who have undergone bariatric surgery. Other studies have found that metformin can very rarely increase the risk of lactic acidosis, particularly in patients who are taking high doses and have risk factors such as renal insufficiency or hepatic disease [14].

New medications such as GLP1 agonists and SGLT2 inhibitors have gained importance in treating patients with type 2 diabetes and PCOS in recent years. Metformin and SGLT2 inhibitors have the benefit of being administered orally compared to GLP1 agonists which are injectable except for oral semaglutide [15]. The GLP1 agonist semaglutide has been shown to cause weight loss and decrease HOMA-IR, basal insulin, and fasting blood glucose in obese patients with PCOS who have previously been unresponsive to lifestyle modifications [16]. Similarly, liraglutide also improved BMI, weight, and waist circumference in obese women with PCOS [17]. In a recent systematic review and meta-analysis, GLP1 agonists, alone or combined with metformin, appear to be more beneficial than metformin alone in reducing BMI, waist circumference, and insulin resistance in overweight and obese women with PCOS [18,19]. The focus of this review is to examine if SGLT2 inhibitors would have a meaningful role in treating PCOS.

1.2. SGLT2 Inhibitors

Sodium/glucose cotransporters (SGLT) are integral membrane proteins that mediate glucose transport across the cell membranes along with related substances and are hence called cotransporters [20]. SGLT-1 proteins are present in the cells lining the small intestine, facilitating absorption of D glucose and D galactose across the luminal brush border membrane. SGLT-2 proteins are predominantly expressed in the epithelial cells lining the proximal convoluted tubules (PCTs) of the kidneys and play a significant role in reabsorbing 90% of the glucose in the glomerular filtrate by lowering the renal threshold for glucose and cotransport sodium (Na+) [20]. The sodium-potassium-ATPase pump in the basolateral membrane of the epithelial cell in the PCT maintains the transport of sodium and glucose (via GLUT-2) back into the blood [20].

In the United States, Canagliflozin, Dapagliflozin, Empagliflozin, Ertugliflozin, and Bexagliflozin are the five FDA-approved SGLT2 inhibitors for treating adults with type 2 diabetes. Licogliflozin (LIK066), is a dual SGLT1 and 2 inhibitor [21]. By blocking the SGLT2 proteins in the proximal convoluted tubules of the kidneys, these medications reduce glucose reabsorption and increase urinary glucose excretion, leading to a reduction in HbA1c [22].

Apart from the above benefits, in a large randomized controlled study that enrolled 7020 patients (EMPA-REG OUTCOME), empagliflozin showed a 38% relative risk reduction in cardiac-related deaths in patients with type 2 diabetes at high risk for cardiovascular events [23]. A meta-analysis published by McGuire et al., showed improved cardiovascular and renal outcomes in type 2 diabetes patients on SGLT2 inhibitors, making it a drug of choice in patients with heart failure [24] and renal failure [25]. The cardioprotective effects of SGLT2 inhibitors in patients with heart failure with low ejection fraction appear to be related to improved endothelial function and vasodilatation, reduced inflammation, enhanced diuresis, and improved myocardial metabolism and efficiency [26]. This group of medications is currently being studied for the treatment of other metabolic disorders including obesity and non-alcoholic fatty liver disease.

2. SGLT2 Inhibitors in PCOS

Because prior research has shown such tremendous benefits for patients with other medical conditions who are started on an SGLT2 inhibitor, there has been an interest in exploring whether this may be a novel treatment option for patients with PCOS [27–30]. In this review, we examine the effects of SGLT2 inhibitors on various outcomes in women with polycystic ovary syndrome.

There have been five randomized clinical trials, Cai et al., 2022 [31], Elkind-Hirsch et al., 2021 [32], Javed et al., 2019 [33], Tan et al., 2022 [34], and Zhang et al., 2022 [35] that used SGLT2 inhibitors in women with PCOS and examined clinical outcomes, published as of end of year 2023. In all of these studies, overweight or obese patients with PCOS were treated with an SGLT2 inhibitor and they had at least one comparison arm. A systematic review and meta-analysis of the effect of these medications on the metabolic parameters in four of these five studies observed significant benefits in body weight, HOMA-IR, and fasting glucose level [30]. Table 1 shows the key characteristics of the randomized controlled trials that utilized SGLT2 inhibitors in women with PCOS.

Table 1. Key characteristics of the randomized controlled trials that utilized SGLT2 inhibitors in women with PCOS.

	Cai et al. [31]	Elkind-Hirsch et al. [32]	Javed et al. [33]	Tan et al. [34]	Zhang et al. [35]
SGLT2 inhibitor	Canagliflozin 100 mg daily	Dapagliflozin 10 mg daily	Empagliflozin 25 mg daily	Licogliflozin 50 mg three times daily	Canagliflozin 100 mg daily (with Metformin 1000 mg twice a day)
Comparison Arm	M	E, E/D, D/M, P/T	M	P	M
Number of participants	C: 33 M: 35	E: 20 D/E: 20 D: 17 D/M: 19 PH/T:16	EM: 19 M: 20	L: 10 P: 10	C/M: 21 M: 20
Study duration (weeks)	12	24	12	2	12
BMI (kg/m^2)	C: 27.26 (25.55 to 28.99) M: 27.95 (26.22 to 29.69)	E: 38.6 ± 1.1 E/D: 39.9 ± 0.9 D: 38 ± 1.1 D/M: 37.6 ± 1.1 P/T: 38.4 ± 1.1	EM: 37.1 ± 6.2 M: 38.7 ± 7.8	38.1 ± 6.3	C/M: 31.11 ± 3.02 M: 29.33 ± 3.19
Age (years)	C: 28.58 (26.72 to 30.43) M: 27.83 (25.97 to 29.68)	E: 30 ± 1.1 E/D: 31 ± 1.4 D: 28 ± 1.5 D/M: 31 ± 1.6 PH/T: 30 ± 1.5	EM: 26.0 (8.0) M: 31.5 (20.0)	27.6 ± 5.3	C/M: 26.38 ± 5.89 M: 25.5 ± 4.36

C = canagliflozin; M = metformin; D = dapagliflozin; EM = empagliflozin; L = licogliflozin; E = exenatide; PH = phentermine; T = topiramate; P = placebo.

3. Effects of SGLT2-Inhibitors on Various Outcomes

3.1. Effect on Menstrual Irregularity

Menstrual irregularity is one of the hallmarks of PCOS, and Metformin helps to induce ovulation in women with PCOS [36]. Both studies that evaluated the effects of

SGLT2 inhibitors on menstrual patterns showed improvement, and one of the two showed statistically significant results. Cai et al. evaluated the impact of both metformin and SGLT2 inhibitors on menstrual irregularity, and at week 12, the number of menstrual cycles per year was increased in both the canagliflozin 1.34 (0.66 to 2.02) and the metformin group 1.37 (0.63 to 2.11), suggesting that canagliflozin is non-inferior to metformin. However, the results were not significant when comparing the two groups [31]. In Zhang et al., improvement in menstrual cycle irregularity was noted in both the canagliflozin/metformin group (80.95%, 17/21) and the metformin group (80.00%; 16/20); however, there was no significant difference seen between the two groups ($p = 0.6228$) [35].

3.2. Biochemical Hyperandrogenism

3.2.1. Total Testosterone

Biochemical hyperandrogenism, elevation of testosterone, DHEAS, and/or androstenedione levels, is one of the diagnostic criteria in PCOS. Nearly 75% of women with PCOS have elevated androgen levels [37]. Combined oral contraceptive pills help to treat biochemical hyperandrogenism by suppressing ovarian androgen production and increasing the production of SHBG (sex hormone-binding globulin), which in turn decreases the free androgen levels. When looking at the effect of SGLT2 inhibitors on hormonal parameters, either alone or in combination with metformin, four out of the five studies showed a decrease in total testosterone [31–33,35] with two of the studies reaching statistical significance [32,35]. In Cai et al., there was an overall reduction in total testosterone in the canagliflozin group and no significant difference ($p = 0.411$) was seen between canagliflozin -0.15 (-0.38 to 0.08) vs. metformin -0.00 (-0.25 to 0.24) groups [31]. Similarly, Elkind-Hirsch et al. showed a statistically significant decrease in total testosterone (TT) when compared to baseline ($p < 0.001$) in the dapagliflozin as well as the other treatment groups including exenatide, exenatide/dapagliflozin, dapagliflozin/metformin, and phentermine/topiramate [32]. In Zhang et al., the canagliflozin/metformin combination decreased total testosterone significantly compared to metformin alone [canagliflozin/metformin: -2.49 ± 1.55 vs. metformin: -2.20 ± 1.30; ($p = 0.0233$)], though both groups demonstrated significantly lower TT levels when compared to baseline ($p < 0.0001$ and $p = 0.0343$, respectively) [35]. In Javed et al., TT levels increased in the empagliflozin group (% baseline change 2.6 (37.0) %) and decreased in the metformin group (% baseline change -14 (33.6)%); although, neither result was statistically significant [33]. Tan et al. demonstrated a non-significant reduction in total testosterone in the licogliflozin group compared to the placebo (9% reduction, 90% CI: 0.77–1.07; $p = 0.340$) [34]. Table 2 reviews the hormonal parameters examined in the studies that utilized SGLT2 inhibitors in women with PCOS.

Table 2. Comparison of the Changes in Hormonal Parameters in the trials that used SGLT2 inhibitors in women with PCOS.

	Cai et al. [31]	Elkind-Hirsch et al. [32]	Javed et al. [33]	Tan et al. [34]	Zhang et al. [35]
SGLT1/2 inhibitor	Canagliflozin	Dapagliflozin	Empagliflozin	Licogliflozin	Canagliflozin (with Metformin)
Total Testosterone	Pre-treatment: 1.78 ng/mL (1.52 to 2.05) LS mean -0.15 (-0.38 to 0.08)	Pre-treatment: 46 ng/dL $\pm$ 5 Post-treatment: 35 ng/dL $\pm$ 4.4 (-11) *	Pre-treatment: 1.6 nmol/L $\pm$ 0.4 Post-treatment: 1.6 nmol/L $\pm$ 0.6	Effect size: 9% decrease in (TR$_{LIK066}$:TR$_{PCB}$) [TT]: 0.91; 90% CI: 0.77–1.07; $p = 0.340$	Pre-treatment: 0.95 ng/mL (0.78–1.08) Post-treatment: 0.53 ng/mL (0.45–0.84) *

Table 2. Cont.

	Cai et al. [31]	Elkind-Hirsch et al. [32]	Javed et al. [33]	Tan et al. [34]	Zhang et al. [35]
Free Androgen Index	n/a	Pre-treatment: 6.7 ± 1.0 Post-treatment: 4.7 ± 0.8 (−2.0) *	Pre-treatment: 10.3 ± 3.0 Post-treatment: 9.4 ± 3.6	n/a	Pre-treatment: 28.62% ± 16.4 Post-treatment: 19.15% ± 13.19 *
DHEAS	Pre-treatment: 261.80 ug/dL (217.77 to 305.83) LS mean −68.96 (−126.36 to −11.55) **	Pre-treatment: 210 mcg/dL ± 22 Post-treatment: 187 mcg/dL ± 24 (−23)	Pre-treatment: 6.1 μmol/L ± 1.6 Post-treatment: 6.2 μmol/L ± 2.1	Effect size: 24% decrease in (TR_{LIK066}:TR_{PCB} [DHEAS]: 0.76; 90% CI: 0.65–0.89; $p = 0.008$ *	n/a
Androstenedione	Pre-treatment: 4.17 ng/mL (3.53 to 4.81) LS mean −0.48 (−1.04 to 0.09)	n/a	Pre-treatment: 5.7 nmol/L ± 1.4 Post-treatment: 5.7 n μmol/L ± 1.9	Effect size: 19% decrease in (TR_{LIK066}:TR_{PCB} [A4]: 0.81; 90% CI: 0.68–0.99; $p = 0.089$)	Pre-treatment: 3.57 ng/mL ± 1.29 Post-treatment: 3.22 ng/mL ± 1.35
SHBG	Pre-treatment 33.76 nmol/L (21.64 to 45.89) LS mean −4.82 (−19.40 to 9.75)	Significantly increased *—no data provided by paper	Pre-treatment: 17.3 nmol/L ± 6.4 Post-treatment: 19.2 nmol/L ± 8.5 *	Effect size: 15% increase in (TR_{LIK066}:TR_{PCB} [SHBG]: 1.15; 90% CI: 0.97–1.36; $p = 0.173$)	Pre-treatment: 13.60 nmol/L (8.55–20.15) Post-treatment: 13.6 nmol/L (9.55–24.10)
Free testosterone	Pre-treatment 2.40 pg/mL (1.92 to 2.88) LS mean 0.30 (−0.30 to 0.89)	n/a	n/a	Effect size: 12% decrease in (TR_{LIK066}:TR_{PCB}[FT]: 0.88; 90% CI: 0.70–1.11; $p = 0.353$)	n/a

DHEAS—dehydroepiandrosterone sulfate; SHBG—sex hormone-binding globulin; FT—free testosterone; A4—androstendione; TR_{LIK066}:TR_{PCB}—ratio of relative changes between licogliflozin and placebo; * statistically significant within-group comparison $p < 0.05$; ** statistically significant compared to the metformin alone group in Cai et al. To convert from ng/dL to nmol/L multiply ng/dL by 0.0347. μIU/mL is equivalent to mU/L. To convert ng/mL to nmol/L multiply the ng/mL by 2.5. To convert μg/dL to μmol/L multiply the μmol/L by 20.7. μg/dL is equivalent to mcg/dL.

3.2.2. Free Androgen Index

In Zhang et al., in the canagliflozin/metformin group, the free androgen index (FAI) at 12 weeks decreased significantly compared to baseline ($p = 0.0457$) but not in the metformin-only group [35]. Additionally, Elkind-Hirsch et al. demonstrated that FAI ($p < 0.001$) significantly decreased in the SGLT2 inhibitor group. In Javed et al., there were non-significant reductions in FAI in both the metformin and empagliflozin groups (−7.0 ± 31.4% baseline change in the empagliflozin group vs. −9.7 ± 34.0% baseline change in the metformin group) [33]. In Tan et al., there was a non-significant reduction in FAI in the licogliflozin group compared to the placebo (21% reduction, 90% CI: 0.58–1.08, $p = 0.204$) [34].

3.2.3. Dehydroepiandrosterone Sulfate

Three out of the four studies that evaluated Dehydroepiandrosterone sulfate (DHEAS) showed a decrease in levels [31,32,34]. One result was statistically significant compared to baseline [34], while one was statistically significant compared to metformin [31]. In Cai et al., there was a reduction in DHEAS levels in the canagliflozin group, but an increase in DHEAS levels in the metformin group (LS mean difference of −68.96 vs. 36.52, respectively, $p = 0.013$) [31]. In Tan et al., the licogliflozin group had a statistically significant decrease in DHEAS levels (effect size of 24%, treatment ratio of licogliflozin to placebo of 0.76 90% CI 0.65–0.89, $p = 0.008$) [34]. In Elkind-Hirsch et al., DHEA-S levels decreased in the SGLT2 inhibitor group when compared to baseline patient parameters; however, the drug effect did not reach statistical significance [32]. Both the empagliflozin and metformin groups in Javed et al. showed an increase in levels of DHEAS compared to baseline (1.0 ± 20.1 and 8.1 ± 15.0%, respectively) but were not statistically significant [33].

3.2.4. Androstenedione

Four studies noted a decrease in androstenedione levels [31,33–35]. In Tan et al. the licogliflozin group showed a reduction in androstenedione levels compared to the placebo (effect size of 19%, treatment ratio of licogliflozin to placebo of 0.81 90% CI 0.68–0.99, $p = 0.089$) [34]. In Javed et al., the empagliflozin group had an overall decrease in androstenedione levels (-2.2 (24.4)% baseline change) while the metformin group had an overall increase in levels (5.6 (59.8)% baseline change) [33]. In Cai et al., there was a decrease in androstenedione levels in the canagliflozin group, while levels slightly increased in the metformin group; although neither was statistically significant (-0.48 (-1.04 to 0.09) vs. 0.04 (-0.49 to 0.56) $p = 0.199$) [31]. In Zhang et al., no significant changes in androstenedione were seen in either the canagliflozin/metformin group, or in metformin alone compared to the baseline [35].

3.2.5. Sex Hormone-Binding Globulin (SHBG)

Two out of five studies that examined SHBG showed a significant increase in levels [32,33].

In Zhang et al., in the metformin group the SHBG (sex hormone-binding globulin) levels increased significantly ($p = 0.0303$), but no changes were observed in the canagliflozin/metformin group [35]. In Javed et al., there was a significant increase in the SHBG levels in the empagliflozin group (9.9 ± 22.6% baseline change, $p = 0.049$) compared to the baseline [33]. The metformin group showed a non-significant increase in levels of SHBG (6.4 ± 25.5%) [33]. In Elkind-Hirsch et al., SHBG levels significantly increased in the dapagliflozin group ($p < 0.001$) [32]. In Cai et al., SHBG levels decreased in both the canagliflozin and metformin groups with no significant difference between the two groups (-4.82 (-19.40 to 9.75) vs. -13.58 (-31.21 to 4.05) $p = 0.472$) [31]. In Tan et al., there was a non-significant increase in SHBG levels in the licogliflozin group compared to the placebo (treatment ratio of licogliflozin to placebo of 1.15 90% CI 0.97–1.36, $p = 0.173$) [34].

3.3. Obesity and Other Anthropometric Indices

Nearly 38–88% of women with PCOS have a BMI in the overweight or obese range [38]. Metformin improves metabolic outcomes in PCOS women and is therefore recommended by international guidelines for women with a BMI > 25 [9]. SGLT2 inhibitors, just like metformin, appear to improve anthropometric indices, with multiple studies showing a decrease in BMI, waist circumference, and hip circumference. In Cai et al., all study participants had a similar decrease in weight (kg) [canagliflozin: -2.82 (-3.97 to -1.66) vs. metformin: -2.68 (-3.93 to -1.43)] and BMI (kg/m^2) [canagliflozin: -1.04 (-1.56 to -0.53) vs. metformin: -0.90 (-1.46 to -0.35)] [31]. Similarly, Javed et al. did not find a statistically significant change in total mass ($p = 0.079$) or BMI ($p = 0.069$) [33]. In Elkind-Hirsch et al., patients in the exenatide/dapagliflozin and phentermine/topiramate groups had greater decreases in BMI compared to patients in other treatment groups [32]. In Zhang et al., there was a statistically significant decrease in both body weight and BMI for patients receiving both canagliflozin and metformin ($p < 0.0001$ and <0.0001, respectively) as well as metformin alone ($p < 0.0001$ and $p < 0.0001$, respectively), but not a statistically significant difference between groups [35]. Tan et al. found that body weight before and after treatment was stable in patients who received licogliflozin (BMI not examined) [34]. Table 3 shows the studies that examined the effects of SGLT2 inhibitors in women with PCOS.

Table 3. Comparison of the changes in anthropometric parameters and BMI in studies that used SGLT2 inhibitors in women with PCOS.

	Cai et al. [31]	Elkind-Hirsch et al. [32]	Javed et al. [33]	Zhang et al. [35]
SGLT2 inhibitor	Canagliflozin	Dapagliflozin	Empagliflozin	Canagliflozin (with Metformin)
BMI (kg/m^2)				
Pretreatment	27.26 (25.55 to 28.99)	38 ± 1.1	37.1 ± 6.2	31.11 ± 3.02
Posttreatment	LS Mean: −1.04 (−1.56 to −0.53)	37.4 ± 1.2 (−0.6) *	36.6 ± 6.0	28.62 ± 2.91 *
Weight (kg)				
Pretreatment	72.94 (67.89 to 77.99)	104 ± 3	102.3 ± 16.6	81.23 ± 9.83
Posttreatment	LS Mean: −2.82 (−3.97 to −1.66)	102.6 ± 4 (−1.4) *	101.5 ± 16.3	75.40 ± 8.68 *
Waist Circumference (cm)				
Pretreatment	92.87 (88.00 to 97.75)	104 ± 3	101.2 ± 9.7	n/a
Posttreatment	LS Mean: −4.05 (−6.18 to −1.91)	101 ± 3.2 (−3)	99.6 ± 9.5 *	
Waist-to-hip ratio				
Pretreatment	0.91 (0.88 to 0.93)	0.81 ± 0.02	n/a	n/a
Posttreatment	LS Mean: −0.02 (−0.04 to 0.00)	0.79 ± 0.017 (−0.02)	n/a	n/a

* $p < 0.05$.

Three studies examined waist and hip circumference. Cai et al. found similar decreases for canagliflozin and metformin in waist circumference (cm) [canagliflozin: −4.05 (−6.18 to −1.91) vs. metformin: −3.27 (−5.54 to −0.99) ($p = 0.629$)] and hip circumference (cm) [canagliflozin: −2.62 (−4.02 to −1.21) vs metformin: −2.93 (−4.42 to −1.44) ($p = 0.767$)] [31]. Elkind-Hirsch et al. only found a statistically significant decrease in waist circumference and waist-to-hip ratio with exenatide plus dapagliflozin and phentermine plus topiramate compared to dapagliflozin with metformin [32]. Finally, Javed et al. found that empagliflozin led to a statistically significant decrease in waist circumference ($p = 0.024$) and hip circumference ($p = 0.013$) compared to the baseline. There was also a statistically significant difference between empagliflozin and metformin for both waist (empagliflozin: −1.6 ± 2.8% vs. metformin: 0.2 ± 2.1%; $p = 0.029$) and hip circumference (empagliflozin: −2.0 ± 3.0% vs. metformin: 1.1 ± 1.9%; $p = 0.001$) [33].

3.4. Effect on Glycemic Indices

Nearly 20–35% of women with PCOS have impaired glucose tolerance and 5–10% have type 2 diabetes [39]. Three out of four studies that examined glycemic indices appear to show statistically significant findings and improvements in insulin resistance. Table 4 reviews measures of glycemic control across four studies. Cai et al. found that canagliflozin led to an increase in homeostatic model assessment insulin sensitivity index (HOMA-ISI) [LS mean 0.42 95% CI (0.23 to 0.62)], along with a decrease in glycated hemoglobin (HbA1c) [LS mean −0.26 95% CI (−0.43 to −0.09)], fasting blood glucose [LS mean −0.23 95% CI (−0.40 to −0.06)], fasting serum insulin [LS mean −7.70 95% CI (−11.46 to −3.94), and postprandial insulin [LS mean −81.43 95% CI (−122.71 to −40.14)] [31]. Tan et al. showed that licogliflozin reduced hyperinsulinemia by decreasing the area under the curve for insulin by 68%, the maximum peak of insulin by 74%, HOMA-IR by 30%, and fasting glucose by 6% [34]. Zhang et al. found a lower area under the curve for glucose and the area under the curve for the insulin-to-glucose ratio in patients who received metformin + canagliflozin vs. metformin alone. However, there were no differences in fasting blood glucose, fasting insulin, area under the curve for insulin, or HOMA-IR [35]. Javed et al. did not find that empagliflozin leads to any changes in insulin sensitivity (insulin, fasting glucose, HOMA-IR) [33].

Table 4. Changes in glycemic indices in the trials that employed SGLT2 Inhibitors in women with PCOS.

	Cai et al. [31]	Elkind-Hirsch et al. [32]	Javed et al. [33]	Zhang et al. [35]
SGLT2 inhibitor	Canagliflozin	Dapagliflozin	Empagliflozin	Canagliflozin (with Metformin)
Hemoglobin A1c (HbA1c)%				
Pretreatment	5.60 (5.37 to 5.83)	n/a	n/a	n/a
Posttreatment	Change from baseline LS mean: −0.26 (−0.43 to −0.09)	n/a	n/a	n/a
HOMA-IR				
Pretreatment	5.33 (3.92 to 6.73)	4.1 ± 0.7	2.6 (2.1)	5.70 (3.38–6.08)
Posttreatment	Change from baseline LS mean: −2.04 (−2.89 to −1.18)	3.4 ± 0.6 (−0.7) *	2.4 (2.7)	3.14 (1.91–4.71) *
FBG				
Pretreatment	5.18 mmol/L (4.99 to 5.38)	98 mg/dL ± 2.3	4.5 mmol/L (0.6)	5.70 mmol/L (5.27–6.02)
Posttreatment	Change from baseline LS mean: −0.23 (−0.40 to −0.06)	93 mg/dL ± 2.1 (−5) *	4.5 mmol/L (0.6)	5.20 mmol/L (4.88–5.35)
FINS				
Pretreatment	22.58 mU/L (16.99 to 28.17)	n/a	12.6 µIU/mL (11.6)	21.5 mU/L (14.35–24.20)
Posttreatment	Change from baseline LS mean: −7.70 (−11.46 to −3.94)	n/a	12.7 µIU/mL (14.4)	12.0 mU/L (8.20–20.15) *

HOMA-IR—homeostatic model assessment of insulin resistance; FBG—fasting blood glucose; FINS—fasting serum insulin. * $p < 0.05$; [31]. To convert from mg/dL to mmol/L divide mg/dL by 18. µIU/mL is equivalent to mU/L.

3.5. Changes in Metabolic Indices

In a limited number of studies, SGLT2 inhibitors have also shown mixed results in impacting metabolic parameters, as seen in Table 5. One out of the four studies that looked at cholesterol found statistically significant decreases in total cholesterol and triglycerides from the baseline with canagliflozin and metformin [35], and one out of two studies that examined blood pressure found statistically significant improvements in systolic (SBP) and diastolic blood pressure (DBP) [32]. In Cai et al., canagliflozin was not found to significantly decrease total cholesterol (mmol/L) [0.17 (−0.05 to 0.39)], LDL cholesterol (mmol/L) [0.22 (0.06 to 0.51)], or increase HDL cholesterol [0.02 (−0.17 to 0.13)]. It did lead to a slight decrease in triglycerides (mmol/L) [−0.36 (−0.54 to −0.17) [31]. Zhang et al. and Javed et al. did not find significant differences in lipid parameters [33,35]. Elkind-Hirsch et al. found that triglycerides were reduced with exenatide/dapagliflozin, but not with dapagliflozin alone [32]. Data on the impact of SGLT2 inhibitors on systolic and diastolic blood pressure are also limited. Out of the five studies reviewed, only two (Elkind-Hirsch et al. [32] and Javed et al. [33]) looked at changes in SBP and DBP. While Elkind et al. found that systolic and diastolic blood pressures were both significantly decreased by all treatments (exenatide, dapagliflozin, exenatide/dapagliflozin, dapagliflozin/metformin, and phentermine/topiramate) ($p < 0.035$) [32], they did not assess differences between treatment groups. Javed et al. found no differences in blood pressure after 12 weeks in patients on empagliflozin compared to metformin [33]. It is important to note that patients in both studies were normotensive before starting the study.

Table 5. Changes in metabolic parameters in the studies that used SGLT2 inhibitors in women with PCOS.

	Cai et al. [31]	Elkind-Hirsch et al. [32]	Javed et al. [33]	Zhang et al. [35]
SGLT2 inhibitor	Canagliflozin	Dapagliflozin	Empagliflozin	Canagliflozin (with Metformin)
Total Cholesterol				
Pretreatment	4.87 mmol/L (4.58 to 5.16)	183 mg/dL ± 6	4.8 mmol/L ± 1.0	4.90 mmol/L ± 0.93
Posttreatment	LS mean: 0.17 mmol/L (−0.05 to 0.39)	186 mg/dL ± 11 (+3.0)	4.7 mmol/L ± 1.1	4.54 mmol/L ± 0.80 *
Triglycerides				
Pretreatment	1.75 mmol/L (1.37 to 2.14)	143 mg/dL ± 21	1.5 mmol/L (1.3)	1.54 mmol/L (1.09–2.01)
Posttreatment	LS mean: −0.36 mmol/L (−0.54 to −0.17)	n/a	1.4 mmol/L (0.9)	1.20 mmol/L (0.84–1.63) *
LDL				
Pretreatment	3.04 mmol/L (2.66 to 3.43)	107 mg/dL ± 6	2.8 mmol/L ± 1.0	3.06 mmol/L ± 0.97
Posttreatment	LS mean: 0.22 mmol/L (0.06 to 0.51)	113.5 mg/dL ± 10 (6.5)	2.7 mmol/L ± 1.1	2.83 mmol/L ± 0.70
HDL				
Pretreatment	1.33 mmol/L (1.12 to 1.54)	44 mg/dL ± 2	1.1 mmol/L ± 0.2	-
Posttreatment	LS mean: 0.02 mmol/L (−0.17 to 0.13)	43 mg/dL ± 2.2 (−1.0)	1.1 mmol/L ± 0.2	-

* $p < 0.05$; [31]. To convert from mg/dL to mmol/L divide mg/dL by 18.

3.6. Side Effects of SGLT2 Inhibitors and Limitations of the RCTs

While SGLT2 inhibitors can have many benefits for patients with PCOS, potential adverse effects must be noted. The side effect profile of SGLT2 inhibitors in these studies appears to be favorable, with primarily mild gastrointestinal symptoms like metformin. The most common adverse effects reported by the studies overall included yeast infections, urinary tract infections, lightheadedness, diarrhea, and flatulence [32,34]. In Cai et al., adverse effects were more common in the metformin group compared to the SGLT2 inhibitor group [31]. In Zhang et al., the most common side effects in the canagliflozin/metformin group were nausea, diarrhea, dizziness, and abdominal pain [35]. Though no serious adverse events were reported in any of the studies, patients with PCOS trialing an SGLT2 inhibitor should be aware of potential side effects, most commonly the gastrointestinal and potentially infectious.

In studies of patients with type 2 diabetes, the use of SGLT2 inhibitors has been associated with an elevated risk of diabetic ketoacidosis (DKA) [40]. In particular, patients are at increased risk of euglycemic DKA or moderately elevated glucose levels. There are two mechanisms behind this described by Liu et al. [41]. First, as SGLT2 inhibitors increase the excretion of urinary glucose, there is a decrease in insulin secretion which can lead to the production of free fatty acids and conversion to ketone bodies, and second, there is also an increase in the secretion of glucagon, leading to the increased production of ketone bodies [41].

Data from the CANVAS Program, which looked at patients with type 2 diabetes and high cardiovascular risk, revealed an increase in the rate of fractures in patients taking SGLT2 inhibitors. In this study, patients taking an SGLT2 inhibitor had a greater rate of all fractures compared to the placebo, as well as a similar trend with low-trauma fractures [42]. One caveat is that most of the research in the literature on SGLT inhibitors has been done on patients with diabetes, and more studies are needed in patients with PCOS to evaluate the side-effect profile in this population.

Because all the patients in the studies that used SGLT2 inhibitors were either overweight or obese, more research is needed to determine if SGLT2 inhibitors are effective for PCOS women with a normal BMI. Another potential limitation was the variability in study length, which was from 2 to 24 weeks. Though all the studies investigated various biochemical parameters, no data were provided regarding clinical hyperandrogenic factors (i.e., hirsutism, acne, alopecia), which would be helpful to assess in further studies. In addition, pregnancy rates and outcomes were not evaluated in these studies.

4. Conclusions

Polycystic ovary syndrome is the most common hormonal disorder in women of childbearing age. Though there is no cure for PCOS, the goal is to manage the symptoms and prevent long-term complications. Insulin resistance and compensatory hyperinsulinemia affect a significant percentage of women with PCOS. SGLT2 inhibitors, by improving glucotoxicity and insulin sensitivity, could play a beneficial role in treating some of the metabolic and hormonal derangements in PCOS. They have been shown to improve menstrual frequency, reduce body weight and total fat mass, lower total testosterone and DHEAS levels, and improve glycemic indices in patients with PCOS. SGLT2 inhibitors, when compared to a placebo or standard of care in patients with PCOS, appear to have a similar effect on improving menstrual cycles as metformin. Given the benefits shown in these studies, SGLT2 inhibitors could be considered a novel treatment strategy for PCOS as they target multiple hormonal, metabolic, and glycemic control-associated abnormalities. Alternatively, for patients who are unable to tolerate or have contraindications to metformin, SGLT2 inhibitors have shown promise to be a viable alternative. Given the limited number of studies that have investigated the benefits of SGLT2 inhibitors in patients with PCOS, larger sample sizes are needed to further evaluate these benefits. In particular, randomized double-blind placebo-controlled trials comparing metformin, SGLT2 inhibitors, and a placebo would be helpful in further distinguishing metabolic, hormonal, glycemic, and clinical outcomes.

Funding: This research received no external funding.

Conflicts of Interest: The authors declare no conflicts of interest.

References

1. Crespo, R.P.; Bachega, T.A.S.S.; Mendonça, B.B.; Gomes, L.G. An Update of Genetic Basis of PCOS Pathogenesis. *Arq. Bras. Endocrinol. Metabol.* **2018**, *62*, 352–361. [CrossRef]
2. Eiras, M.C.; Pinheiro, D.P.; Romcy, K.A.M.; Ferriani, R.A.; Dos Reis, R.M.; Furtado, C.L.M. Polycystic Ovary Syndrome: The Epigenetics Behind the Disease. *Reprod. Sci.* **2022**, *29*, 680–694. [CrossRef] [PubMed]
3. Ilie, I.R. Chapter Four—Neurotransmitter, Neuropeptide and Gut Peptide Profile in PCOS-Pathways Contributing to the Pathophysiology, Food Intake and Psychiatric Manifestations of PCOS. In *Advances in Clinical Chemistry*; Makowski, G.S., Ed.; Elsevier: Amsterdam, The Netherlands, 2020; Volume 96, pp. 85–135. [CrossRef]
4. Liao, B.; Qiao, J.; Pang, Y. Central Regulation of PCOS: Abnormal Neuronal-Reproductive-Metabolic Circuits in PCOS Pathophysiology. *Front. Endocrinol.* **2021**, *12*, 667422. [CrossRef] [PubMed]
5. McCartney, C.R.; Campbell, R.E. Abnormal GnRH Pulsatility in Polycystic Ovary Syndrome: Recent Insights. *Curr. Opin. Endocr. Metab. Res.* **2020**, *12*, 78–84. [CrossRef] [PubMed]
6. Diamanti-Kandarakis, E.; Dunaif, A. Insulin resistance and the polycystic ovary syndrome revisited: An update on mechanisms and implications. *Endocr. Rev.* **2012**, *33*, 981–1030. [CrossRef] [PubMed]
7. Barber, T.M. Why are women with polycystic ovary syndrome obese? *Br. Med. Bull.* **2022**, *143*, 4–15. [CrossRef] [PubMed]
8. Moghetti, P.; Tosi, F.; Bonin, C.; Di Sarra, D.; Fiers, T.; Kaufman, J.-M.; Giagulli, V.A.; Signori, C.; Zambotti, F.; Dall'Alda, M.; et al. Divergences in Insulin Resistance Between the Different Phenotypes of the Polycystic Ovary Syndrome. *J. Clin. Endocrinol. Metab.* **2013**, *98*, E628–E637. [CrossRef] [PubMed]
9. Teede, H.J.; Misso, M.L.; Costello, M.F.; Dokras, A.; Laven, J.; Moran, L.; Piltonen, T.; Norman, R.J. Recommendations from the International Evidence-Based Guideline for the Assessment and Management of Polycystic Ovary Syndrome. *Hum. Reprod.* **2018**, *33*, 1602–1618. [CrossRef]
10. Vitek, W.; Alur, S.; Hoeger, K.M. Off-Label Drug Use in the Treatment of Polycystic Ovary Syndrome. *Fertil. Steril.* **2015**, *103*, 605–611. [CrossRef]
11. Forslund, M.; Melin, J.; Alesi, S.; Piltonen, T.; Romualdi, D.; Tay, C.T.; Witchel, S.; Pena, A.; Mousa, A.; Teede, H. Different Kinds of Oral Contraceptive Pills in Polycystic Ovary Syndrome: A Systematic Review and Meta-Analysis. *Eur. J. Endocrinol.* **2023**, *189*, S1–S16. [CrossRef]
12. Abdalla, M.A.; Shah, N.; Deshmukh, H.; Sahebkar, A.; Östlundh, L.; Al-Rifai, R.H.; Atkin, S.L.; Sathyapalan, T. Impact of Metformin on the Clinical and Metabolic Parameters of Women with Polycystic Ovary Syndrome: A Systematic Review and Meta-Analysis of Randomised Controlled Trials. *Ther. Adv. Endocrinol. Metab.* **2022**, *13*, 20420188221127142. [CrossRef]

13. Aroda, V.R.; Edelstein, S.L.; Goldberg, R.B.; Knowler, W.C.; Marcovina, S.M.; Orchard, T.J.; Bray, G.A.; Schade, D.S.; Temprosa, M.G.; White, N.H.; et al. Long-term Metformin Use and Vitamin B12 Deficiency in the Diabetes Prevention Program Outcomes Study. *J. Clin. Endocrinol. Metab.* **2016**, *101*, 1754–1761. [CrossRef] [PubMed]
14. Shurrab, N.T.; Arafa, E.-S.A. Metformin: A Review of Its Therapeutic Efficacy and Adverse Effects. *Obes. Med.* **2020**, *17*, 100186. [CrossRef]
15. Hughes, S.; Neumiller, J.J. Oral Semaglutide. *Clin. Diabetes* **2020**, *38*, 109–111. [CrossRef] [PubMed]
16. Carmina, E.; Longo, R.A. Semaglutide Treatment of Excessive Body Weight in Obese PCOS Patients Unresponsive to Lifestyle Programs. *J. Clin. Med.* **2023**, *12*, 5921. [CrossRef] [PubMed]
17. Tian, D.; Chen, W.; Xu, Q.; Li, X.; Lv, Q. Liraglutide monotherapy and add on therapy on obese women with polycystic ovarian syndromes: A systematic review and meta-analysis. *Minerva Medica* **2022**, *113*, 542–550. [CrossRef] [PubMed]
18. Ma, R.; Ding, X.; Wang, Y.; Deng, Y.; Sun, A. The therapeutic effects of glucagon-like peptide-1 receptor agonists and metformin on polycystic ovary syndrome: A protocol for systematic review and meta-analysis. *Medicine* **2021**, *100*, e26295. [CrossRef] [PubMed]
19. Lyu, X.; Lyu, T.; Wang, X.; Zhu, H.; Pan, H.; Wang, L.; Yang, H.; Gong, F. The Antiobesity Effect of GLP-1 Receptor Agonists Alone or in Combination with Metformin in Overweight/Obese Women with Polycystic Ovary Syndrome: A Systematic Review and Meta-Analysis. *Int. J. Endocrinol.* **2021**, *2021*, 6616693. [CrossRef]
20. Sano, R.; Shinozaki, Y.; Ohta, T. Sodium–Glucose Cotransporters: Functional Properties and Pharmaceutical Potential. *J. Diabetes Investig.* **2020**, *11*, 770–782. [CrossRef]
21. Teo, Y.N.; Ting, A.Z.H.; Chong, E.Y.; Tan, J.T.A.; Syn, N.L.; Chia, A.Z.Q.; Ong, H.T.; Cheong, A.J.Y.; Li, T.Y.-W.; Poh, K.K.; et al. Effects of Sodium/Glucose Cotransporter 2 (SGLT2) Inhibitors and Combined SGLT1/2 Inhibitors on Cardiovascular, Metabolic, Renal, and Safety Outcomes in Patients with Diabetes: A Network Meta-Analysis of 111 Randomized Controlled Trials. *Am. J. Cardiovasc. Drugs* **2022**, *22*, 299–323. [CrossRef]
22. Pinto, L.C.; Rados, D.V.; Remonti, L.R.; Viana, M.V.; Leitão, C.B.; Gross, J.L. Dose-Ranging Effects of SGLT2 Inhibitors in Patients with Type 2 Diabetes: A Systematic Review and Meta-Analysis. *Arq. Bras. Endocrinol. Metabol.* **2022**, *66*, 68–76. [CrossRef]
23. Zinman, B.; Wanner, C.; Lachin, J.M.; Fitchett, D.; Bluhmki, E.; Hantel, S.; Mattheus, M.; Devins, T.; Johansen, O.E.; Woerle, H.J.; et al. Empagliflozin, Cardiovascular Outcomes, and Mortality in Type 2 Diabetes. *N. Engl. J. Med.* **2015**, *373*, 2117–2128. [CrossRef]
24. Wahinya, M.; Khan, Z. Sodium-Glucose Cotransporter-2 (SGLT2) Inhibitor Therapy for the Primary and Secondary Prevention of Heart Failure in Patients with and without Type 2 Diabetes Mellitus: A Systematic Review. *Cureus* **2023**, *15*, e37388. [CrossRef]
25. McGuire, D.K.; Shih, W.J.; Cosentino, F.; Charbonnel, B.; Cherney, D.Z.I.; Dagogo-Jack, S.; Pratley, R.; Greenberg, M.; Wang, S.; Huyck, S.; et al. Association of SGLT2 Inhibitors with Cardiovascular and Kidney Outcomes in Patients with Type 2 Diabetes. *JAMA Cardiol.* **2021**, *6*, 148–158. [CrossRef]
26. Chen, S.; Coronel, R.; Hollmann, M.W.; Weber, N.C.; Zuurbier, C.J. Direct Cardiac Effects of SGLT2 Inhibitors. *Cardiovasc. Diabetol.* **2022**, *21*, 45. [CrossRef]
27. Lempesis, I.G.; Apple, S.J.; Duarte, G.; Palaiodimos, L.; Kalaitzopoulos, D.R.; Dalamaga, M.; Kokkinidis, D.G. Cardiometabolic Effects of SGLT2 Inhibitors on Polycystic Ovary Syndrome. *Diabetes/Metab. Res. Rev.* **2023**, *39*, e3682. [CrossRef] [PubMed]
28. Somagutta, M.R.; Jain, M.; Uday, U.; Pendyala, S.K.; Mahadevaiah, A.; Mahmutaj, G.; Jarapala, N.; Gad, M.A.; Srinivas, P.M.; Sasidharan, N.; et al. Novel Antidiabetic Medications in Polycystic Ovary Syndrome. *Discoveries* **2022**, *10*, e145. [CrossRef] [PubMed]
29. Pruett, J.E.; Romero, D.G.; Cardozo, L.L.Y. Obesity-Associated Cardiometabolic Complications in Polycystic Ovary Syndrome: The Potential Role of Sodium-Glucose Cotransporter-2 Inhibitors. *Front. Endocrinol.* **2023**, *14*, 951099. [CrossRef]
30. Sinha, B.; Ghosal, S. A meta-analysis of the effect of sodium glucose cotransporter-2 inhibitors on metabolic parameters in patients with polycystic ovary syndrome. *Front. Endocrinol.* **2022**, *13*, 830401. [CrossRef] [PubMed]
31. Cai, M.; Shao, X.; Xing, F.; Zhang, Y.; Gao, X.; Zeng, Q.; Dilimulati, D.; Qu, S.; Zhang, M. Efficacy of canagliflozin versus metformin in women with polycystic ovary syndrome: A randomized, open-label, noninferiority trial. *Diabetes Obes. Metab.* **2021**, *24*, 312–320. [CrossRef]
32. Elkind-Hirsch, K.E.; Chappell, N.; Seidemann, E.; Storment, J.; Bellanger, D. Exenatide, Dapagliflozin, or Phentermine/Topiramate Differentially Affect Metabolic Profiles in Polycystic Ovary Syndrome. *J. Clin. Endocrinol. Metab.* **2021**, *106*, 3019–3033. [CrossRef]
33. Javed, Z.; Papageorgiou, M.; Deshmukh, H.; Rigby, A.S.; Qamar, U.; Abbas, J.; Khan, A.Y.; Kilpatrick, E.S.; Atkin, S.L.; Sathyapalan, T. Effects of Empagliflozin on Metabolic Parameters in Polycystic Ovary Syndrome: A Randomized Controlled Study. *Clin. Endocrinol.* **2019**, *90*, 805–813. [CrossRef] [PubMed]
34. Tan, S.; Ignatenko, S.; Wagner, F.; Dokras, A.; Seufert, J.; Zwanziger, D.; Dunschen, K.; Zakaria, M.; Huseinovic, N.; Basson, C.T.; et al. Licogliflozin versus Placebo in Women with Polycystic Ovary Syndrome: A Randomized, Double-Blind, Phase 2 Trial. *Diabetes Obes. Metab.* **2021**, *23*, 2595–2599. [CrossRef] [PubMed]
35. Zhang, J.; Xing, C.; Cheng, X.; He, B. Canagliflozin Combined with Metformin versus Metformin Monotherapy for Endocrine and Metabolic Profiles in Overweight and Obese Women with Polycystic Ovary Syndrome: A Single-Center, Open-Labeled Prospective Randomized Controlled Trial. *Front. Endocrinol.* **2022**, *13*, 1003238. [CrossRef] [PubMed]
36. Penzias, A.; Bendikson, K.; Butts, S.; Coutifaris, C.; Falcone, T.; Fossum, G.; Gitlin, S.; Gracia, C.; Hansen, K.; La Barbera, A.; et al. Role of metformin for ovulation induction in infertile patients with polycystic ovary syndrome (PCOS): A guideline. *Fertil. Steril.* **2017**, *108*, 426–441. [CrossRef] [PubMed]

37. Huang, A.; Brennan, K.; Azziz, R. Prevalence of hyperandrogenemia in the polycystic ovary syndrome diagnosed by the National Institutes of Health 1990 criteria. *Fertil. Steril.* **2010**, *93*, 1938–1941. [CrossRef] [PubMed]
38. Barber, T.M.; Hanson, P.; Weickert, M.O.; Franks, S. Obesity and Polycystic Ovary Syndrome: Implications for Pathogenesis and Novel Management Strategies. *Clin. Med. Insights Reprod. Health* **2019**, *13*, 1179558119874042. [CrossRef] [PubMed]
39. Salle, K.E.S.; Wickham, E.P.; Cheang, K.; Essah, P.A.; Karjane, N.W.; Nestler, J.E. Glucose intolerance in polycystic ovary syndrome—A position statement of the Androgen Excess Society. *J. Clin. Endocrinol. Metab.* **2007**, *92*, 4546–4556. [CrossRef]
40. Marilly, E.; Cottin, J.; Cabrera, N.; Cornu, C.; Boussageon, R.; Moulin, P.; Lega, J.-C.; Gueyffier, F.; Cucherat, M.; Grenet, G. SGLT2 Inhibitors in Type 2 Diabetes: A Systematic Review and Meta-Analysis of Cardiovascular Outcome Trials Balancing Their Risks and Benefits. *Diabetologia* **2022**, *65*, 2000–2010. [CrossRef]
41. Liu, J.; Li, L.; Li, S.; Wang, Y.; Qin, X.; Deng, K.; Liu, Y.; Zou, K.; Sun, X. Sodium-Glucose Co-Transporter-2 Inhibitors and the Risk of Diabetic Ketoacidosis in Patients with Type 2 Diabetes: A Systematic Review and Meta-Analysis of Randomized Controlled Trials. *Diabetes Obes. Metab.* **2020**, *22*, 1619–1627. [CrossRef]
42. Neal, B.; Perkovic, V.; Mahaffey, K.W.; de Zeeuw, D.; Fulcher, G.; Erondu, N.; Shaw, W.; Law, G.; Desai, M.; Matthews, D.R.; et al. Canagliflozin and Cardiovascular and Renal Events in Type 2 Diabetes. *N. Engl. J. Med.* **2017**, *377*, 644–657. [CrossRef] [PubMed]

Disclaimer/Publisher's Note: The statements, opinions and data contained in all publications are solely those of the individual author(s) and contributor(s) and not of MDPI and/or the editor(s). MDPI and/or the editor(s) disclaim responsibility for any injury to people or property resulting from any ideas, methods, instructions or products referred to in the content.

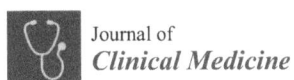

Article

Semaglutide Treatment of Excessive Body Weight in Obese PCOS Patients Unresponsive to Lifestyle Programs

Enrico Carmina * and Rosa Alba Longo

Endocrinology Unit, University of Palermo School of Medicine, 90144 Palermo, Italy
* Correspondence: enricocarmina28@gmail.com

Abstract: In spite of the widespread use of lifestyle modifications programs, many patients with PCOS are obese and prevalence of obesity in PCOS remains high. In this study, we present the data on the use of semaglutide, an incretin mimetic drug, in obese PCOS patients who were unresponsive to a lifestyle modification program. Twenty-seven obese patients with a diagnosis of PCOS, who did not reduce their body weight by a lifestyle modification program, were included in this study and treated by semaglutide, 0.5 mg subcutaneously once a week. After three months of treatment, an improvement in body weight with a mean decrease in body weight of 7.6 kg and a mean BMI loss of 3.1 was observed, while very few side effects were reported. Almost 80% of the studied obese PCOS patients obtained at least a 5% decrease in their body weight. Only a few patients (22%) obtained a decrease in body weight lower than 5% and were considered non-responsive to semaglutide, at least at the used doses. These patients presented a more severe obesity than responsive patients. Independently of results on body weight, and in patients who did not obtain a 5% decrease in their body weight, insulin basal values decreased, and HOMA-IR improved. Fasting blood glucose normalized in 80% of semaglutide-treated IFG PCOS women. In patients who were responsive to semaglutide (weight loss > 5%), the treatment was continued for additional three months. Weight loss slowed but continued and, at the end of the six months of therapy, the mean body weight loss was 11.5 kg and mean BMI reduced from 34.4 to 29.4. A total of 80% of responsive patients normalized menstrual cycles. In conclusion, treatment with semaglutide, at low doses, significantly reduces body weight in almost 80% of obese PCOS patients who were unresponsive to a previous lifestyle plan. It is often associated with the normalization of menstrual cycles, and these important results are obtained with very few side effects.

Keywords: PCOS; obese PCOS; semaglutide; weight loss; impaired fasting glucose; insulin resistance

Citation: Carmina, E.; Longo, R.A. Semaglutide Treatment of Excessive Body Weight in Obese PCOS Patients Unresponsive to Lifestyle Programs. *J. Clin. Med.* **2023**, *12*, 5921. https://doi.org/10.3390/jcm12185921

Academic Editor: Błażej Męczekalski

Received: 9 August 2023
Revised: 7 September 2023
Accepted: 11 September 2023
Published: 12 September 2023

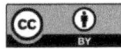

Copyright: © 2023 by the authors. Licensee MDPI, Basel, Switzerland. This article is an open access article distributed under the terms and conditions of the Creative Commons Attribution (CC BY) license (https://creativecommons.org/licenses/by/4.0/).

1. Introduction

Obesity is common in polycystic ovary syndrome (PCOS) [1–3] and is associated with severe insulin resistance, metabolic alterations and cardiovascular complications [2–6]. It strongly affects the long-term prognosis of PCOS patients [2,3,6]. In obese PCOS patients, lifestyle modification programs that include diet and physical exercise are considered first-line treatment and many studies have shown that these programs may improve the clinical presentation and long-term prognosis of the syndrome [2,3]. However, many patients with PCOS remain obese, and the prevalence of obesity in PCOS is higher than in the general population [1–3,6].

In the past, drugs that improve insulin resistance, like metformin, have shown only a modest ability to improve body weight in obese PCOS patients [2,7,8]. Better results have been obtained with products that mimic intestinal incretins and, in particular, the glucagon-like peptide 1 (GLP-1) effect, improving not only insulin production but also reducing appetite and energy intake [9]. Liraglutide, a GLP-1 mimetic product, may reduce body weight in obese subjects [10] and has been used in obese PCOS patients with mixed results [11,12]. Most meta-analyses report that many obese PCOS patients treated by liraglutide lose more than 5% of their body weight, with a total weight loss of 4–6 kg [11]. These results are not really satisfactory because most patients remain obese, and side effects are common and determine a high withdrawal rate [11,12].

More recently, semaglutide, a new incretin mimetic product, has shown the ability to more consistently reduce body weight in obese type 2 diabetic patients as well as in obese nondiabetic subjects [12–17]. However, data on obese PCOS patients are almost non-existent and it is unclear whether semaglutide may be used to reduce body weight in this disorder and what doses of the drug should be used to avoid side-effects.

In this study, we present data on use of low doses (0.5 mg once a week subcutaneously) of semaglutide in 27 obese PCOS patients who were unresponsive to a lifestyle modification program. Our data show that this treatment reduces body weight in most obese PCOS patients.

2. Materials and Methods

Twenty-seven obese (body mass index (BMI) kg/m^2, ≥30) patients with a diagnosis of PCOS who were unresponsive to a lifestyle modification program were included in this study. All these patients were referred between 2021 and 2022 because of obesity, hyperandrogenism and menstrual disorders, and were initially treated for three months with a lifestyle program (low-fat hypocaloric diet, a personalized program of physical exercise and psychological support) but did not reduce body weight (body weight loss lower than 5%).

The diagnosis of PCOS was based on Rotterdam criteria, with two out of three of the following criteria: chronic anovulation, clinical or biologic hyperandrogenism, and/or polycystic ovaries on ultrasound after the exclusion of other medical disorders [2]. All studied patients presented phenotype A PCOS (chronic anovulation, hyperandrogenism and polycystic ovaries) [2,4].

In all patients, serum levels of total testosterone (T), 17-hydroxy-progesterone (17OHP), fasting insulin and fasting glucose were determined on days 3–5 of the cycle. An oral glucose test (OGTT, 75 g of glucose) was performed with measurement of blood glucose at 30, 60 and 120 min. In non-menstruating women, blood samples were obtained after withdrawal bleeding after progestogen administration.

Anovulation was defined as serum progesterone < 3 ng/mL (<9.54 nmol/L). Clinical hyperandrogenism was defined as the presence of hirsutism. Hirsutism was assessed by Ferriman–Gallwey–Lorenzo scores [18], and patients with scores higher than 6 were considered hirsute. Adult acne and female-pattern hair loss were not considered a sign of hyperandrogenism if androgen levels were normal [19,20]. Biochemical hyperandrogenism was defined as serum testosterone > 34 ng/dL.

Total testosterone was determined by mass spectrometry after liquid chromatography (LC/MS) assay while 17OHprogesterone and serum insulin were measured by specific RIAs using previously described methods [21,22]. Insulin sensitivity was evaluated by the quantitative HOMA-IR method (glucose mg/dL × insulin mU/mL/405) [23]. In all patients, serum 17OH progesterone values were determined to exclude the existence of Non-Classic Congenital Adrenal Hyperplasia [24]. In some patients, because of clinical suspicion, urinary free cortisol, and serum prolactin and TSH were measured by commercial RIA methods to exclude other endocrine conditions.

In all assays, intra-assay and inter-assay coefficients of variation did not exceed 6% and 15%, respectively.

Transvaginal pelvic ultrasound was performed using a transducer frequency of 8–10 MHz and the presence of polycystic ovaries was established by the finding of an increased number of follicles, each of which measured 2–10 mm in diameter, and/or increased ovarian size [25].

No patient had received any medication for at least 3 months before the study, and all patients gave informed consent for this evaluation. The treatment with semaglutide and the research protocol obtained institutional approval from the ethical committee of our university (2021/22).

The various values of the women with PCOS were compared to those of 65 normal ovulatory women. These controls were drawn from the same population and did not report complaints of hyperandrogenism or menstrual irregularities.

All studied obese PCOS patients were treated by semaglutide, 0.5 mg subcutaneously once a week for three months. During this period, side effects were recorded each month while, at the end of the three months of treatment, body weight, BMI and FGL scores were reassessed, fasting blood glucose and serum insulin were re-evaluated and HOMA-IR was calculated again.

In responsive patients (weight loss > 5%), the semaglutide treatment was prolonged at the same dose for an additional three months and, at the end of the six months of therapy, body weight, BMI, FGL scores, fasting blood glucose and serum insulin were re-assessed and menstrual cycle characters and side effects were recorded.

Statistical Analysis

Statistical analyses were performed using Statview 5.0 (SAS Institute, Cary, NC, USA). Because several values were not normally distributed, a log transformation was necessary to obtain a normal distribution. Analysis of variance (ANOVA), followed by Tukey tests, were performed to assess differences in clinical and biochemical parameters between basal conditions and three and six months of treatment with semaglutide. The accuracy of parameters used to discriminate between basal and post-treatment values were evaluated using ROC curve analyses. Differences in reliability between different parameter values were assessed by Tukey multiple comparison tests. $p < 0.05$ was considered statistically significant. All results are reported as mean $\pm$ SD.

3. Results

All studied PCOS patients were obese (BMI range 30.4–47.9) and 33% of patients presented moderate (BMI > 35 < 40) or severe (BMI > 40) obesity. As shown in Table 1, the studied cohort of PCOS patients had significantly ($p < 0.01$) increased values of BMI, FGL scores, total testosterone, 17OH Progesterone, fasting glucose, insulin, HOMA-IR and triglycerides and significantly ($p < 0.01$) lower levels of HDL-cholesterol compared to normal controls. No differences in total cholesterol and LDL cholesterol values between patients and controls were observed. All studied patients reported irregular (oligomenorrhea or secondary amenorrhea) menses.

Table 1. Some clinical and hormonal data of 27 obese PCOS patients and 65 normal controls.

	PCOS Patients	Controls
Age (yrs.)	30 $\pm$ 9	29 $\pm$ 3
BMI (kg/m^2)	35.7 $\pm$ 6 **	23 $\pm$ 4
FGL index	10 $\pm$ 2 **	3 $\pm$ 1
LH/FSH ratio	1.7 $\pm$ 0.5 **	1.1 $\pm$ 0.4
Total testosterone (ng/dL)	53 $\pm$ 15 **	22 $\pm$ 5
17-OH-Progesterone (ng/mL)	1.2 $\pm$ 0.4 **	0.8 $\pm$ 0.2
Fasting glucose (mg/dL)	98 $\pm$ 12 **	78 $\pm$ 9
Insulin (mU/mL)	16 $\pm$ 7 **	9 $\pm$ 3
HOMA-IR	4 $\pm$ 2 **	1.2 $\pm$ 0.3
Total Cholesterol (mg/dL)	171 $\pm$ 22	168 $\pm$ 20
HDL Cholesterol (mg/dL)	46 $\pm$ 8 **	55 $\pm$ 5
LDL Cholesterol (mg/dL)	108 $\pm$ 17	105 $\pm$ 15
Triglycerides (mg/dL)	94 $\pm$ 21 **	65 $\pm$ 18

** $p < 0.01$ versus controls.

Fifteen PCOS patients (55.6%) had fasting values of blood glucose higher than 100 mg/dL (IFG, increased fasting glucose, patients), while four patients (all with increased fasting glucose) presented impaired glucose tolerance (blood glucose > 140 mg/dL and <200 mg/dL at 120 min after OGTT). No patients were affected by type 2 diabetes.

After semaglutide treatment for three months, BMI, body weight, fasting glucose, insulin and HOMA-IR values significantly ($p < 0.01$) decreased. The mean weight loss was 7.6 ± 3 kg (range 2–12 kg) and mean BMI loss was 3.1 ± 1 (range 0.9–4.6). % body weight loss was 8.9 ± 3.7 (range 2.8–14.6%). Fasting glucose, insulin and HOMA-IR decreased significantly ($p < 0.01$) and twelve IFG PCOS patients (80%) showed normal fasting blood glucose, while in the remaining three IFG patients (20%) the values of fasting glucose improved (decrease of at least 10 mg/dL) but remained higher than 100 mg/dL.

% weight loss negatively correlated with basal BMI ($p < 0.01$) and basal body weight ($p < 0.05$) but not with basal blood glucose or insulin or HOMA-IR values. No correlations were found between decrease in fasting glucose or insulin or calculated HOMA-IR and basal BMI, body weight, glucose, insulin, or HOMA-IR.

Six patients (22.2%) lost less than 5% of their body weight and were considered unresponsive to semaglutide, while twenty-one patients lost more than 5% of their body weight and were considered responsive to semaglutide. Nine responsive patients lost more than 10% of their body weight and were considered highly responsive to semaglutide. In Table 2, some characters of highly responsive and non-responsive PCOS patients were compared. PCOS patients who did not respond to semaglutide presented with a significantly ($p < 0.01$) higher BMI than PCOS patients who lost > 10% of their body weight after treatment with semaglutide.

Table 2. Basal BMI, fasting glucose, insulin and HOMA-IR in PCOS patients treated by semaglutide and divided according to their response to the therapy.

	Highly Responsive PCOS Patients (Weight Loss > 10%)	Non-Responsive PCOS Patients (Weight Loss < 5%)
Number of patients	9	6
BMI (kg/m^2)	32 ± 5 **	40 ± 5
Fasting glucose (mg/dL)	94 ± 11	102 ± 11
Insulin (mU/mL)	14.9 ± 2.9	17.8 ± 10
Homa-IR	3.6 ± 0.5	4.6 ± 2

** $p < 0.01$ versus non responsive PCOS patients.

Twenty-one obese PCOS patients who were responsive (weight loss > 5%) to semaglutide therapy continued the treatment with this product at the same dose for an additional three months. In Table 3, the results of the treatment on BMI, and glucose metabolism are shown. In these responsive PCOS patients, the additional three months of treatment with semaglutide induced a small further decrease in body weight (mean weight loss −2.5 kg) with a total weight loss of 11.5 kg after six months of therapy (Table 3). No further changes in fasting glucose, insulin or HOMA-IR were found. In these responsive patients, menstrual disorders improved, with fifteen PCOS women (71% of responsive patients) achieving normal menses. No significant changes in FGL scores were observed.

Treatment with semaglutide, 0.5 mg once a week for up to six months induced few side effects, with nine patients (33%) reporting morning nausea and two patients complaining of sporadic vomiting. No patient withdrew from the therapy because of side effects.

Table 3. Changes in BMI, body weight, fasting glucose, insulin, and insulin resistance (HOMA-IR) (mean ± SD) in 21 obese PCOS women responsive (weight loss > 5%) to semaglutide treatment (0.5 mg subcutaneously once a week).

	Basal	After 3 Months of Treatment with Semaglutide	After 6 Months of Treatment with Semaglutide
BMI (kg/m^2)	34.4 ± 5.9	30.8 ± 5 **	29.4 ± 5 **
Body weight (kg)	85 ± 15	76 ± 16 **	73.5 ± 15 **
Fasting glucose (mg/dL)	97 ± 12	90 ± 8 **	90 ± 6 **
Insulin (mU/mL)	17 ± 7	11 ± 5 **	11 ± 5 **
HOMA-IR	3.5 ± 2	2.5 ± 1 **	2.4 ± 0.8 **

** $p < 0.01$ versus basal values.

4. Discussion

In this study, we evaluated the effect of low doses (0.5 mg subcutaneously once a week) of semaglutide on body weight and insulin and glucose blood levels in 27 obese PCOS women who were unresponsive to a lifestyle program. All PCOS patients presented a classic form of PCOS (phenotype A: chronic anovulation, hyperandrogenism and polycystic ovaries) and were treated by 0.5 mg of semaglutide subcutaneously once a week. No specific lifestyle plan was added to the pharmacologic treatment, but patients were told to maintain a normal food intake and a regular physical activity.

Our results show an improvement in body weight, with a mean decrease in body weight of 7.6 kg and a mean BMI loss of 3.1. Almost 80% of obese PCOS patients who were unresponsive to a lifestyle plan, obtained an at least 5% decrease in their body weight and this was associated with a significant improvement in basal glucose and insulin resistance (calculated by HOMA-IR). Only a few patients (22%) showed a decrease in body weight of lower than 5% and were considered non-responsive to semaglutide, at least at the used doses.

The mean weight loss observed after treatment with semaglutide was larger than that reported with metformin [2,7,8] or liraglutide [9–12] and was obtained using low doses of the product with very few side effects. Independently of results on body weight, and also in patients who did not reach a 5% decrease in their body weight, insulin basal values decreased, and HOMA-IR improved in all treated patients. Fasting blood glucose normalized in 80% of semaglutide-treated IFG PCOS women, with the remaining few IFG PCOS patients obtaining a decrease of at least 10 mg/100 mL of their fasting blood glucose. This suggests that semaglutide, independently of its effect on body weight, may represent a good alternative to metformin for improving insulin resistance and preventing type 2 diabetes in PCOS.

Interestingly, comparing patients who were unresponsive to semaglutide therapy with patients who were highly responsive (weight loss > 10%), we found that unresponsive patients were significantly more obese (mean BMI 40 versus 32, $p < 0.01$). This may suggest that, in severely obese patients, higher doses of semaglutide are needed. Consistently with this, in most studies on the general population, higher doses of semaglutide (1 mg or more once a week) have been used for the treatment of obesity [13–17]. However, it should be noted that many patients with severe obesity present a genetic form of obesity that may not be sensitive to drugs that mimic an incretin effect [26,27].

In patients who were responsive to semaglutide (weight loss > 5%), the treatment was continued for an additional three months. Weight loss slowed but continued and, at the end of the six months of therapy, the mean body weight loss was 11.5 kg and mean BMI reduced from 34.4 to 29.4. This very good treatment result was associated with an improvement in menstrual cycles, which, in almost 80% of the responsive patients, became normal. All this was obtained with very few side effects.

Of course, other studies are needed, but these initial results look very promising and suggest that semaglutide may become a very important tool for the treatment of obese PCOS patients.

In conclusion, treatment with semaglutide at low doses significantly reduces body weight in almost 80% of obese PCOS patents who were unresponsive to a previous lifestyle plan. It is often associated with the normalization of menstrual cycles and these important results are obtained with very few side effects. The best results are obtained in patients with mild obesity, while patients with severe obesity are generally unresponsive to the product, at least at the used doses. Independently of the effects on body weight, semaglutide treatment improves insulin resistance and may normalize fasting glucose in IFG PCOS patients.

Author Contributions: Conceptualization, E.C. and R.A.L.; Methodology, E.C.; software, E.C.; validation, E.C. and R.A.L.; format analysis, E.C.; investigation, E.C.; resources, E.C.; data curation, E.C.; writing—original draft preparation, E.C.; writing—review and editing, E.C.; visualization, E.C.; supervision, E.C.; project administration, E.C. All authors have read and agreed to the published version of the manuscript.

Funding: This research received no external funding.

Institutional Review Board Statement: The research protocol obtained institutional approval from the ethical committee of university of Palermo (2021/22).

Informed Consent Statement: Informed consent was obtained from all subjects.

Data Availability Statement: Data supporting results can be found at the office of Prof. Carmina.

Conflicts of Interest: The authors declare no conflict of interest.

References

1. Carmina, E.; Legro, R.S.; Stamets, K.; Lowell, J.; Lobo, R.A. Difference in body weight between American and Italian women with Polycystic Ovary Syndrome: Influence of the diet. *Hum. Reprod.* **2003**, *11*, 2289–2293. [CrossRef] [PubMed]
2. Azziz, R.; Carmina, E.; Chen, Z.; Dunaif, A.; Laven, J.S.; Legro, R.S.; Lizneva, D.; Natterson-Horowitz, B.; Teede, H.J.; Yildiz, B.O. Polycystic ovary syndrome. *Nat. Rev. Dis. Primers* **2016**, *2*, 16057. [CrossRef] [PubMed]
3. Teede, H.J.; Misso, M.L.; Costello, M.F.; Dokras, A.; Laven, J.; Moran, L.; Piltonen, T.; Norman, R.J. International PCOS Network. Recommendations from the international evidence-based guideline for the assessment and management of polycystic ovary syndrome. *Fertil. Steril.* **2018**, *110*, 364–379. [CrossRef] [PubMed]
4. Carmina, E.; Chu, M.C.; Longo, R.A.; Rini, G.B.; Lobo, R.A. Phenotypic Variation in Hyperandrogenic Women Influences the Findings of Abnormal Metabolic and Cardiovascular Risk Parameters. *J. Clin. Endocrinol. Metab.* **2005**, *90*, 2545–2549. [CrossRef] [PubMed]
5. Essah, P.A.; Nestler, J.E.; Carmina, E. Differences in dyslipidemia between American and Italian women with polycystic ovary syndrome. *J. Endocrinol. Investig.* **2008**, *31*, 35–41. [CrossRef] [PubMed]
6. Carmina, E.; Lobo, R.A. Comparing Lean and Obese PCOS in Different PCOS Phenotypes: Evidence That the Body Weight Is More Important than the Rotterdam Phenotype in Influencing the Metabolic Status. *Diagnostics* **2022**, *12*, 2313. [CrossRef] [PubMed]
7. Naderpoor, N.; Shorakae, S.; de Courten, B.; Misso, M.L.; Moran, L.J.; Teede, H. Metformin and lifestyle modification in polycystic ovary syndrome: Systematic review and meta-analysis. *Hum. Reprod. Update* **2015**, *21*, 560–574. [CrossRef] [PubMed]
8. Apovian, C.M.; Aronne, L.J.; Bessesen, D.H.; McDonnell, M.E.; Murad, M.H.; Pagotto, U.; Ryan, D.H.; Still, C.D. Pharmacological Management of Obesity: An Endocrine Society Clinical Practice Guideline. *J. Clin. Endocrinol. Metab.* **2015**, *100*, 342–362. [CrossRef]
9. Näslund, E.; Barkeling, B.; King, N.; Gutniak, M.; Blundell, J.E.; Holst, J.J.; Rössner, S.; Hellström, P.M. Energy intake and appetite are suppressed by glucagon-like peptide-1 (GLP-1) in obese men. *Int. J. Obes. Relat. Metab. Disord.* **1999**, *23*, 304–311. [CrossRef]
10. Mehta, A.; Marso, S.P.; Neeland, I. Liraglutide for weight management: A critical review of the evidence. *J. Obes. Sci. Pract.* **2017**, *3*, 3–14. [CrossRef]
11. Ge, J.J.; Wang, D.J.; Song, W.; Shen, S.M.; Ge, W.H. The effectiveness and safety of liraglutide in treating overweight/obese patients with polycystic ovary syndrome: A meta-analysis. *J. Endocrinol. Investig.* **2022**, *45*, 261–273. [CrossRef] [PubMed]
12. Jensterle, M.; Herman, R.; Janež, A. Therapeutic Potential of Glucagon-like Peptide-1 Agonists in Polycystic Ovary Syndrome: From Current Clinical Evidence to Future Perspectives. *Biomedicines* **2022**, *10*, 1989. [CrossRef] [PubMed]
13. Singh, G.; Krauthamer, M.; Bjalme-Evans, M. Wegovy (Semaglutide): A New Weight Loss Drug for Chronic Weight Management. *J. Investig. Med.* **2022**, *70*, 5–13. [CrossRef] [PubMed]

14. Rubino, D.; Abrahamsson, N.; Davies, M.; Hesse, D.; Greenway, F.L.; Jensen, C.; Lingvay, I.; Mosenzon, O.; Rosenstock, J.; Rubio, M.A.; et al. STEP 4 Investigators. Effect of Continued Weekly Subcutaneous Semaglutide vs. Placebo on Weight Loss Maintenance in Adults with Overweight or Obesity: The STEP 4 Randomized Clinical Trial. *JAMA* **2021**, *325*, 1414–1425. [CrossRef] [PubMed]
15. Wadden, T.A.; Bailey, T.S.; Billings, L.K.; Davies, M.; Frias, J.P.; Koroleva, A.; Lingvay, I.; O'Neil, P.M.; Rubino, D.M.; Skovgaard, D.; et al. STEP 3 Investigators. Effect of Subcutaneous Semaglutide vs Placebo as an Adjunct to Intensive Behavioral Therapy on Body Weight in Adults with Overweight or Obesity: The STEP 3 Randomized Clinical Trial. *JAMA* **2021**, *325*, 1403–1413. [CrossRef] [PubMed]
16. Rubino, D.M.; Greenway, F.L.; Khalid, U.; O'Neil, P.M.; Rosenstock, J.; Sørrig, R.; Wadden, T.A.; Wizert, A.; Garvey, W.T.; The STEP 8 Investigators. Effect of Weekly Subcutaneous Semaglutide vs Daily Liraglutide on Body Weight in Adults with Overweight or Obesity without Diabetes: The STEP 8 Randomized Clinical Trial. *JAMA* **2022**, *327*, 138–150. [CrossRef] [PubMed]
17. Phillips, A.; Clements, J.N. Clinical review of subcutaneous semaglutide for obesity. *J. Clin. Pharm. Ther.* **2022**, *47*, 184–193. [CrossRef]
18. Hatch, R.; Rosenfield, R.L.; Kim, M.H.; Tredway, D. Hirsutism: Implications, etiology, and management. *Am. J. Obstet. Gynecol.* **1981**, *140*, 815–830. [CrossRef]
19. Carmina, E.; Azziz, R.; Bergfeld, W.; Escobar Morreale, H.F.; Futterweit, W.; Huddleston, H.; Lobo, R.A.; Olsen, E. Female pattern hair loss and androgen excess: A report from the multidisci-plinary Androgen Excess and PCOS committee. *J. Clin. Endocrinol. Metab.* **2019**, *104*, 2875–2891. [CrossRef]
20. Carmina, E.; Dreno, B.; Lucky, W.A.; Agak, W.G.; Dokras, A.; Kim, J.J.; Lobo, R.A.; Tehrani, F.R.; Dumesic, D. Female Adult Acne and Androgen Excess: A Report From the Multidisciplinary Androgen Excess and PCOS Committee. *J. Endocr. Soc.* **2022**, *6*, bvac003. [CrossRef]
21. Carmina, E. Prevalence of idiopathic hirsutism. *Eur. J. Endocrinol.* **1998**, *139*, 421–423. [CrossRef] [PubMed]
22. Carmina, E.; Longo, R.A. Increased Prevalence of Elevated DHEAS in PCOS Women with Non-Classic (B or C) Phenotypes: A Retrospective Analysis in Patients Aged 20 to 29 Years. *Cells* **2022**, *11*, 3255. [CrossRef] [PubMed]
23. Carmina, E.; Stanczyk, F.; Lobo, R.A. Evaluation of hormonal status. In *Jerome Strauss Robert Barbieri Antonio Gargiulo: Yen & Jaffe's Reproductive Endocrinology*, 8th ed.; Elsevier: Amsterdam, The Netherlands, 2018; Chapter 34; pp. 887–915.
24. Carmina, E.; Dewailly, D.; Escobar-Morreale, H.F.; Kelestimur, F.; Moran, C.; Oberfield, S.; Witchel, S.F.; Azziz, R. Non-classic congenital adrenal hyperplasia due to 21-hydroxylase deficiency revisited: An update with a special focus on adolescent and adult women. *Hum. Reprod. Updat.* **2017**, *23*, 580–599. [CrossRef] [PubMed]
25. Dewailly, D.; Lujan, M.; Carmina, E.; Cedars, M.; Laven, J.; Norman, R.; Escobar Morreale, H. Definition and significance of polycystic ovarian morphology: A task force report from the Androgen Excess and Polycystic Ovary Syndrome Society. *Hum. Reprod. Update* **2014**, *20*, 334–352. [CrossRef] [PubMed]
26. Pigeyre, M.; Yazdi, F.T.; Kaur, Y.; Meyre, D. Recent progress in genetics, epigenetics and meta-genomics unveils the pathophysiology of human obesity. *Clin. Sci.* **2016**, *130*, 943–986. [CrossRef] [PubMed]
27. Masood, B.; Moorthy, M. Causes of obesity: A review. *Clin. Med.* **2023**, *23*, 284–291. [CrossRef]

Disclaimer/Publisher's Note: The statements, opinions and data contained in all publications are solely those of the individual author(s) and contributor(s) and not of MDPI and/or the editor(s). MDPI and/or the editor(s) disclaim responsibility for any injury to people or property resulting from any ideas, methods, instructions or products referred to in the content.

MDPI
St. Alban-Anlage 66
4052 Basel
Switzerland
www.mdpi.com

Journal of Clinical Medicine Editorial Office
E-mail: jcm@mdpi.com
www.mdpi.com/journal/jcm

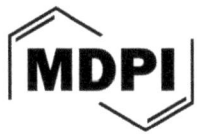

Disclaimer/Publisher's Note: The statements, opinions and data contained in all publications are solely those of the individual author(s) and contributor(s) and not of MDPI and/or the editor(s). MDPI and/or the editor(s) disclaim responsibility for any injury to people or property resulting from any ideas, methods, instructions or products referred to in the content.